W9-ARZ-866

Medical Assistant Exam Prep

Sixth Edition

ALSO FROM KAPLAN

Anatomy Coloring Book
Anatomy Flashcards
ATI TEAS Strategies, Practice & Review with 2 Practice Tests
National Registry Paramedic Examination Strategies, Practice & Review
Nursing School Entrance Exams

Medical Assistant Exam

Prep

Sixth Edition

Practice Test + Proven Strategies

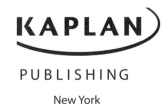

PUBLISHING

New York

This publication is designed to provide accurate information in regard to the subject matter covered as of its publication date, with the understanding that knowledge and best practice constantly evolve. The publisher is not engaged in rendering medical, legal, accounting, or other professional service. If medical or legal advice or other expert assistance is required, the services of a competent professional should be sought. This publication is not intended for use in clinical practice or the delivery of medical care. To the fullest extent of the law, neither the Publisher nor the Editors assume any liability for any injury and/or damage to persons or property arising out of or related to any use of the material contained in this book.

RMA® is a registered trademark of American Medical Technologists (AMT), which neither sponsors nor endorses this book.

CMA® is a registered trademark of the American Association of Medical Assistants (AAMA), which neither sponsors nor endorses this book.

© 2017 by Kaplan, Inc.

Published by Kaplan Publishing, a division of Kaplan, Inc.
750 Third Avenue
New York, NY 10017

All rights reserved. The text of this publication, or any part thereof, may not be reproduced in any manner whatsoever without written permission from the publisher.

10 9 8 7 6 5 4 3 2 1

ISBN-13: 978-1-5062-2349-0

Kaplan Publishing books are available at special quantity discounts to use for sales promotions, employee premiums, or educational purposes. For more information or to purchase books, please call the Simon & Schuster special sales department at 866-506-1949.

Contents

KAPLAN

For Test Changes or Late-Breaking Developments

kaptest.com/publishing

The material in this book is up-to-date at the time of publication but the test makers may have instituted changes to the tests since that date. Be sure to carefully read the materials you receive when you register for the test. If there are any important late-breaking developments—or any changes or corrections to the Kaplan test preparation materials in this book—we will post that information online at kaptest.com/publishing.

About the Editor

Nancy Szwydek, MPH, RN, RHIA, RMA, CMAC, CRAT, has more than 40 years' experience working in the health care field in both clinical and administrative capacities. She is currently director of quality assurance for Kaplan Campus Health, overseeing the health programs of 11 Kaplan campuses. She is also online department chair for the Health Information Management, Health Informatics, and Billing & Coding programs at Kaplan University. In addition, Ms. Szwydek is an accreditation peer reviewer for MAERB/CAAHEP and an item and module writer for medical assisting exams for a national credentialing organization. For over 10 years, Ms. Szwydek served as chair of the Medical Assisting program at Kaplan University, where she was instrumental in completing the first self-study program and achieving programmatic accreditation for the program through CAAHEP.

Ms. Szwydek holds a master of public health degree and a certified medical assistant certificate (CMAC). She is a registered nurse, a registered health information administrator (RHIA), a registered medical assistant (RMA), and a certified rhythm analysis technician (CRAT).

Kaplan thanks the following experts for their contributions to this book:

Diann L. Martin, PhD, RN

Joanna Holly, MS, RN, CNA

Kathleen A. Locke, CMA

Margaret Riley, BSN, RN

Kari Williams, BS, DC

How to Use This Book

If you are reading this book, the chances are good that you are preparing for your CMA or RMA exam. You probably have completed, or soon will complete, a program of study in medical assisting. Congratulations on your decision to seek certification or registration. In addition to demonstrating your expertise, these credentials are becoming increasingly important to employers. While the exams may seem daunting, this book can help you prepare. Just follow the program of study outlined here.

STEP 1: READ PART 1 (BASICS)

Chapter 1 contains information on test eligibility, registration, and content: the what, where, when, why, and how of the CMA and RMA exams. In Chapter 3, you will find Kaplan's special test strategies and advice for the day of the exam. You can trust Kaplan to bring you the best strategies and the most up-to-date information on your test.

STEP 2: TAKE THE DIAGNOSTIC TEST

The 30-question diagnostic test will help you determine where your strengths and weaknesses lie. You can use this information to shape your approach to the review chapters, spending more time with the topics that need more review. Because the exams cover a broad range of content, this focused approach will help you make the most of your study time.

STEP 3: READ THE REVIEW CHAPTERS

Chapters 4 through 17 review the general, administrative, and clinical topics on the CMA and RMA exams. Each chapter concludes with review questions to help you gauge what you have learned. Be sure to read the answer explanations for all questions, including those you answered correctly. You often can pick up new information on many topics while reading about why incorrect answer choices are incorrect.

STEP 4: TAKE THE FULL-LENGTH PRACTICE TEST

When you are nearing your exam date, take Kaplan's full-length practice exam. This exam mimics the format of the actual CMA exam and also provides great practice for the RMA exam. It will help you build your stamina for the real test and give you a good sense of your level of preparation. Detailed answer explanations follow the exam, and these can help you understand why you got off track on a particular question.

The Resources section in the back of this book contains a wealth of information on searching for jobs and links to professional organizations and publications.

Best of luck on your exam, and best wishes in your career as a medical assistant!

Basics

Chapter 1: **Trends in Medical Assisting**

OCCUPATIONAL OUTLOOK

The United States Department of Labor anticipates the supply of medical assistant jobs to increase by 23 percent between 2014 and 2024. This growth is much faster than average, with almost 139,000 jobs available. Job growth for medical assistants is attributed to an aging "baby boom" population and an increase in preventive care initiatives. Acute and chronic diseases will result in increased office visits, and physicians will seek additional medical assistants to perform clinical and administrative duties in order to see more patients.

MEDICAL ASSISTANTS TODAY—WHY CREDENTIALING MATTERS

Medical assisting is one of the fastest-growing occupations in the United States today. Rapid growth in the demand for health care makes this profession a great choice for people who want to get into the medical field. The greatest demand will be for medical assistants who have formal education and credentials in the field.

Medical assistants are trained to assist in physician practices, clinics, and other health care facilities in both administrative and clinical duties. A medical assistant's role is flexible, yet the best option for employment is to complete formal training and seek credentials that validate his or her knowledge and expertise. Most physicians and other employers prefer to hire medical assistants who have graduated from an approved or accredited program of study. These programs range from diploma programs lasting a year to associate degree programs lasting two years. The sites for training include vocational and technical schools as well as community colleges and universities. While formal training is not mandatory, it is highly recommended and it is required to become credentialed as either a certified medical assistant or a registered medical assistant. Programs of study for medical assistants generally cover the following topics:

- Anatomy and physiology
- Medical terminology
- Record keeping
- Insurance processing and billing/coding of claims
- Laboratory testing and specimen procurement
- Clinical and diagnostic procedures
- Pharmacology
- Office practices and procedures
- Medical law and ethics
- First aid and emergency care
- Pharmacology
- Nutrition
- Electronic medical records

The education program also includes a practical externship experience in a medical office.

Medical assistants work to keep the offices of health care professionals running smoothly and serve the needs of the patients. Currently about 59 percent of medical assistants work in physicians' offices; about 15 percent work in state, local, or private hospital environments; 10 percent work in offices of other health care practitioners such as nurse practitioners, chiropractors, and podiatrists; and the remaining 7 percent work in outpatient care centers. Though no states currently license or individually regulate medical assistant practice, duties may vary on a state-by-state basis. Some states do require special training for certain duties to be performed by the medical assistant. Some common duties of medical assistants include:

- Acquiring health and medical history information from patients
- Obtaining vital signs, including temperature, pulse, respiration, and blood pressure
- Preparing patients for examinations and tests
- Assisting physicians with examinations, treatments, and procedures
- Performing venipuncture and capillary puncture
- Collecting and preparing laboratory specimens
- Performing basic office-based laboratory tests
- Sterilizing and preparing medical equipment
- Providing patient instruction on diet, medications, preparation for tests, and other health information
- Performing electrocardiograms
- Purchasing and maintaining inventory of supplies and office equipment
- Scheduling appointments
- Assisting with pharmacy orders and refills as directed by the physician
- Managing patient phone contacts and computerized patient management systems
- Preparing billing, coding, and insurance claims

- Managing mail and correspondence for the office
- Administering medications via injection or nonparenteral routes
- Documenting in the electronic medical record

MEDICARE AND MEDICAID EHR INCENTIVE PROGRAMS

Incorporating electronic records can be costly, and providers may be resistant to implementing them. Recognizing this, the Centers for Medicare and Medicaid (CMS) spearheaded an initiative to provide incentives to health care providers for incorporating electronic medical records. This incentive program was classified as "meaningful use" and consisted of three stages, with financial incentives offered for implementation at each stage. The third and final stage was completed in 2014. As of 2015, approximately 87 percent of physicians had implemented some degree of EHRss into their practices.

Stage 1 involved capturing data and sharing with other professionals or the patient.

Stage 2 involved an advanced clinical process, including computerized provider order entry (CPOE). By law, anyone entering medication, laboratory, and radiology orders into an electronic record must be credentialed. This incentive has led employers to make credentialing a prerequisite for employment; in other words, in many workplaces medical assistants must already possess a professional credential to be eligible for hire. Although credentialing has long been available for medical assistants, it was widely regarded as a voluntary "extra" in the past. The medical assistant in today's healthcare, however, should anticipate the need to become credentialed in order to secure employment.

Stage 3 focused on improved outcomes, including providing patients with a means of engaging in their own care. The provider had to meet at least two of the following goals: patient electronic access to their health records, secure messaging between patients and providers, and a collection of patient-generated health data (through devices such as Fitbit or mobile apps). Additionally, thresholds for computerized physician order entry (CPOE) were increased for items such as laboratory and diagnostic testing. To be eligible for this stage of incentive payments, physicians were required to order 60 percent of tests electronically and to send 80 percent of prescriptions to the pharmacy electronically.

FOCUS ON PROFESSIONALISM

Attire and Personal Presentation

Medical assistants' appearance should signal a clean, safe environment for patients. Choosing appropriate attire and being well-groomed are extremely important. Guidelines to follow include:

- Wear scrubs that are clean and neatly pressed.
- Wear clean, closed-toed shoes, avoiding flashy colors.
- Keep hair clean, natural-colored, and pulled away from the face.

- Avoid excessive jewelry and strong fragrance.
- Keep nails trim (no long or false fingernails) and use natural or light-colored polish, or no polish.
- Hide visible tattoos.

Communication

Careful attention to the variety of verbal and nonverbal forms of communication that you engage in helps to create an overall positive client experience. Greet patients in a courteous, respectful manner as they arrive to help them feel comfortable. It is important to address patients formally by their title and last name, such as "Mr. Sanchez" or "Ms. Bestock," and to avoid overly familiar terms such as "Honey" or "Sweetie," which patients may find disrespectful.

Take care to provide instruction to patients in terms they can understand. Doing so will help patients understand and implement their treatment plan or instructions. When preparing correspondence to providers and/or patients, write formal letters using standard formatting and correct grammar and punctuation; these qualities communicate professionalism. Finally, never diagnose a patient, and never assure a patient that "everything will be all right." Although it is important to be honest and ethical, do not work beyond your scope of practice.

Dependability

- Be punctual; arrive on time. The office depends on the medical assistant for an effective work flow. Punctuality and dependability help to avoid unnecessary interruptions.
- Follow direction: Pay attention to detail in your clinical and administrative duties. Make notes of progress and steps taken so you always know where your projects stand.

Confidentiality

Medical assistants have access to a large amount of sensitive patient information that may include diagnosis, insurance concerns, and family issues. Consequences of failure to abide by standards of confidentiality are serious. Such a lapse could result not only in job loss but also legal action. Adhering to strict confidentiality standards is imperative not only in the workplace, but also in public: Patient information should never be divulged. Do not make copies of records unless instructed, because doing so risks sharing information with unauthorized individuals. Assure that phone conversations are private, and be cautious when faxing or emailing information. Always note to the recipient that such information is confidential.

Empathy

Patients in the health care environment are often frightened and vulnerable. Although you should never intrude and ask patients for details unless instructed to by the health care provider, you should treat all patients and their families with respect and kindness. This affirms that you do care about their health and well-being. Actively listen to the patient, and convey serious concerns to the provider.

Critical Thinking

Thinking critically means making clear, reasoned judgments and acting on them. The medical assistant plays a crucial role in the efficient functioning of an office and performing patient triage. Critical thinking involves:

- Problem-solving skills
- Foresight and anticipation
- Having the knowledge and skills needed in your profession
- Strong communication skills
- Thoroughness and attention to detail

Being a Team Player

Everyone involved in health care serves a vital role in ensuring that patients receive the best care possible and that the goals of the organization are achieved. As an important member of the health care team, the medical assistant must be able to function as part of a cohesive unit in order to meet patient needs and achieve goals.

EMERGING DISEASES AND PUBLIC HEALTH CONCERNS

Emerging diseases are conditions that are either brand new to a population or occurred in the past but undergo a marked increase in incidence. The Centers for Disease Control and Prevention (CDC) and the World Health Organization (WHO) are very proactive in sharing concerns with the health care community should an emerging disease present a threat to a population or geographic region. As important members of the health care team, medical assistants should be knowledgeable about these diseases in order to educate patients and to treat them according to a provider's orders.

As of 2016, the WHO identified a list of the top 10 emerging diseases. Many of the listed diseases are not present in the United States, including Marburg hemorrhagic fever, Lassa fever, Middle East respiratory syndrome coronavirus (MERS-CoV), severe acute respiratory syndrome (SARS), Nipah virus disease, Rift Valley fever, and chikungunya. However, ease of travel makes the chance of spread across continents a potential threat.

Other diseases have been noted in the United States, and medical assistants should be familiar with these conditions as well.

Zika Disease

Zika is caused by a virus and presents with symptoms unlikely to result in death or hospitalization. However, the results can be devastating for a developing fetus—leading to severe birth defects if a pregnant female is infected. The virus has also been connected to Guillain-Barré syndrome. Zika is transmitted through the bite of an infected mosquito. Other means of spreading the disease are through pregnant female to fetus, blood transfusions, and transmission through sex partners.

Mild symptoms, which develop 3–14 days after exposure, include fever, rash, joint pain, and red eyes. These symptoms can last several days to a week. There is no vaccine available to prevent the infection, so preventing Zika means preventing mosquito bites. Protect the skin by wearing insect repellent, shirts with long sleeves, and long pants. Discourage the presence of mosquitoes by eliminating areas of stagnant water—such as outdoor buckets—where mosquitoes breed.

Candida auris

Candida auris is an emerging drug-resistant fungus that has been found in the United States and is known to spread throughout health care organizations. Invasive circulatory *Candida auris* has the potential to be fatal: It has resulted in death in approximately 60 percent of infected patients. Patients tend to experience fever and chills with little or no response to antifungal treatment; sepsis, organ failure, and coma are extreme symptoms that can occur if the infection becomes invasive. Standard and contact precautions are extremely important to prevent the spread of this condition. Daily sanitation of equipment will aid in preventing colonization on exam tables and other pieces of office equipment and furniture. *Candida auris* can be diagnosed through laboratory testing of blood and/or urine.

Ebola Virus Disease

Ebola is transmitted to humans from animals and can then be transferred by human-to-human contact through broken skin or mucous membranes. Although the disease originally was found in Central Africa, it has found its way into other countries, including the United States. Ebola is fatal if left untreated. Although there are currently no licensed vaccines to treat the condition, there are a few candidates undergoing evaluation.

The incubation period for Ebola varies, and symptoms may occur anywhere from 2 to 21 days after exposure. Fever, fatigue, muscle pain, headache, and sore throat are among the early symptoms; these are followed by vomiting, diarrhea, rash, and impaired kidney and liver function. Supportive care (consisting of hospitalization, rehydration, rest, and medication aimed at symptomatic relief) is the treatment of choice.

Whooping Cough (Pertussis)

More than 2 million children under the age of three do not receive the series of vaccines recommended by the Department of Health and Human Services because of either lack of access to health care services or parental choice to refuse immunization. Although whooping cough had never been eradicated, its incidence had greatly decreased. However, it is now increasing.

This highly contagious bacterial disease is spread through coughing or sneezing (droplet transmission). Educating adults on how to avoid transmitting the bacteria to children is essential, because adults can spread the disease without even realizing they are infected. Good hand hygiene, covering the nose and mouth when coughing or sneezing, and avoiding kissing children on the lips are proactive ways to prevent spread of the disease. Further steps to prevent the spread of infection are avoiding contact with infants when experiencing respiratory symptoms, ensuring infants are vaccinated based on the regular schedule, and instructing adults to receive pertussis vaccine as part of the tetanus/diphtheria booster. Medical assistants should be familiar with the recommended vaccination schedule and should continue to monitor and educate patients on these vaccines. The current schedule can be retrieved through the Centers for Disease Control and Prevention at https://www.cdc.gov/vaccines/schedules/hcp/imz/child-adolescent.html.

Anthrax

Anthrax has been used as a bioterrorism agent in the past, and in the event of a bioterrorism attack it would likely be used again: This microbe can be produced in a lab, persists in the environment, and remains undetected when being introduced. It takes only a small quantity of the bacteria to cause illness. Inhalation of the spores is the most severe exposure, which can lead to death unless treated quickly.

Anthrax symptoms range from breathing difficulties to gastrointestinal upset and fever. A two-month course of antibiotics may be necessary to treat those exposed to the bacteria. While a vaccine is available, it is not typically used in the general public and is not FDA-approved for postexposure treatment. Public awareness that this type of infection is possible, along with prompt reporting of signs and symptoms, will help to detect outbreaks of anthrax.

Shingles

Patients with shingles experience painful blisters. Although shingles is not life-threatening, it can lead to complications including skin infections, neurological issues, and (if the outbreak is near or in the eyes) visual disturbances.

Implementation of the varicella vaccine has greatly reduced the chance of developing shingles. However, individuals who have had chickenpox retain the varicella zoster virus, which causes shingles, in their bodies. An estimated one in four adults over the age of 50 will develop shingles, and the risk of getting the disease increases with age. The illness is contagious in immunosuppressed patients and unvaccinated individuals who come in contact with shingles lesions. Older adults should be encouraged to receive the shingles vaccine.

Other Notable Diseases

In recent decades, HIV/AIDS, meningococcal meningitis, hepatitis, and other diseases have been important public health concerns. Medical assistants must be aware of diseases that pose a threat to public health. To maximize your safety and the safety of your patients, continue to keep your knowledge up-to-date by monitoring medical journals and the CDC website.

Chapter 2: **Overview of the Exams**

PROFESSIONAL CREDENTIALS

If you are wondering whether you should become certified or formally credentialed, the answer is yes! By being formally certified, you will have an edge in the job market and greater options for both a higher salary and continued professional growth. It is in your best interest to be certified in your field.

Table 2.1 gives an overview of the organizations that currently credential medical assistants. These credentialing agencies are approved by the National Commission for Certifying Agencies (NCCA) and are known and recognized by health care employer groups.

Organization Name	Credential Offered	Term of Credential	Exam Fees	Notes
American Association of Medical Assistants (AAMA)	CMA	5 years	$125 recent grads & members, $250 others	Not-for-profit membership & certification organization (annual dues $25–$40 student, $77–$107 regular; varies by state)
American Medical Technologists (AMT)	RMA	3 years	$95 initial, $70 subsequent	Not-for-profit membership & certification organization (annual dues $50)
National Healthcareer Association (NHA)	CCMA	2 years	$149	For-profit certification agency
National Center for Competency Testing (NCCT)	NCMA	1 year	$90 student, $135 regular	For-profit certification agency
American Medical Certification Association (AMCA)	CMAC	2 years	$139	For-profit certification agency

Table 2.1—Certification Sponsoring Organizations

The American Association of Medical Assistants (AAMA) awards the Certified Medical Assistant (CMA) credential. Applicants must graduate from an approved medical assistant program and complete a certification examination. CMAs are required to renew their credential every five years through continuing education or by retaking the exam.

The American Medical Technologists (AMT) is a nonprofit certification agency and membership organization representing a variety of allied health care professionals. The AMT awards the Registered Medical Assistant (RMA) credential to candidates who pass a computerized test that can be taken at a variety of locations in the United States and Canada.

The National Healthcareer Association (NHA) is a for-profit certification agency that offers the Certified Clinical Medical Assistant (CCMA) credential. To take the test, candidates must have completed either a medical assistant training program or at least 12 months of work as a medical assistant. CCMAs must renew their credential every two years through continuing education.

The National Center for Competency Testing (NCCT) is a for-profit agency that awards the National Certified Medical Assistant (NCMA) credential. To take the test, candidates must have completed either an approved medical assistant training program or at least two years of on-the-job training under the direction of a physician. NCMAs must renew their credential annually through continuing education.

Finally, the American Medical Certification Association (AMCA) is a for-profit agency that awards multiple credentials, including Clinical Medical Assistant Certification (CMAC). To qualify for this exam, students must graduate from an approved training program for medical assistants or have two or more years of current experience in the field. Credential renewal can be accomplished through completion of 10 continuing education units every two years or by retaking the exam.

WHAT TO EXPECT ON THE EXAMS

CMA Testing

The CMA test is developed and administered by the National Board of Medical Examiners (NBME) under an agreement with the AAMA. Membership in the AAMA is not a requirement to sit for the examination. To become a CMA, the candidate must achieve a passing score on the entire examination. Each candidate receives a percentile ranking and performance score on the three areas of content covered in the test. These areas include Cognitive, Psychomotor, and Affective domains.

Test Format

The CMA test is a computer based, multiple-choice test consisting of questions that have "one best answer" from a group of five options. The test includes 200 items—180 are scored, 20 are pre-tested. The random pre-test questions do not count toward your score.

The questions are formatted as incomplete statements or questions followed by choices that complete the statement or that answer the question. Options other than the best answer may be partially correct, but you will be asked to select the *best answer* to each question. Some questions will require that you identify body parts or anatomical regions from an illustration or diagram. You are required to achieve a passing score on each section of the test to become certified. You will receive an unofficial pass or fail result right away. Confirmation of your score will also be mailed to you within 12 weeks of your test date.

CMA Test Content

The AAMA provides a detailed content outline of the subjects covered in each section of the CMA test: general knowledge, administrative knowledge, and clinical knowledge. You should complete a thorough and general review of the content areas as they are outlined. The test is designed to measure your comprehensive knowledge of the medical assistant subject matter and your ability to apply this knowledge in practice. For information on the CMA exam, including the most up-to-date content outlines and exam registration information, visit the AAMA website at aama-ntl.org.

General:

Medical terminology

Anatomy and physiology

Psychology

Professionalism

Communication

Medicolegal guidelines and requirements

Administrative:

Data entry

Equipment

Computer concepts

Records management

Screening and processing mail

Scheduling and monitoring appointments

Resource information and community services

Maintaining the office environment

Office policies and procedures

Practice finances

Clinical:

Principles of infection control

Treatment areas

Patient preparation and assisting the physician

Patient history interview

Collecting and processing specimens and diagnostic testing

Preparing and administering medications

Emergencies and emergency preparation

First aid

Nutrition

Test Eligibility and Registration

To be eligible to take the CMA exam, you must complete an application and file all required documents. You must be graduating from, or be a graduate of, an accredited medical assistant program and you may need to have a copy of your official transcripts and your date of graduation. The transcript must have the seal of the registrar from your program. You must have attended a program accredited by either the Commission on Accreditation of Allied Health Education Programs (CAAHEP), or the Accrediting Bureau of Health Education Schools (ABHES). A listing of accredited programs can be found on the AAMA website (aama-ntl. org/medassisting/caahep_prgs.aspx).

The CMA examination packet contains pertinent policies for test registration, fee information, eligibility information, and a list of examination locations. To request a package, contact the AAMA via phone, fax, or mail, or log on to the AAMA website.

American Association of Medical Assistants
20 N. Wacker Drive, Suite 1575
Chicago, IL 60606
Phone: 1-312-899-1500
Fax: 1-312-899-1259
Fax-on-demand (request an application): 1-312-899-6813
aama-ntl.org

The CMA examination is offered throughout the year at locations throughout the United States. When you apply, you will receive instructions for making an appointment at one of the 200 nationwide testing centers closest to you.

Payment for the examination must accompany the application. At the present time, the fee is $125 for current and recent (within one year) graduates. Nonrecent graduates or CMAs seeking recertification must pay $250 to take the exam, but those who are AAMA members can take the test for $125. Accepted forms of payment include credit cards, certified checks, and money orders. Registration fees are nonrefundable. However, for a $65 fee, candidates may transfer their testing eligibility period to the next available 90-day testing period. Requests must be submitted in writing to the AAMA Certification Department at least 30 days prior to the end of the original testing period. Only one transfer is allowed per candidate. If you are applying for an initial certification exam, you will not be required to submit a copy of your official transcript with the application. However, your eligibility for certification will be verified through communication with the educational institution. Applicants for recertification must submit their

CMA certificates and proof of current provider level CPR certification. Note that if information or material is missing, your application for the test will not be processed.

If you need special accommodations for test day, you must include a written petition along with your application and test fees. Your request should include a diagnosis by a health professional whose credentials also must be included. The petition should state how you are limited by your condition and provide examples. See aama-ntl.org for detailed information. Your application processing time is approximately 30 days following your submission of all application materials. You will receive notification of your score approximately 10 weeks after you take the exam.

Recertification

The AAMA requires that the CMA credential be recertified every five years. To maintain certification, the CMA must either complete a recertification examination or a continuing education requirement.

CMAs may choose to recertify by taking the same exam used for initial certification. To follow this route, you must submit an application at least 90 days before the first day of your testing month.

Another option for recertification is through completion of continuing education credit. The AAMA requires 60 continuing education credits during the prior 5 years to maintain continuous certification. The continuing education option calls for 30 hours of continuing education that has been approved by the AAMA. You will be expected to complete 10 hours each of administrative credit, clinical credit, and general credit. In addition, 20 hours of variable credits combined from any of the topic areas can be applied to your continuing education requirement. You will need to submit information about the programs that you attended, including the site of the program, the length of the program, the topic, and any proof of attendance and approval by the AAMA.

The AAMA website contains a list of approved continuing education programs (aama-ntl.org/recertified/how.aspx). In addition, the AAMA offers continuing education programs online, in its printed journals, and at its national membership conference. The AAMA will assist member CMAs by maintaining an online database that accumulates their completed continuing education credits on an ongoing basis. Applicants who seek recertification by continuing education should apply for recertification at least 90 days in advance of the expiration of their current CMA certification. The application for certification by continuing education can be downloaded from the AAMA website (aama-ntl.org/recertified/how.aspx).

Every CMA can decide whether to recertify by exam or continuing education. For some people, the prospect of taking a standardized test under timed, proctored conditions is no big deal. These individuals may decide the planning and time commitment required for continuing education is not worth it. Other people may see recertification via continuing education as a reward for the educational and professional development activities they would have undertaken anyway. They may be less comfortable with standardized testing.

RMA Testing

Exam Format

The RMA test is conducted by the American Medical Technologists (AMT). Like the CMA exam, this test is intended to evaluate entry-level competencies of medical assistants. It assesses the skills and knowledge needed to perform the medical assistant's job duties, as designated by subject matter experts. The RMA test consists of 200 multiple-choice questions with four answer choices for each item. Candidates have three hours to complete the test. As in the CMA exam, you are expected to select the one best answer for each item. You will be required to recall facts, understand medical illustrations, solve problems, and interpret information from case studies. The RMA exam can be taken on paper or on a computer. For more information about these options, see Chapter 3.

If you take the test by computer, your score will appear immediately. If you take the pencil-and-paper test, your results will arrive by mail six to eight weeks after you take the exam. A score of 70 or above is required for passing the test. A scaled scoring system is used and a score of 70 does not relate to the number of items scored correctly or the percentage of correct answers on the test. Students who fail the examination will be given detailed information about the areas in which weak test performance was noted. In this way, students can focus their study in preparing to test again. Students who have to retake the exam must complete the entire examination.

Exam Content

Similar to the CMA exam, the RMA exam covers three areas of content that include general medical assisting knowledge (about 43 percent of the test items), administrative knowledge (about 23 percent of the test items), and clinical aspects of medical assisting (about 35 percent of the test items).

The RMA candidate handbook contains an outline for the content areas covered in the exam. These content areas are more general than those of the CMA exam, but the exam itself covers essentially the same material with less emphasis on administrative competencies. See the AMT website for more information (amt1.com). Following are the content areas covered by the RMA exam.

> **General:**
>
> Anatomy and physiology
>
> Medical terminology
>
> Medical law
>
> Bioethics
>
> Human relations
>
> Patient education

Administrative:

Insurance

Financial bookkeeping

Medical receptionist/secretarial

Clinical:

Asepsis

Sterilization

Instruments

Vital signs

Physical examination

Clinical pharmacology

Minor surgical procedures

Therapeutic modalities

Laboratory procedures

EKGs

First aid

Test Eligibility and Registration

To take the RMA exam, you must be at least 18 years old and a high school graduate from an accredited school or approved equivalent. You must also meet one of the following medical assistant education requirements:

1. Be a graduate of an accredited medical assisting program as determined by CAAHEP or ABHES.

2. Be a graduate of a medical assisting program in a college or postsecondary school that is accredited by a regional accrediting commission or by a group that is approved by the U.S. Department of Education.

3. Complete a formal medical services training program of the U.S. Armed Forces.

In lieu of these educational requirements, applicants are eligible to take the exam if they have five years of experience in medical assisting. No more than two of these years may have been as an instructor in a medical assisting program.

The RMA examination is offered in two formats. One is administered on a computer-based testing system under contract with Pearson VUE test centers. These VUE test centers are located at several hundred sites throughout the United States and the U.S. territories. A list of centers can be found at pearsonvue.com/amt. In addition, the AMT offers pencil-and-paper testing at the VUE test centers. The computer-based and paper exams have the same form and content. To apply for the RMA exam, you must apply to the AMT registrar and receive an approval letter authorizing your eligibility to take the exam. A $90 fee is required with the application. Applications are available on the AMT website (amt1.com). You also may contact AMT by phone, fax, or mail:

American Medical Technologists
10700 West Higgins Road
Park Ridge, IL 60018
Phone: 1-847-823-5169 or 1-800-275-1268
Fax: 1-847-823-0458
Email: mail@americanmedtech.org
Website: americanmedtech.org

Once you receive the authorization to test, if you are taking the computer-based test, you may log on to the Pearson VUE website at pearsonvue.com/amt to schedule an exam time and test location. Exams are available year-round by appointment. You also may sign up for the pencil-and-paper version of the exam, which also is administered at Pearson VUE test centers on certain dates and times. You may receive a refund or reschedule your test if you notify the test center at least one day in advance. As with the CMA exam, if you require special accommodations, you must request them in writing.

You should plan to arrive at the site at least 30 minutes in advance to check in and you will need to bring two forms of identification. A primary form of identification must be an official document containing a signature and a photo ID. Examples include a passport, photo driver's license, employee ID card, or a military ID. The other source of personal identification may include a credit card or other item. In addition to identification, you will need to bring your approval letter to the exam site.

The AMT board reserves the right to cancel any exam scores if, in their opinion, there is reason to question the validity of a score. The board also reserves the right to investigate conduct that occurred during the exam. Specific scores may be canceled due to behaviors such as copying, using notes, removing test materials, or helping others during the exam. If the board exercises their rights in canceling your score, you will be given a chance to retake the test without any penalty or additional fees. Significant score increases upon retesting may also be investigated.

You may retake the test no sooner than three months after a failed test and no later than two years following your application date. The fee for retesting is $60. You can retake the examination up to three times if you fail. You must complete a new application if you fail the exam on your second retake. If you require a second retake, you will be asked to submit evidence of retraining or additional training.

You may ask that your initial answer sheet be rescored if you get a failing score on the RMA exam. You must request the rescoring in writing within 60 days of the release of your results to the AMT and pay a fee to have this processed. Your test will be rescored by hand. The AMT notes that their scoring procedures are quality checked on a regular basis and they state that it is unlikely that rescoring will change the examination results.

You have the right to appeal a failing score. If you wish to review the exam, you must submit a written request within 60 days of the release of your original scores. You will then be granted an opportunity to review your test with an AMT representative present. For details of this process, refer to AMT's *Candidate Handbook.*

Deciding Between the Computer-Based and Paper Exams

The AMT recommends that candidates contact the AMT registrar in their discipline to help them decide whether to take the exam on the computer or on paper. Some advantages of the computer exam include the fact that you get your score immediately at the end of your test instead of having to wait several weeks. There is no danger of accidentally skipping a line on your answer sheet and incorrectly gridding the rest of your test. Candidates also find that the computer-based exam takes less time than the paper exam because they do not have to deal with test booklets and answer sheets. Individuals who are less comfortable with computers will want to take the paper-and-pencil exam. Skipping questions and returning to them later is easier on the paper exam. The AMT's practice materials are on paper, so it is easier to become familiar with this version of the exam. Ultimately, you must decide for yourself which option is best for you.

CCMA Testing

The Certified Clinical Medical Assistant (CCMA) exam is administered by the National Healthcareer Association (NHA). The exam lasts 1 hour and 50 minutes and has 110 items, 100 of which count toward your score. (The 10 unscored items are pre-test questions that the NHA is trying out for future exams.) Questions are in the following three content areas: medical office procedures (50 percent of test items), financial procedures (30 percent), and risk management (20 percent). To maintain certification, CCMAs must complete 10 hours of NHA-approved continuing education credits every two years.

Test Eligibility and Registration

To be eligible to take the CCMA exam, you must meet both the following requirements:

1. Possess a high school diploma or equivalent recognized in the state where you live. If you do not currently meet this requirement but will do so within 12 months, you may be eligible for provisional CCMA certification.

2. Successfully complete either a medical assistant training program or a minimum of one year of supervised work experience as a medical assistant. (Be prepared to provide documentation of this training or work experience upon request.)

Once you create a profile online at nhanow.com, you can register for the examination and schedule your exam date at a PSI testing location. NHA sends a confirmation email when the application is processed.

National Healthcareer Association
11161 Overbrook Road
Leawood, KS 66211
800-499-9092
nhanow.com
info@nhanow.com

NCMA Testing

The National Certified Medical Assistant (NCMA) exam is administered by the National Center for Competency Testing (NCCT). It is a three-hour exam with 150 scored items in the following five content categories: medical office management (about 19 percent of test items), medical terminology (about 11 percent), pharmacology (about 11 percent), anatomy and physiology (about 11 percent), and medical procedures (about 47 percent). To maintain certification, NCMAs must complete 14 hours of NCCT-approved continuing education credits annually.

Test Eligibility and Registration

To be eligible to take the NCMA, you must meet one of the following requirements:

1. Be a current student in a Medical Assistant program approved by NCCT.
2. Have graduated from a NCCT-approved medical assistant program within the past five years.
3. Have logged two years of verifiable experience as a medical assistant within the past five years.
4. Have completed medical assistant training or its equivalent during U.S. military service within the last five years.

Application for NCMA must be completed online at ncctinc.com at least 14 days prior to testing. Registration is valid for one year after NCCT receives your application and payment. Testing takes place at approved public testing sites throughout the United States and is generally given in electronic format.

National Center for Competency Testing
7007 College Blvd., Suite 385
Overland Park, KS 66211
Phone: 800-875-4404
Fax: 913-498-1243
ncctinc.com

CMAC Testing

Certified Medical Assistant Certification (CMAC) is administered by the American Medical Certification Association (AMCA). The exam lasts 3 hours and 15 minutes and consists of 200 questions testing knowledge of phlebotomy, EKG, anatomy and physiology, law and ethics, safety and infection control, patient care, medical office administration, and health care systems. To maintain certification, CMACs must complete 10 hours of continuing education every two years.

Test Eligibility and Registration

To sit for an AMCA test, you must be 18 years old, possess a high school diploma or equivalent, and meet one of the following requirements:

1. Graduate from a training program that maps to the blueprint of an AMCA certification exam (proof of completion is required).

2. Have two or more years of work experience and be currently working in that field. Candidates must provide proof of employment/experience in the form of a written letter and high school diploma or equivalent. Letters, which should include daily responsibilities and tasks performed as part of your role, must be verified, written on company letterhead, and signed by an authorized party.

Once you have established an account, you can test at an approved location or through ProctorU, which is a virtual proctoring method. This option involves additional fees but offers candidates the opportunity to test from a home location.

American Medical Certification Association
194 Route 46 East
Fairfield, NJ 07866
888-960-2622
Fax: 973-582-1801
www.amcaexams.com

Chapter 3: **Test-Taking Skills and Study Strategies**

This chapter will provide you with strategies for taking the CMA and RMA credentialing exams. First, you will receive general advice to improve your test performance. Then you will learn about test-specific strategies based on guidelines the AAMA and the AMT offer to test takers. Finally, this chapter will present advice for the day of the test. Remember, by reviewing the information in this book and taking the practice exam, you are preparing to do your best on the medical assisting exam.

GENERAL TEST PREPARATION

Many medical assistant students find test taking to be stressful. This section will provide the tools to support your success on the exam. Most important, know the content the test covers. Be prepared before the test by keeping up with your work and devising a study schedule. You have completed a full program of study and it is unlikely that last-minute cramming will be effective in preparing for the exam.

You may want to begin your review by taking the diagnostic test in this book or using practice test questions prepared by the AAMA or AMT. This will help you benchmark your knowledge and identify content areas for focused review. This book includes content-specific review chapters that cover all areas tested on both the CMA and RMA exams. Each chapter ends in review questions to help clarify your knowledge of that content area. In addition, this book includes a full-length CMA practice test. Take this comprehensive test using the time frame that you will be given for the actual exam. Note that the answers and explanations following the end-of-chapter review questions, diagnostic test questions, and the full-length practice test questions contain not only the correct answer, but also a content summary that identifies the best answer and rationale for selection of this answer. Be sure to read these explanations, even for questions you answered correctly. If your study time is limited, this method will ensure that you cover relevant content without having to refer back to your class notes or textbooks.

The certifying board of the American Association of Medical Assistants provides detailed information about the CMA exam in *A Candidate's Guide to the AAMA CMA Certification/ Recertification Examination*. This publication is available for download from the AAMA website or by contacting the organization (see Chapter 1 for contact information). The AAMA recommends that the best way to prepare for the exam is a general yet thorough review of the subject matter. AAMA chapters in certain areas sponsor exam study groups. Check the AAMA website or contact the organization by phone to learn more.

The AMT publishes a *Candidate Handbook* containing detailed information about exam policies along with a set of practice test items. This handbook is available through the AMT at amt1.com.

CMA/RMA EXAM STRATEGIES

Consider the Question Before Looking at the Answers

Read each test item carefully before you select an answer. People often make mistakes because they fail to read the test question in detail, especially with questions containing "not" or "except." Also, try to think of what the answer should be based on your knowledge of test content before you look at the answer choices. You will be less likely to choose an incorrect but attractive answer.

Use Process of Elimination

With most multiple-choice questions, you will be able to eliminate one or more of the answer options readily. Cross them off on the exam book and improve your odds of selecting the best answer for each test item.

Pace Yourself

Avoid spending too much time on any single test item. Circle test items that may require extra time and come back to them after you have finished the rest of the exam. Wear a watch and pace yourself through each of the three test sections: general, administrative, and clinical. Set up checkpoints during the exam to help your pacing.

Answer Every Question

Mark a response for each item. All items are scored equally and no points are subtracted for incorrect answers. Do not leave any items blank. If you do not know the answer to a particular question, eliminate as many answers as possible and make an educated guess.

Mark Up Your Test Booklet

If you are taking a pencil-and-paper exam, it may be helpful to make notes in the test booklet next to specific responses, such as "true" or "false" or "unsure." This will save you time if you have to come back to a particular question.

Be Careful with Your Answer Sheet

If you are taking a paper-based test, make sure that you fill in the computer-scored answer sheet carefully and that you are not skipping any items or getting your answer sheet out of sync with the correct test item. Do not make any stray marks on the answer sheet. Fill in the circle using a No. 2 pencil and if you erase or change a test response, do so clearly and with care. If you leave an item blank because you need more time or want to come back to it, make sure to circle the question in your test booklet so that you will come back to the correct item on the answer sheet.

If you finish the exam with extra time, go back and make sure that you have answered each test item and that your answer sheet is properly completed. Look to make sure that you did not leave any blanks, and that you have selected only one response to each question.

Watch for Questions Containing "Not" or "Except"

Remember to watch out for questions phrased as negative statements (e.g., "Each of the following is correct EXCEPT"). The negative word may be printed in uppercase letters.

Practice Doing Calculations in Your Head

Calculators are not permitted in the test center and scratch paper will not be provided. When you take practice tests, do so without using scratch paper to simulate actual test conditions.

Look Away at Times

Taking the test on the computer leads to eye muscle fatigue. If you stare at the screen for the entire duration of the exam, you may develop a headache that will impede concentration. Give your eyes a short break every ten or fifteen minutes by focusing on a distant object, such as the door to the testing room. (Make sure you do not appear to be looking at another candidate's computer screen.)

ON THE DAY OF THE EXAM

Make sure that you get plenty of sleep the night before the exam. Wear comfortable clothing and dress in layers, because you won't know how hot or cold the examination room will be. Wear a watch and be prepared to check your speed and time allotment during the test to pace your progress. Eat a good breakfast so you will not be hungry during the exam. During breakfast, read something to warm up your brain. You do not want the test to be the first thing you read that day.

Arrive at the test center in plenty of time to register and receive instructions. Make sure that you bring your approval letter and required identification material. For both the CMA exam and the paper-and-pencil RMA exam, you will need two No. 2 pencils with erasers. Make sure that you do not bring any notes, calculators, phones, or other unacceptable materials to the test location.

No reference materials are allowed in the exam room. No electronic equipment (including cell phones, pagers, and calculators) is allowed in the test center.

Communication between examinees is not permitted during the exam. An examinee that is detected trying to give or obtain aid shall be subject to invalidation of scores. You must obtain permission from the test proctor to leave the testing room. You will be given permission only for using the restroom. Only one examinee may leave the room at a time. No smoking, eating, or drinking is allowed in the examination room.

Finally, face your test with energy and confidence. Remember that you have prepared well using this book, sample materials from the test makers, and your textbooks and class notes. Now you are ready for success.

PART TWO

Diagnostic Test

HOW TO TAKE THE DIAGNOSTIC TEST

The following short diagnostic quiz will test your knowledge of the basic content areas on the CMA and RMA exams and help you focus your study time. Give yourself 24 minutes for the quiz. Find a quiet place where you will not be disturbed, and mark your answers on the answer sheet using a No. 2 pencil.

After the test, you will find an answer key, answers and explanations, and a correlation chart. When you score your test, compare any incorrect answers to the correlation chart to see which topics give you the most difficulty. You should focus your review on these subjects, particularly if your study time is limited. Be sure to read the answer explanations for all questions, including those you answered correctly. You can pick up important information from reading another person's explanation of why the incorrect answers are incorrect.

Best of luck!

ANSWER SHEET

1. Ⓐ Ⓑ Ⓒ Ⓓ Ⓔ
2. Ⓐ Ⓑ Ⓒ Ⓓ Ⓔ
3. Ⓐ Ⓑ Ⓒ Ⓓ Ⓔ
4. Ⓐ Ⓑ Ⓒ Ⓓ Ⓔ
5. Ⓐ Ⓑ Ⓒ Ⓓ Ⓔ
6. Ⓐ Ⓑ Ⓒ Ⓓ Ⓔ
7. Ⓐ Ⓑ Ⓒ Ⓓ Ⓔ
8. Ⓐ Ⓑ Ⓒ Ⓓ Ⓔ
9. Ⓐ Ⓑ Ⓒ Ⓓ Ⓔ
10. Ⓐ Ⓑ Ⓒ Ⓓ Ⓔ
11. Ⓐ Ⓑ Ⓒ Ⓓ Ⓔ
12. Ⓐ Ⓑ Ⓒ Ⓓ Ⓔ
13. Ⓐ Ⓑ Ⓒ Ⓓ Ⓔ
14. Ⓐ Ⓑ Ⓒ Ⓓ Ⓔ
15. Ⓐ Ⓑ Ⓒ Ⓓ Ⓔ

16. Ⓐ Ⓑ Ⓒ Ⓓ Ⓔ
17. Ⓐ Ⓑ Ⓒ Ⓓ Ⓔ
18. Ⓐ Ⓑ Ⓒ Ⓓ Ⓔ
19. Ⓐ Ⓑ Ⓒ Ⓓ Ⓔ
20. Ⓐ Ⓑ Ⓒ Ⓓ Ⓔ
21. Ⓐ Ⓑ Ⓒ Ⓓ Ⓔ
22. Ⓐ Ⓑ Ⓒ Ⓓ Ⓔ
23. Ⓐ Ⓑ Ⓒ Ⓓ Ⓔ
24. Ⓐ Ⓑ Ⓒ Ⓓ Ⓔ
25. Ⓐ Ⓑ Ⓒ Ⓓ Ⓔ
26. Ⓐ Ⓑ Ⓒ Ⓓ Ⓔ
27. Ⓐ Ⓑ Ⓒ Ⓓ Ⓔ
28. Ⓐ Ⓑ Ⓒ Ⓓ Ⓔ
29. Ⓐ Ⓑ Ⓒ Ⓓ Ⓔ
30. Ⓐ Ⓑ Ⓒ Ⓓ Ⓔ

DIAGNOSTIC TEST

Time: 24 minutes

DIRECTIONS (Questions 1–30): All of the following questions and incomplete statements are followed by five answer choices. For each question, select the single answer that best answers the question or completes the statement. Fill in the corresponding circle on your answer sheet.

1. The threat of touching someone without permission is called

    (A) invasion of privacy

    (B) battery

    (C) assault

    (D) slander

    (E) libel

2. Which of the following terms refers to a condition of insufficient blood-clotting cells?

    (A) Erythrocytopenia

    (B) Hypovolemia

    (C) Thrombocytopenia

    (D) Erythrocytosis

    (E) Thrombophlebitis

3. Which of the following foods does NOT represent carbohydrates?

    (A) Oats

    (B) Corn

    (C) Lettuce

    (D) Milk

    (E) Fish

4. According to Dr. Elisabeth Kübler-Ross, most individuals who experience the impending death of a loved one will initially experience which of the following emotions as part of the grieving process?

    (A) Bargaining

    (B) Empathy

    (C) Acceptance

    (D) Denial

    (E) Grief

5. Which of the following refers to the portion of the brain responsible for balance and movement?

    (A) Cerebrum

    (B) Brain stem

    (C) Medulla oblongata

    ✗ (D) Hippocampus

    (E) Cerebellum

6. Which of the following items is NOT part of effective communication?

    (A) Sender

    ✓ (B) Receiver

    (C) Message

    (D) Noise

    (E) Feedback

7. The artery that carries oxygenated blood to the body pumped from the left ventricle is called the

    (A) pulmonary vein

    (B) aorta

    (C) superior vena cava

    (D) pulmonary artery

    (E) inferior vena cava

8. Therapeutic communication differs from normal, everyday communication in that it

    (A) involves medical terms

    (B) is only used by therapists

    (C) involves special skills

    (D) can only be used in the office

    (E) only includes nonverbal communication

9. Which of the following is NOT true about arbitration?

    (A) It can prevent a lengthy trial.

    (B) Both parties must agree to it.

    (C) It is not binding.

    (D) A third party attempts to bring settlement.

    (E) It may be used in malpractice cases.

10. Which of the following is the term for "fast heartbeat"?

    (A) Tachypnea
    (B) Tachyphagia
    (C) Bradycardia
    (D) Tachycardia
    (E) Bradypnea

11. A medical assistant would use word processing software to create which of the following?

    (A) Superbills
    (B) A record of all patients and their addresses
    (C) An inventory of the office supplies
    (D) Appointment schedules
    (E) Transcriptions

12. Before seeing the physician, patients should not have to wait longer than

    (A) 30 minutes
    (B) 1 hour
    (C) 10 minutes
    (D) 5 minutes
    (E) 15 to 20 minutes

13. An outguide is a(n)

    (A) place marker
    (B) tab
    (C) binder
    (D) file sorter
    (E) file jacket

14. Which of the following data entry notes has a misplaced comma?

    (A) The patient, a 25-year-old Caucasian woman, complained of chest pains.
    (B) The culture, did not grow any bacteria.
    (C) Dr. Smith, Dr. Brown, and Dr. Jones were present.
    (D) The doctor tried to reach the patient, but she was not at home.
    (E) The patient's blood pressure, heartbeat, and pulse were normal.

15. Before choosing to which facility to refer a patient, always verify the patient's

    (A) insurance

    (B) income

    (C) transportation

    (D) age

    (E) address

16. When opening and processing mail, the medical assistant should consider which of the following items as fifth priority?

    (A) Catalogs

    (B) Magazines and newspapers

    (C) All first-class mail

    (D) Airmail

    (E) Registered mail

17. All filing equipment must be located

    (A) in the physician's personal office

    (B) in the reception area

    (C) within easy reach of patients

    (D) in a secure area

    (E) in the exam room

18. A disadvantage of the wave scheduling system is that

    (A) patients may have a long wait before seeing the physician

    (B) patients become annoyed because they have appointments at the same time

    (C) it prevents the medical assistant from pulling the patient's chart

    (D) it assumes that two patients will actually be seen by the doctor within the same time frame

    (E) it can cause appointments to be overbooked

19. A record of all employees and their earnings, deductions, and other information is called

    (A) employee earnings

    (B) payroll tasks

    (C) accounts payable

    (D) payroll register

    (E) employee financial listing

20. The policy section of the policy and procedures manual includes the

    (A) chain of command for the office
    (B) patients' names and numbers
    (C) specialists' names and addresses
    (D) office hours
    (E) physician's home address

21. Which of the following reflects the ability of the kidneys to concentrate urine?

    (A) Ketones
    (B) Specific gravity
    (C) pH
    (D) Protein
    (E) Odor

22. Which of the following actions should the medical assistant NOT take when preparing the patient for an exam?

    (A) Inform the patient about how the exam will be done.
    (B) Witness any consent that is necessary prior to the exam.
    (C) Reassure the patient that everything will be okay.
    (D) Allow the patient to verbalize concerns and ask questions about the exam.
    (E) Assist the patient to get into gown and draping.

23. Tympanic thermometers are used to measure temperature in/on the

    (A) mouth
    (B) ear
    (C) rectum
    (D) forehead
    (E) arm

24. The physician asks the medical assistant to give Ativan 2 mg to the patient. A vial reads 1 mg per 1 mL. Which of the following doses would the medical assistant administer?

    (A) 1 mL
    (B) 2 mL
    (C) 1 mg
    (D) 1/2 mL
    (E) 3/4 mL

25. Symptoms of shock include

    (A) edema
    (B) hypertension and a bounding pulse
    (C) chest pain radiating down the left arm
    (D) hypotension and a weak thready pulse
    (E) nausea and vomiting

26. A wound that does not heal as expected due to infection is said to heal by

    (A) first intention
    (B) debridement
    (C) wet to dry dressings
    (D) second intention
    (E) surgical intervention

27. Which of the following represents the morphology of cocci bacteria?

    (A) Rod
    (B) Spiral
    (C) Spherical
    (D) Coiled
    (E) Spirochete

28. The three most important factors in performing a hand wash are

    (A) friction, soap, and warm running water
    (B) antibacterial soap, length of time spent, and hot water
    (C) length of time spent, type of soap, running water
    (D) position of the hands, friction, and temperature of the water
    (E) availability of feet controls for soap, cold water, length of time spent

29. When an elderly patient in a crowded waiting room falls unconscious, a medical assistant's first action should be to

    (A) call 911
    (B) call the physician to check the patient
    (C) start rescue breathing
    (D) check the patient's airway
    (E) start CPR

30. If the physician is performing a routine bimanual pelvic exam, which of the following will the medical assistant have available?

    (A) Sterile gloves and speculum

    (B) Overhead light source and water-soluble lubricant

    (C) Biopsy tray and sterile gloves

    (D) Exam gloves and water-soluble lubricant

    (E) Hemocult card and exam gloves

ANSWER KEY

1. C
2. C
3. E
4. D
5. E
6. D
7. B
8. C
9. C
10. D
11. E
12. E
13. A
14. B
15. A
16. B
17. D
18. B
19. D
20. D
21. B
22. C
23. B
24. B
25. D
26. D
27. C
28. A
29. D
30. D

ANSWERS AND EXPLANATIONS

1. **C**

   The threat of touching someone without permission is assault (C), while the actual touching without permission is battery (B). Slander (D) is defaming a person using the spoken word. Libel (E) is writing harmful, untrue things about another person. Invasion of privacy (A) is allowing another person to see or hear another person's medical information without explicit permission from the patient.

2. **C**

   The suffix that means "lack of" is *-penia*. That eliminates all answers except choices (A) and (C). An erythrocyte is a red blood cell and thrombocyto means "blood clot cell." The correct answer is thrombocytopenia. Erythrocytopenia (A) means insufficient red blood cells. Hypohematosis (B) is a condition of low blood volume. Erythrocytosis (D) means a condition of red cells. Thrombophlebitis (E) means inflammation of clots in the vein.

3. **E**

   Carbohydrates are fruits, vegetables, grains, and dairy foods. Oats (A) and corn (B) are examples of grains. Lettuce (C) is a vegetable and milk (D) is representative of dairy. Fish (E) is a protein.

4. **D**

   In working with hundreds of dying patients and their families, Kübler-Ross found that the most common initial reaction upon learning of their condition was denial (D). Bargaining (A), such as saying, "I will be a better person if my mother lives," is a subsequent stage. Acceptance of loss and death (C) is the final stage of the grieving process. Empathy (B) is not a component of Kübler-Ross's conceptual model. Grief (E) is the work of the entire multistage emotional experience of loss and death. The stages of denial, bargaining, anger, and acceptance may reoccur in different sequences for different individuals.

5. **E**

   The cerebellum is the part of the brain responsible for balance and movement. The cerebrum (A) is the portion of the brain for thought and personality. The brain stem (B) contains the medulla oblongata (C) and is responsible for basic functions like breathing and respiration. The hippocampus (D) is part of the diencephalon and is responsible for long-term memory.

6. **D**

   A complete communication event is comprised of a sender (A), a receiver (B), a message (C), and feedback (E). Physical or emotional noise (D) serves as a barrier to effective communication.

KAPLAN

7. **B**

The aorta carries oxygenated blood to the body as the left ventricle pumps it out. The superior vena cava (C) and inferior vena cava (E) return deoxygenated blood to the right side of the heart. The pulmonary artery (D) carries blood from the right side of the heart to the lungs. The pulmonary vein (A) returns oxygenated blood to the left ventricle.

8. **C**

Therapeutic communication involves a set of skills and talents including active listening, reflection, and observation of both verbal and nonverbal communication. None of the other items correctly explain or define therapeutic communication.

9. **C**

Arbitration differs from mediation in that it is binding when both parties agree to accept it in place of a trial. Both mediation and arbitration can be used to prevent lengthy and expensive trials. A third person or panel attempts to impartially offer a settlement.

10. **D**

The suffix for beat is *-cardia*. The prefix meaning fast is *tachy-*. Tachypnea (A) means fast breathing. Tachyphagia (B) means fast eating or swallowing, bradycardia (C) means slow heartbeat, and bradypnea (E) means slow breathing.

11. **E**

Word processing software is the software used to create memos, reports, transcripts, and letters. This software allows you to set up margins to create a professional document. Superbills would be created with a financial database or billing software system. Patient names and addresses, supply inventories, and appointment schedules would be created with spreadsheet software such as Excel. This leaves item (E) as the best answer to this question.

12. **E**

Patients do not want to wait any longer than 20 minutes to see the physician. Thirty minutes (A) is too long to wait. An hour wait (B) is far too long to see a physician. Ten minutes (C) would be an ideal time, but it does not give the patient enough time with the physician. Five minutes (D) is an unrealistic time to wait.

13. **A**

An outguide is used as a marker for the medical chart when it is removed from the file cabinet. A tab (B) is used inside the chart. A binder (C) is used to hold papers. File sorters (D) are to separate a grouping of charts. File jackets (E) are envelopes that the medical file can fit into.

14. **B**

There should not be a comma in this sentence. All of the other sentences are correct.

15. **A**

The specialist to which you want to send the patient may not accept the patient's insurance.

16. **B**

Fifth-priority mail includes magazines and newspapers. Sixth-priority mail includes catalogs (A). Third-priority mail includes all first class mail (C). Second-priority mail includes airmail (D). Top-priority mail includes registered mail (E).

17. **D**

Medical records must be kept in a secure area so other patients cannot see private information. It is not necessary to store records in the physician's office (A). A reception area (B) may not be secure enough. Having patients' medical records within easy reach of patients (C) can tempt someone to look at another patient's chart. Having patients' charts in the exam room (E) will also tempt a patient to read another's chart.

18. **B**

A problem with wave scheduling is patients who arrive at the same time and expect to be seen at their appointment time will be unhappy if they are made to wait.

19. **D**

The payroll register (D) is a list of all employees and their earnings, deductions, and other information. Employee earnings (A) are salaries or wages, plus indirect forms of payment. Payroll tasks (B) include calculating the amount of wages or salaries paid and amounts deducted from employees' earnings. Accounts payable (C) is amounts charged with suppliers or creditors that remain unpaid. The employee financial listing (E) is the list that contains the appropriate information concerning the employees' deductions and earnings. Each employee will have his or her own list with deductions and earnings on it.

20. **D**

Office hours would be listed in the policy portion of the policy and procedure booklet. Chain of command for the office (A) is not listed in the policy booklet. The physician would be the head of the office. Patients' names and numbers (B) would be listed in the database, not in the policy and procedures booklet. Specialists' names and addresses (C) would be listed in the database. The physician's home address (E) would not be included in the policy and procedures booklet.

21. **B**

Specific gravity is defined as the weight of a substance compared with the weight of an equal volume of distilled water. This measures the amount or concentration of dissolved substances in the urine sample. The range of specific gravity varies and depends on the patient's fluid intake. Ketones (A) are by-products of fat metabolism and will present in the urine of a patient restricting calories and carbohydrates. Choice C (pH) is an abbreviation for potential hydrogen ion concentration. This will determine if the urine is acidic or alkaline. Protein (D), primarily albumin, can be secreted in minute amounts by the kidneys. Nonpathological presentation of protein can be associated with excessive exercise, exposure to extremes in temperature, or emotional stress. Consistent presentation is associated with renal disease. The odor (E) of urine is usually not recorded, but can indicate many conditions. The aromatic odor of urine does not specifically measure the concentration of urine.

22. **C**

The medical assistant should not tell the patient that everything will be okay. This can be construed as a guarantee of results and become a legal issue. If the outcome of the exam is not favorable for the patient, the patient will lose faith in the medical treatment team. The medical assistant should give the patient information (A) and allow him or her to verbalize concerns and ask questions (D). The medical assistant can witness consents (B) if the patient is aware of the procedure being done and understands the consent form. The medical assistant would assist the patient with gowning and draping as needed (E).

23. **B**

Tympanic thermometers measure the temperature using the tympanic membrane in the inner ear.

24. **B**

The correct amount is 2 mL. The medical assistant would calculate the desired 2 mg divided by the available 1 mg, and multiply by the delivery vehicle of 1 mL.

25. **D**

Regardless of the cause of shock, symptoms always include hypotension and a weak and thready pulse due to the inability of the body to deliver enough oxygen to supply the body's needs.

26. **D**

Wounds that have damaged tissues, are infected, kept open on purpose, or fail to heal normally heal by second intention or from the bottom of the wound to the top. First intention (A) is normal wound healing in which a three-phase repair process allows the wound to come together and the tissues to repair. Wet to dry dressings (C) and debridement (B)

are methods of treatment of wounds that heal by second intention. Surgical intervention (E) may be necessary for wounds that are severely damaged.

27. **C**

Cocci are round or spherical in shape and can occur alone or in pairs and clusters. Bacilli are rod shaped (A) and can have round, straight, or pointed ends. Spirilla are spiral shaped (B) and are usually motile. Tightly coiled (D) spirals are called spirochetes. Spirochete (E) bacteria are usually tightly coiled spirilla.

28. **A**

Water should be running and the temperature should be comfortably warm, but not hot (to prevent damage to the skin). Friction is necessary to dislodge bacteria from the skin and nails.

29. **D**

Checking the patient's airway should be the first priority. Rescue breathing (C) or CPR (E) should not be attempted until lack of respiration and heartbeat have been established. Another person should be sent to notify the physician (B) and to call 911 (A) if needed.

30. **D**

Exam gloves are used for a pelvic exam. Unless there are special circumstances, a pelvic exam is not a sterile procedure. A water-soluble lubricant is used for the exam. The light source (B) should be a gooseneck lamp that is adjustable. A speculum (A) may be used, but is not necessary for a bimanual exam. The hemocult card (E) would be used to test a stool specimen for blood and might be done with a rectal exam. A biopsy tray (C) would not be necessary for a simple pelvic exam.

USING YOUR DIAGNOSTIC TEST RESULTS IN YOUR REVIEW

Use this chart to see which subjects you should emphasize in your review. Find the numbers of the questions you answered incorrectly and look at the corresponding topics. When you begin working through the subject review chapters in this book, first go to the topics that are difficult for you.

Review Chapter	Area of Study	Question Number
4	Medical terminology	2, 10
5	Anatomy and physiology, body systems	5, 7
6	Nutrition	3
7	Psychology	4
8	Patient communication	6, 8
9	Professional and legal knowledge	1, 9
10	Office administration, scheduling, making appointments	12, 18
10	Office administration, scheduling, referrals and follow-up care	15
10	Office administration, office policies and procedures	20
10	Office administration, data entry	14
10	Office administration, computers and other equipment	11
10	Office administration, records management	13, 17
10	Office administration, mail processing and screening	16
11	Financial management	19
12	Patients in the clinical setting, principles of infection control	28
12	Patients in the clinical setting, treatment area preparation	23
12	Patients in the clinical setting, patient preparation	22
12	Patients in the clinical setting, assisting the physician during exams	30
13	Laboratory work	21
14	Medications	24
15	Minor surgery	26
16	Emergencies, recognition and response	25
16	Emergencies, first aid	29

PART THREE

CMA/RMA Exam Review

Chapter 4: **Medical Terminology**

The field of medicine involves an often complex and highly descriptive language. Many of the terms are unfamiliar to the general public. As a medical assistant, you will be using these terms regularly in your work, and you should be ready to assist patients by translating the terms into common language. In this chapter, you will review how to break down terms into parts for easier understanding, and you will review strategies for word building that aid in communicating medical terms to others. Common terms used in a variety of body systems and clinical practice settings will be defined. In addition, you will review abbreviations that are used commonly in medical practice.

USE OF MEDICAL TERMINOLOGY

Medical terms are used in documents such as clinical records, medical reports, and insurance correspondence. It is often better to avoid medical terms when speaking directly to a patient or conducting patient education. Most patients would be confused if we asked them, "Do you have rhinorrhea?" It is more efficient to ask if a patient has had a runny nose. Be aware that you will be called upon to translate medical terms for your patients.

OVERVIEW OF WORD COMPONENTS

One important method to understand complex medical words is to break them down into recognizable components. A list of common word parts along with examples follows.

1. Prefix: comes at the beginning of a word

   Example: In *peri/nat/o/logy*, *peri-* is the prefix

2. Suffix: comes at the end of a word

   Example: In *peri/nat/o/logy*, *-ology* is the suffix

3. Word root: body of the word

   Example: In *peri/nat/o/logy, nat* is the word root

4. Combining form: body of the word with a vowel

   Example: In *peri/nat/o/logy, nat/o* is a combining form

Linking elements together builds words that describe medical conditions, procedures, diseases, and structures. Structures usually have a Latin background, while procedures, processes, and diseases come from Greek words.

WORD BUILDING

There are a few word-building rules that can help either build or translate a new or unfamiliar term. (Remember, however, there are many exceptions to rules in constructing words.)

1. The combining vowel is usually "o." It is used to join word roots together to form a term.

    Example: cardi/o/gram. When the second word begins with a vowel, as in the term *gastr/ectomy,* no joining vowel is used.

2. Prefixes rarely are altered with a combining vowel to join to word roots.

    Example: hyper/emesis, hyper/trophy

3. Words are constructed in relation to the body's structure. When more than one root appears in a word, they are connected in order from head to toe or from the inside organ outward.

    Example: Gastr/o/intestine/al means pertaining to the stomach and intestine. *Cephal/o/pelvic* means pertaining to the head and pelvis. *Ot/o/rhin/o/laryng/o/logist* means one who studies the ear, nose, and throat.

4. The root word is the foundation of the word.

    Example: erythr/o/cyte

5. A suffix used in a medical term usually describes a procedure or action. When attempting to translate a word, you should be able to begin at the end.

    Example: cardi/o/logy means the study of the heart; *proct/o/scop/y* is the process of using an instrument to look into the anus.

6. To make singular medical terms plural, you need to use different endings based on how the singular word ends. Table 4.1 lists some examples of singular and plural medical terms.

Singular form	Replace ending with	Plural form
carcinoma	-mata	carcinomata
bacterium	-a	bacteria
corpus	-i	corpi
metastasis	-ses	metastases
coccus	-i	cocci
index	-ices	indices
amoeba	-ae	amoebae
thorax	-aces	thoraces
myopathy	-ies	myopathies
pelvis	-es	pelves

Table 4.1—Forming Plurals

TRANSLATING A WORD FOR MEANING

Remember, the word root is the main meaning of the word and the prefix and suffix help to clarify what the root means. To translate a word, begin at the end. Then, move to the first word. Lastly, translate the word in the middle. For example:

1. *poly/dips/ia* (ia) condition of (poly) many (dips) thirst
2. *an/iso/cyt/osis* (osis) condition of (an) un (iso) equal (cyt) cells
3. *orth/o/dont/ist* (ist) specialist in (orth) straightening (dont) teeth
4. *micr/o/scop/ic* (ic) pertaining to (micro) small (scop) instrument for looking
5. *tachy/card/ia* (ia) condition of (tachy) fast (card) heart

COMMON WORD COMPONENTS

Prefixes

Common prefixes include the following. As part of your review, it may be helpful to test yourself with flashcards on these items.

Directions:

above: supra-, super-, epi-, ultra-, hyper-

against: anti-, contra-

around: peri-before: pre-, pro-, ante-

behind: retro-, dors/o, poster/o

below: infra-, sub-, hypo-

between: inter-

inside: endo-

middle: mid-

near: para-

outside: exo-, ecto-, extra-

side: later/o

through: dia-, per-

within: intra-

Number:

1/10: deci-

1/100: centi-

1/1000: milli-

1000: kilo-

first: primi-, proto-

four: quadr-

half: semi-, hemi-

none: nulli-

one: uni-, mono-

two: diplo-, bi-

three: tri-

Description:

after: post-

bad: mal-

beyond: meta-

both: ambi-, amphi-

different: hetero-

difficult or poor: dys-

double: ambi-, amphi-

easy: eu-

equal: iso-

false: pseudo-

fast: tachy-large: macro-

many: multi-, poly-

same: homo-

slow: brady-

small: micro-

unequal: aniso-

without: a-, an-

Suffixes

Common suffixes used in medical terms include the following:

blood: -emia

bursting forth: -rrhexis

cell: -cyte

condition: -osis, -iasis, -ia, -ism

to crush: -tripsy

to cut into: -tomy

cutting instrument: -tome

destroy: -lysis

disease of: -pathy

drooping: -ptosis

enlargement: -megaly

enzyme-related: -ase

fear: -phobia

flow or discharge: -rrhea

formation: -genesis

hardening: -sclerosis

herniation: -cele

infestation: -iasis

inflammation: -itis

instrument to examine: -scope

instrument to measure: -meter

instrument to record data: -graph

involuntary movement: -spasm

kill: -cide

lack of: -penia

live birth: -para

madness: -mania

make a new opening: -ostomy

measurement: -metry

morbidity or unhealthy condition: -ia

narrowing: -stenosis

nutrition/development: -trophy

one who: -er

pain: -algia, -dynia

pertaining to: -ic, -al, -otic, -ac, -ar, -ous, -ical

picture: -gram

pregnancy: -gravida

process of: -y

recording of data: -graphy

to remove or cut out: -ectomy

resembling: -oid:

seizure: -lepsy

small in size: -ule, -ole

softening: -malacia

specialist: -ist

staying in one place: -stasis

stone: -lith

stretching: -ectasia

study of: -logy

surgical fixation: -pexy

surgical puncture: -centesis

to surgically repair: -plasty

swelling: -edema

treatment: -therapy

tumor: -oma:

vomiting: -emesis

washing: -clysis

Word Roots

Common word roots and combining forms used in medical terms are listed here. They are arranged by the pertinent body system.

Digestive:

first part of small intestine: duoden/o

second part of small intestine: jejun/o

third part of small intestine: ile/o

esophagus: esophag/o

gall bladder: cholecyst/o

gums: gingiv/o

intestine: enter/o

large intestine: col/o

lips: cheil/o

liver: hepat/o

mouth: stomat/o

pyloric valve: pylor/o

rectum: proct/o, rect/o

sigmoid colon: sigmoid/o

stomach: gastr/o

teeth: dent/o, dont/o

throat: pharyng/o

tongue: gloss/o, lingu/o

Urinary:

bladder: cyst/o

kidney: nephr/o, ren/o

opening: meat/o

renal pelvis: pyel/o

stone: lith/o

sugar: gluc/o, glyc/o

ureter: ureter/o

urethra: urethr/o

urine: ur/o

Reproductive:

birth: nat/o

breast: mast/o, mamm/o

fallopian tube: salping/o

foreskin: phim/o

menstruation: men/o

milk: lact/o

navel: oomphal/o

ovary: oophor/o

penis: pen/o, balan/o

prostate: prostate/o

testicle: orchid/o, orchi/o

uterus: hyster/o, uter/o

vagina: colp/o

Color:

black: melan/o

blue: cyan/o

green: chlor/o

purple: purpur/o

red: erythr/o

white: leuk/o

yellow: xanth/o

Muscles and Bones:

ankle: tars/o

back: lumb/o

bone marrow: myel/o

bone: oste/o

bursa: burs/o

cartilage: chrondr/o

extremities: acr/o

fingers/toes: phalang/o

foot: pod/o, ped/o

hand: chir/o

joint: arthr/o

movement: kinesi/o

muscle: my/o

neck: cervic/o

ribs: cost/o

spine: rachi/o, spondyl/o

sternum: stern/o

straight: orth/o

synovial: synov/o

tendon: tend/o, tendin/o

wrist: carp/o

General:

abdomen: lapar/o

beginning/formation: arche/o, gen/o

body: corp/o

breathing: pne/o

cancer: carcin/o

child: pedi/a

dead: necr/o

death: thanat/o

disease: path/o

fixed: ankyl/o

heat: pyr/o, therm/o

opening: meat/o

pus: py/o

rod-shaped bacteria: bacill/o

round bacteria: cocc/o

swallowing: phag/o

think: gnos/o

tumor: onc/o

water: hydr/o

women: gynec/o

Nervous System and Special Senses:

brain: encephal/o

cerebrum: cerebr/o

cornea: kerat/o

covering on brain: mening/o

ear drum: myring/o, tympan/o

ear: ot/o

eye: ophthalm/o

eyelid: blephar/o

head: cephal/o

hearing: phon/o

iris: irid/o

nerve: neur/o

pupil: core/o

smell: osm/o

speech: phas/o

spinal cord: myel/o

taste: gust/o, geus/o

tears: lacrim/o

vision: op/o

white of eye: scler/o

Skin/Connective:

fat: lip/o

fungus: myc/o

gland: aden/o

hair: trich/o, pil/o

nail: onych/o

porridge-like: ather/o

skin: dermat/o, cutan/o

sweat: hidr/o

Heart/Lungs:

artery: arteri/o

blood: hem/o, hemat/o

branch/forked: furc/o

bronchus: bronchi/o

chest: thorac/o

clot: thromb/o

diaphragm: phren/o

heart: cardi/o

larynx: laryng/o

lung: pneumon/o, pulmon/o

nose: rhin/o, nas/o

trachea: trache/o

vein: phleb/o, ven/o

vessel: vas/o, angi/o

SPECIALTY PRACTITIONERS

Physicians who have extra training or experience in select specialties may choose to limit their practice to certain types of patients. Knowing the specialty areas can help in making referrals. The following terms indicate a variety of different medical specialists.

Cardiologist: specializes in cardiac disease

Dermatologist: specializes in skin disease

Endocrinologist: specializes in glandular disease

Epidemiologist: specializes in tracking causes of disease

Gastroenterologist: specializes in treatment of the stomach and intestine

Gastrologist: specializes in treatment of stomach

Gerontologist: specializes in the treatment of elderly

Gynecologist: specializes in treatment of women's reproduction

Hematologist: specializes in blood diseases

Hospitalist: specializes in treating people when hospitalized

Immunologist: specializes in immunity and immune disorders

Nephrologist: specializes in kidney disease

Neurologist: specializes in treatment of nervous system

Obstetrician: specializes in pregnancy and delivery of babies

Oncologist: specializes in treating cancer

Ophthalmologist: specializes in treating eye disease

Orthopedist: specializes in bones and joints

Otolaryngologist: specializes in ears and throat disease

Pathologist: specializes in tissue diseases

Pediatrician: specializes in care of children

Perinatologist: specializes in care of high-risk pregnancy

Proctologist: specializes in disease occurring in anus and rectum

Psychiatrist: specializes in mental disorders

Pulmonologist: specializes in lung disease

Radiologist: specializes in radiography and interpreting X-rays

Rheumatologist: specializes in arthritis and joint disease

Urologist: specializes in urinary and male reproductive disease

PRONUNCIATION TIPS

When you are working with medical terms, you can use some general tips to ensure correct pronunciation. These tips include the following.

1. The emphasis in pronunciation shifts to the syllable containing the combining vowel.

   Example: proctoscopy

   In this word, the "to" is emphasized.

2. The letter *y* can function as a combining vowel.

   Example: bradypnea

3. The letters *g* and *c* have a soft sound before *e, i,* or *y.*

   Example: laryngitis, cervical

4. The letters *g* and *c* have a hard sound before all other letters.

   Example: acromegaly, cardiac, gastric

5. The letter p is silent when paired with *s* or *n.*

   Example: -pnea, psoriasis

6. The letters *ae* or *oe* are pronounced with a long *e* sound.

   Example: amoeba

USE OF REFERENCES

Occasionally, you will be given a word that you are not familiar with, and you will not know the correct spelling, pronunciation, or meaning. On such occasions, health care personnel refer to special dictionaries that define medical terms in detail. There are many different dictionaries available, but they are similarly organized. The primary reference portion on terms is organized in alphabetical order. The top of each page has guide words indicating the first and last word on the page. Each entry has a pronunciation guide and tells the origin of the word. A definition or description follows. Additional word sources are suggested to find additional facts. It is important that you become familiar with the use of medical dictionaries to check on spelling and other information.

Most medical dictionaries have reference information following the medical terms. There is usually a lab value reference guide, dietary information, first aid information, addresses of health-related organizations, vitamin and mineral charts, and anatomical figures depicting bones, muscles, and organs.

EASILY MISSPELLED WORDS

Some words become easier to spell once you have a foundation in medical terminology. Many are confusing because of double letters. Other problems occur with similar-sounding words that have different meanings. You need to know the meaning of each word in order to use it correctly, and you should practice spelling these words correctly. Following is a list of commonly misspelled words.

accommodation: adjustment
alopecia: loss of hair

anesthesia: without sensation

anorexia: without appetite

anxiety: nervousness

asthma: breathing disorder

callus: hard, thickened skin

cartilage: connective tissue

cataract: vision disorder

cesarean: abdominal surgery for birth

chlamydia: a type of sexually transmitted disease

cholesterol: a steroid widely distributed in the tissues of animals

circumcision: removal of foreskin

diabetes mellitus: endocrine disorder

diaphragm: membrane to facilitate breathing

diarrhea: loose, watery stool

distal: farther away from point of insertion

emphysema: chronic lung disease

enema: bowel infusion

enuresis: bed wetting

feces: stool

feminine: having the qualities of a woman

flatus: gas

glaucoma: eye disease

goiter: enlarged thyroid

gonorrhea: a type of sexually transmitted disease

hemorrhage: excessive bleeding

hemorrhoid: swollen rectal vein

incision: cut into body

inflammation: swelling and redness

larynx: voice box

menstruation: female monthly discharge

migraine: severe headache

mucous: adjective that describes secretion

mucus: noun meaning thick wet secretion

myasthenia: muscle disease with flaccid muscles

influenza: viral respiratory disease

palpation: touching and pressing patient

palpitation: irregular heartbeat

pancreas: endocrine and digestive organ

paralysis: inability to move

paraplegia: inability to move legs

pneumonia: severe respiratory disease

procedure: medical activity

prostate: male reproductive organ

prostrate: lying face down without movement

pruritis: itching

psychiatrist: physician who treats mental illness

quadriplegia: inability to move arms or legs

sagittal: plane running through body to divide it into left and right

scarring: thickening of skin tissue

supination: lying on back

suppuration: healing

syphilis: a type of sexually transmitted disease

testicle: male gonad

tongue: muscle in mouth used for taste and speech

trachea: windpipe

unconscious: not awake and alert

uterus: female reproductive organ

viral: pathogen

virile: sexual

vomiting: emesis

ABBREVIATIONS

Unacceptable Abbreviations

By the early 2000s, health practitioners were witnessing a high volume of errors in interpretation of medical abbreviations and symbols. In 2005, in an effort to reduce these errors, the Joint Commission began to require its member hospitals and outpatient centers to avoid the use of certain abbreviations that were previously acceptable. (The Joint Commission is the foremost healthcare standards–setting body in the United States.) For example, the abbreviation "qd" once was commonly used, but today, you must write out the word *daily*. Unfortunately, you still may see these older, ambiguous abbreviations and symbols in clinical records or in use by practitioners who refuse to make changes necessary for patient safety.

The following table lists terms that must be written out completely to prevent medical errors. (For the complete list of "do not use" medical abbreviations, including any updates, see the Joint Commission's website: www.jointcommission.org/topics/patient_safety.aspx.) Your office should have a list of approved abbreviations for use in patient records and other documents.

Terms	No longer acceptable	Use instead
Ear terms	AD, AS, AU	Write out
Eye terms	OD, OS, OU	Write out
Discontinue and discharge	D/C, dc, DC	Write out
Subcutaneous	SC, SQ	subQ or subC
Every other day	qod	Write out
Daily	qd	Write out
Morphine sulfate	MS, MSO$_4$	Write out
Magnesium sulfate	MgSO$_4$	Write out
Microgram	μg	mcg or micrograms
Trailing zero	X.0 mg	Write X mg
Lack of leading zero	.X mg	Write 0.X mg
International units	IU	Write out
Units	U or u	Write out

Table 4.2—Unacceptable Abbreviations

If you are reading a medical order and have even a slight concern about what you are reading, verify the order with the prescribing physician.

Acceptable Abbreviations

The following abbreviations are still considered acceptable and frequently used in charting.

Prescriptions:

ac = before eating

Ad lib = as desired

B.I.D. = twice a day

g = grams

gr = grains

mcg = micrograms

mL or ml = milliliters

p.o. = by mouth

pc = after eating

prn = as needed

Q.I.D. = four times a day

STAT = immediately

T or Tbs = tablespoon

t or tsp = teaspoon

T.I.D. = three times a day

Chemistry:

Ca = calcium

Fe = iron

H_2O = water

K = potassium

Na = sodium

NS = normal saline

Disease:

ADD = attention deficit disorder

ADHD = attention deficit hyperactivity disorder

AIDS = auto immune deficiency syndrome

ALS = amyotrophic lateral sclerosis (commonly known as Lou Gehrig's disease)

ARDS = adult respiratory distress syndrome

ASHD = arteriosclerotic heart disease

BP = blood pressure

BPH = benign prostatic hypertrophy

CA = cancer

CAD = coronary artery disease

CHF = congestive heart failure

COPD = chronic obstructive pulmonary disease

CVA = cerebral vascular attack

DM = diabetes mellitus

GC = gonorrhea

GERD = gastroesophageal reflux disease

HTN = hypertension

IBS = irritable bowel syndrome

IDDM = insulin-dependent diabetes mellitus

MI = myocardial infarction

MR = mental retardation

MS = multiple sclerosis

MVP = mitral valve prolapse

NIDDM = non-insulin-dependent diabetes mellitus

PAT = paroxysmal atrial tachycardia

PID = pelvic inflammatory disease

PTSD = post-traumatic stress disorder

PUD = peptic ulcer disease

RA = rheumatoid arthritis

RDS = respiratory distress syndrome

SOB = shortness of breath

STD = sexually transmitted disease

TAH = total abdominal hysterectomy

TIA = transient ischemic attack

TURP = transurethral resection of prostate

URI = upper respiratory infection

UTI = urinary tract infection

VD = venereal disease

VSD = ventricular septal defect

Procedures and Labs:

ABG = arterial blood gas

BS = blood sugar

CABG = coronary artery bypass graft

CBC = complete blood count

CK = creatinine kinase

CPR = cardiopulmonary resuscitation

CT/CAT scan = computer tomography diagnostic procedure

D&C = dilation and curettage

EKG/ECG = electrocardiogram

ESR = sedimentation rate

ESWL = extracorporeal shock wave lithotripsy

FBS = fasting blood sugar

FHT = fetal heart tones

HCT = hematocrit

Hct/hgb = hematocrit and hemoglobin

Hgb A1c = glycosylated hemoglobin

I&D = incision and drainage

IVP = intravenous pyelogram

KUB = x-ray of kidney, ureter, and bladder

LP = lumbar puncture

MRI = magnetic resonance imaging

PE = physical exam

PT = protime

PTT = partial thromboplastin time

ROM = range of motion

T&A = tonsillectomy and adenoidectomy

VS = vital signs

WNL = within normal limits

Clinical Records:

Bx = biopsy

CNS = central nervous system

CSF = cerebral spinal fluid

Dx = diagnosis

EDC = estimated date of confinement

ENT = ear, nose, and throat

FUO = fever of undetermined origin

GI = gastrointestinal

HEENT = head, eyes, ears, nose, and throat

I&O = intake and output

IM = intramuscular

IV = intravenous

LMP = first day of last menstrual period

LOC = level of consciousness

N&V = nausea and vomiting

NKA = no known allergies

OB = obstetrics

Ob/gyn = obstetrics and gynecology

OT = occupational therapy

OTC = over the counter

PERRLA = pupils equal round reactive to light and accommodation

PT = physical therapy

Px = physical

Rx = prescription

subQ or subC = subcutaneously (the Joint Commission no longer approves SQ or SC)

Sx = symptoms

Tx = treatment

VS = vital signs

REVIEW QUESTIONS

1. Which of the following means "condition of excessive sweating"?

   (A) Hidromegaly

   (B) Hyperhydria

   (C) Megalohidria

   (D) Hyperhidrosis

   (E) Hidrohyposis

2. Which of the following is the plural for "bursa"?

   (A) Bursum

   (B) Bursies

   (C) Bursi

   (D) Bursae

   (E) Bursaces

3. Which of the following is a combining form meaning "disease"?

   (A) *carcin/o*

   (B) *path*

   (C) *-pathy*

   (D) *carcin*

   (E) *path/o*

4. Which is INCORRECTLY spelled?

   (A) Diarrhea

   (B) Hemorrhage

   (C) Cataract

   (D) Vomiting

   (E) Diaphram

5. Which of the following is the best description of a nullipara?

   (A) A woman who is pregnant for the first time

   (B) A woman who never gave birth to a live child

   (C) A woman who has never had a child

   (D) A woman pregnant with her ninth child

   (E) A woman who has never been pregnant

6. What order is most appropriate when determining the meaning of a medical term?

   (A) Combining form, suffix, prefix

   (B) Prefix, root, suffix

   (C) Prefix, suffix, root

   (D) Root, suffix, prefix

   (E) Suffix, prefix, root

7. Which of the following terms means "excision of the gallbladder"?

   (A) Cholecystectomy

   (B) Cholecystostomy

   (C) Cholecystotomy

   (D) Cholecystogram

   (E) Cholecystography

8. *Xanth/o* is a color term that means

   (A) blue

   (B) green

   (C) red

   (D) white

   (E) yellow

9. An ENT would most likely use which of the following abbreviations when recording the results of the patient's eye examination?

   (A) HEENT

   (B) PERRLA

   (C) RDS

   (D) ADHD

   (E) GERD

10. The emergency room patient reports pain occurring around the navel. The provider writing the patient note may use what term to describe the location of the pain?

    (A) Epigastric

    (B) Hypogastric

    (C) Hypochondriac

    (D) Iliac

    (E) Periumbilical

ANSWERS AND EXPLANATIONS

1. **D**

   Remember that to translate any medical word, you should begin by dividing it into word parts.

   Hidr/o/megaly

   Hyper/hydr/ia

   Megal/o/hidr/ia

   Hyper/hidr/osis

   Hidr/o/hyp/osis

   Take each word in the answers and look at the suffix. We can eliminate hidromegaly (A) because the suffix is not "condition." *Megaly* means enlargement.

   Now we look at the first part of the word to find a word meaning "excessive." We can eliminate *megal* (enlargement) and *hidr* (sweat), leaving us to consider what is between the prefix and suffix.

   Hyper/hydr/ia

   Hyper/hidr/osis

   Hidr/o is the word root for sweat or perspiration. Hydr/o means "water." Therefore, the correct answer is hyperhidrosis.

2. **D**

   Remember the rules for making plurals. The word ends in the letter *a*. Drop the *a* and add *ae*.

3. **E**

   Path/o is a combining form of word-building meaning "disease." (A) is also a combining form, but it refers to cancer or neoplasm. *Path* (B) is not a combining form of word-building. (C) is a suffix, and (D) is a prefix.

4. **E**

   Diaphragm is the correct spelling. The letter *g* is silent.

5. **B**

   Begin by dividing the word into parts: nulli/para. *Para* means "live births." *Nulli* means none or no. Therefore, the correct answer is (B). Remember that choice (A) is not necessarily correct because a nullipara may have had a stillborn child, abortion, or miscarriage.

6. **D**

When interpreting medical terms, it is most effective to look first at the suffix and/or word ending, followed by the prefix, and then the word root (which may include two or more root words). To analyze the word *pericolitis* using this method, for example, you would break it into its components *peri* + *col* + *itis* (prefix + root + suffix), then interpret it as "inflammation around the colon" ("inflammation" from the suffix *-itis*, "around" from the prefix *peri-*, and "the colon" from the root *col*).

7. **A**

All these terms are related to the gallbladder but mean different things. The suffix, or word ending, is what differentiates them. Cholecystostomy (B) is the process of making an opening (*-ostomy*) in the gallbladder. Cholecystotomy (C) is simply cutting into (*-otomy*) the gallbladder. Cholecystogram (D) is the visible record (*-gram*) of a gallbladder—that is, the x-ray or sonogram. Cholecystography is the process of conducting an x-ray on the gallbladder.

8. **E**

Colors are often used in medical records to describe appearance and provide clues to diagnosis. *Xanth/o* is a yellow color; it is also referred to as jaundice. Yellow is often associated with liver, gallbladder, and/or pancreatic conditions. The medical term for blue (A) is *cyan*, and blue color in the body would indicate a decrease in oxygenation. For example: The patient was cyanotic. The medical term for green (B) is *chlor/o*. In young women, anemia may give a greenish-yellow appearance to the skin and therefore referred to as chloroanemia. The medical term for red (C) is *erythro*; it describes a blushing color (erythema) or a red blood cell (erythrocyte). The medical term for white (D) is *leuk/o*; for instance, leukemia is a disease of white blood cells.

9. **B**

PERRLA is an abbreviation recording that stands for "pupils equal, round, and reactive to light and accommodation." HEENT (A) is an abbreviation that the ENT would use, but it refers to more than just the eyes; it stands for "head, eyes, ears, nose, and throat." RDS (C) is an abbreviation for the condition respiratory distress syndrome. ADHD (D) refers to attention deficit hyperactivity disorder, a behavior disorder and not part of the eye exam. GERD (E) is an abbreviation that stands for gastroesophageal reflux disease.

10. **E**

The abdomen is a large area and often requires more localization of pain, lesions, and procedures. Since *peri-* means "around" and *umbilical* means refers to the navel, periumbilical (E) is the correct answer. The epigastric area (A) is the mid to upper region of the abdomen, on top of the stomach. (The prefix *epi-* means "upon," and *gastric* refers to the stomach.) The hypogastric region (B) is the lower section of the abdomen. (The prefix *hypo-* means "below.") The lateral upper sections of the abdomen below the cartilage of the ribs are referred to as the right and left hypochondriac regions (C). (The prefix *hypo-* means "below," and the root *chrondr* refers to cartilage.) The iliac area (D) is the lower area of the abdomen along the flaring part (*ilium*) of the hip bone.

Chapter 5: **Anatomy and Physiology**

You will need to have an understanding of the structures and functions of the human body in your work as a medical assistant. In this chapter, you will review the major body systems, how they function in the normal patient, and the key changes that disease and illness cause in the human body.

Listed in the following table are the major body systems, their unique function in maintaining a state of wellness, and the organs that make up each system. All systems are needed to maintain a state of homeostasis for normal body function.

ORGANIZING THE BODY AS A WHOLE

System	Function	Sample of Involved Organs
Musculoskeletal	Support and shape/movement	Bones, muscles, tendons, ligaments
Nervous/ Sensory	Translate input and make decisions	Brain, spinal cord, nerves/sensory organs
Circulatory/ Cardiovascular	Transportation of oxygen, hormones, and nutrients	Blood vessels, capillaries, heart
Endocrine	Turn functions on and off	Glands such as pituitary, thymus, thyroid, adrenal, pancreas
Reproductive	Continuation of species, human sexual function	Ovaries, testes, uterus, penis, fallopian tubes, prostate
Integumentary	Protection of internal organs	Skin, hair, nails
Lymphatic	Protection from infection	Lymph vessels, spleen, tonsils
Digestive	Intake and absorption of nutrients	Mouth, teeth, esophagus, stomach, intestines, liver, gall bladder, pancreas
Respiratory	Intake of oxygen and output of waste	Mouth, nose, trachea, bronchi, lungs, alveoli
Excretory	Output of waste	Kidney, ureter, urethra, bladder

Table 5.1—Functions of Body Systems

The human body is made up of 10 body systems, each of which has a specific function. Each body system is made up of organs that work together toward that function. Each organ is made of various tissues. Tissues are made of cells. The smallest unit of the body is the cell, which is visible only under a microscope. Cells are made up of organelles.

Organelles and Cellular Structure

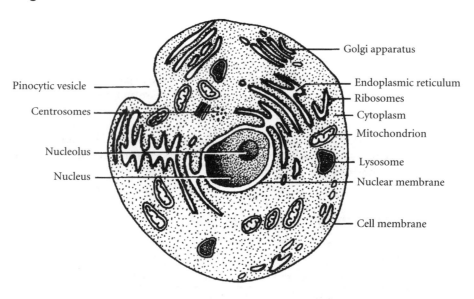

Figure 5.1—Eukaryotic Cell

The typical cell has a variety of organelles that carry out the processes necessary for cellular life. Every cell has a covering called the cell membrane. Each cell has an individual shape and is filled with a colloidal filling called cytoplasm. The key organelle in the cell is the nucleus. It is where the genetic material resides and proteins are made. These proteins are called ribosomes. They are responsible for the growth and development of the cell. They move away from the nucleus and out into the cell with the assistance of a folded membrane called the endoplasmic reticulum. Energy for this and other operations in the cell is produced by mitochondria. The mighty mitochondria are the cell's power plants. These multifunctional units move throughout the entire cell to devour foreign particles or other dead organelles. They move to the edges of the cell and open up the cell membrane to complete pinocytosis (cell drinking) and phagocytosis (cell eating).

Like people, cells move. The Golgi apparatus (also called as Golgi body) is another folded membrane that is used for transportation within the cell. The tips of a Golgi body pinch off and transport mucus through the cytoplasm. Cilia are hair-like appendages that wave back and forth pushing along secretions or particles. Flagella are tail-like appendages that whip through fluids much like swim fins and help propel the cell. A sperm cell is a good example of a cell with flagella.

Reproduction in the cell is carried out through the centriole. When reproduction takes place, the centriole separates and each part goes to an opposite end of the cell. Spindle fibers form between the two centriole pieces and chromosomes gravitate to either end of the cell. Gradually, the cell divides into two identical daughter cells. This process is called mitosis.

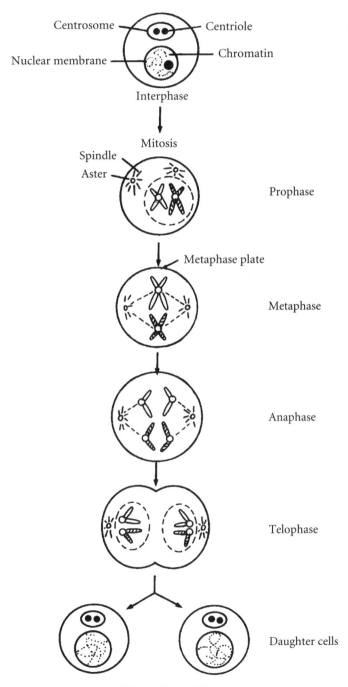

Figure 5.2—Mitosis

Tissue

The organs of the body can be comprised of four layers of tissues. The layers are described in Table 5.2.

Type	Function	Description
Epithelial	Covers and lines	Found as skin, glands, and lining of organs
Connective	Joins together	Identified by type of matrix: • **Hard:** found in bone • **Liquid:** found in blood • **Fibrous:** found in tendon • **Soft:** found in areolar tissue
Muscle	Contracts	Types: • **Cardiac:** found in heart • **Smooth:** found in vessels and organs • **Skeletal:** found in voluntary muscles
Nervous	Carries electric potential	Neurons pick up potential and pass it on to subsequent neurons

Table 5.2—Types of Tissues

There are times when aberrant tissue growth appears. That tissue is called a neoplasm or tumor. If the tissue does not spread beyond the original site, it is benign. However, if the abnormal tissue growth spreads to other areas of the body, the neoplasm is malignant. Malignant epithelial tissue is called a carcinoma. Malignant connective tissue is called a sarcoma. Cancer is detected through tests such as MRI (magnetic resonance imaging), CT scan (computer tomography), lab tests such as PSA (prostatic specific antigen), or biopsy and cell studies (pap smear). Treatment for cancer may require chemotherapy, radiation, surgery, or immunotherapy. The aim of treatment is to destroy the aberrant cell growth.

These seven warning signs of cancer should alert a person to seek a physician's assessment:

1. Lump or mass

2. Change in mole (nevus)

3. Chronic cough or hoarseness

5. Persistent indigestion

5. Unexplained bleeding

6. Sore that does not heal

7. Change in bowel or bladder habits

Describing the Body and Location of Body Parts

To communicate with other members of the health care team, health care professionals use standard terms to describe the body. Anatomical position is the standard visualization of the human body to delineate direction and relative position of body planes.

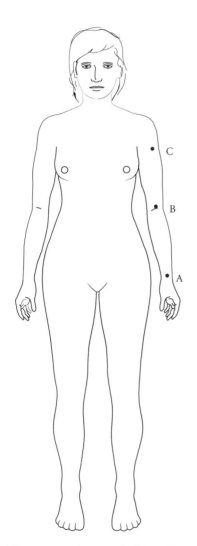

Figure 5.3—Anatomical Position

Term	Meaning	Example
Superior	Above	The nose is superior to the chin
Inferior	Below	The lips are inferior to the nose
Ventral/ Anterior	Belly side	The breasts and knees are on the ventral/anterior side of the body
Dorsal/ Posterior	Back side	The buttocks and knuckles are on the dorsal/posterior side of the body
Distal	Greatest distance away from a point of insertion	(See Figure 5.3) Lesion A is distal from the shoulder
Proximal	Closest to a point of insertion	(See Figure 5.3) Lesion C is proximal to the shoulder
Lateral	Away from the midline	The ears are lateral to the nose
Medial	Toward the midline	The nose is medial to the ears

Table 5.3—Terms Indicating Direction

The body is often divided into body cavities.

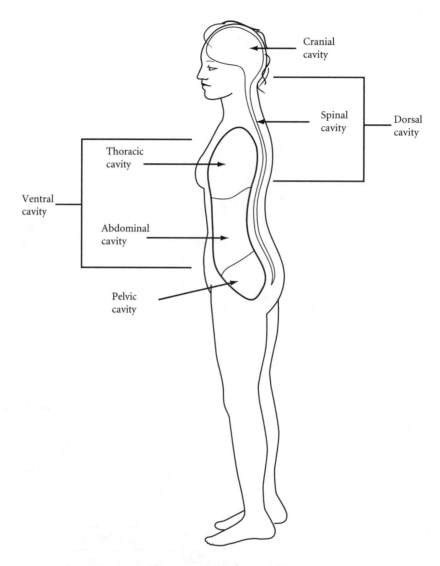

Figure 5.4—Body Cavities

Additionally, the body is divided into planes. Pictures and views of the body are presented through these planes to show different organs.

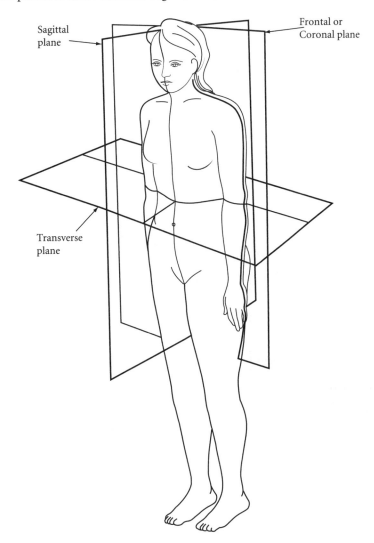

Figure 5.5—Planes

The abdomen is divided into regions to help identify the location of pain or lesions. Remember right and left are always oriented from the patient's perspective.

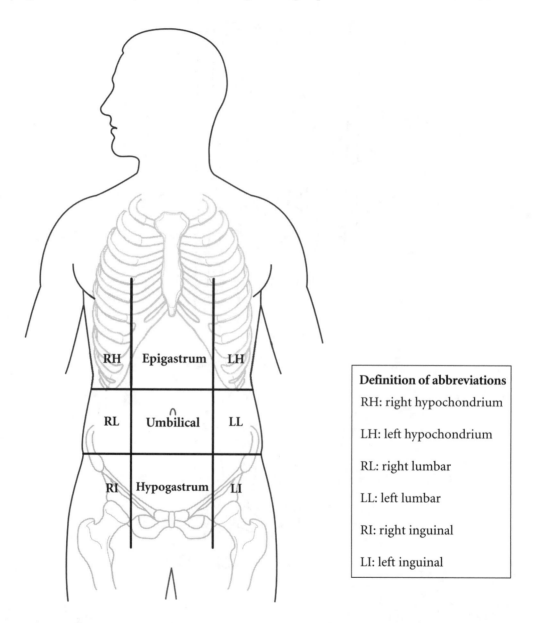

Definition of abbreviations
RH: right hypochondrium
LH: left hypochondrium
RL: right lumbar
LL: left lumbar
RI: right inguinal
LI: left inguinal

Figure 5.6—Regions of Abdomen

BODY SYSTEMS

Integumentary

The integumentary system comprises the skin and body coverings, such as hair and nails. The functions of the integumentary system include:

1. Provision of a protective barrier from foreign invaders
2. Regulation of body temperature
3. Reception of information through pressure receptors
5. Linings for body cavities and organs

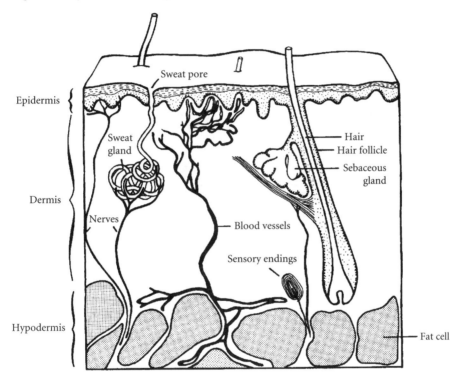

Figure 5.7—Human Skin

The outer layer, or the epidermis, is made up of two sublayers: the stratum corneum (horny layer) and the stratum germinativum (growing layer). The dermal and subcutaneous layers contain accessory structures. Sebaceous glands produce the sebum that moisturizes our skin and scalp. Sudoriferous glands produce perspiration to help regulate body temperature. Ceruminous glands in the lining of the ear produce earwax (cerumen) to provide the ear canal with lubrication and cleaning. It also protects the ear from some bacteria and fungi. In the following list are some potential signs and symptoms noted in a physical exam of the skin, the clinical name associated with each symptom, and the disease state or clinical problem that may be the cause of the symptom.

Color	Name	Indication
Blue	Cyanosis	Lack of oxygen or profusion of the cells
Red	Erythema	Fever, blush, burn, or infection
White	Pale	Anemia
Orange	Cirrhosis	Liver or pancreatic disorder
Gray	Ashen	Serious illness, death
Brown-orange	Bronze	Adrenal problems
Purple	Ecchymosis	Bruising or deep tissue injury
Yellow	Jaundice	Bile problems involving liver, gallbladder, or pancreas

Table 5.4—Skin Exam Signs and Symptoms

In examining a patient's skin, you may note a variety of lesions, marks, or discolorations. Table 5.5 identifies some commonly observed skin blemishes.

Blemish	Description	Example
Papule	Small elevation	Wart
Macule	Flat	Freckle
Vesicle	Papule with clear fluid	Blister, chicken pox
Pustule	Papule with pus	Pimple, boil
Nevus	Brown elevation	Mole
Nodule	Lump under skin	Sebaceous cyst
Decubitus	Ulceration	Pressure sore
Avulsion	Tissue torn out	Dog bite
Excoriation	Tissue rubbed off	Scrape or rubbing of two skin surfaces
Laceration	Cut with clean edges	Knife cut
Fissure	Torn by use at a site of pressure	Rectal fissure
Tear	Ragged edges	Skin shearing from friction
Puncture	Small surface area but deep wound	Stab wound

Table 5.5—Common Skin Blemishes

Table 5.6 lists common skin diseases that you may see in your practice. The list includes a description of the pertinent observations that you would make for each disease.

Disease	Description
Dermatitis	Inflamed, irritated skin
Eczema	Erythema, scaling, and itching due to allergic reaction
Psoriasis	Overgrowth of epidermis resulting in silvery scales
Verruca (wart)	Benign, fleshy tumor caused by virus
Herpes simplex	Viral lesion with water vesicles; Type I: nose and mouth, Type II: genitalia
Tinea pedis (athlete's foot)	Fungus flourishes in warm, moist, dark places; causes scaling, itching, and burning to feet and between toes
Tinea cruritis (jock itch)	Fungus that flourishes in groin and other skin folds; causes burning and redness
Tinea corporis (ringworm)	Red lesions in a circular pattern blanched in the center caused by fungus, *not* a worm
Impetigo	Golden crusts on oozing lesions, bacterial, spread through direct contact or with personal items like towels or bed clothing
Furuncle (boil)	Staph infection in hairy area of body such as groin, neck, or armpit; common in diabetics or those w/impaired immunity; needs systemic antibiotic
Carbuncle	Group of furuncles
Basal cell carcinoma	Shiny pearl-like lesion due to overexposure to sun
Squamous cell carcinoma	Reddened patch of skin that will not heal due to overexposure to sun
Melanoma	Large, asymmetrical, dark, malignant mole that swiftly spreads through body and can be terminal
1st degree burn	Redness, such as sunburn
2nd degree burn	Blisters and redness
3rd degree burn	Full thickness damage through skin into nerves and muscles

Table 5.6—Skin Diseases

Musculoskeletal System

The purpose of the musculoskeletal system is to provide support to and enable movement of the body. Bones function as levers for doing work. Bones also serve as a storehouse for calcium and the site for manufacturing of red blood cells. Additionally, bones often serve to protect soft organs. For example, the rib cage protects the heart and lungs while the cranium protects the brain.

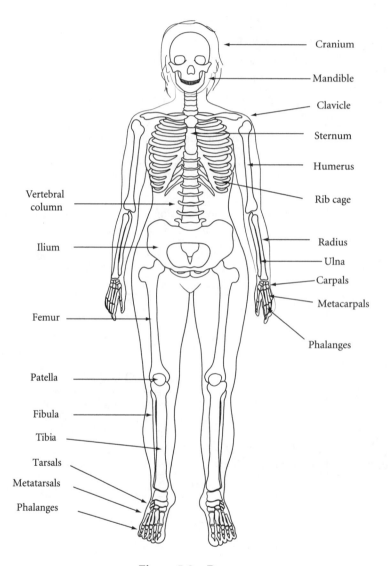

Figure 5.8—Bones

KAPLAN

The human body has two parts to the skeletal system. The axial skeleton is the skull, spinal column, shoulders, and hips. It is the axis or center of the skeleton. Our appendages, arms and legs, hang off the axial skeleton. They make up the appendicular skeleton. Many of the skeletal muscles are attached to the appendicular skeleton by tendons. Overuse or abuse of these muscles may cause tendonitis. Bones are joined together with ligaments at joints. Injuries to ligaments and tendons (strains and sprains) are very painful and slow to heal.

Bones in the body are made of two types of material. Cancellous or spongy bone is a lighter-weight bone composed of a meshwork filled with red marrow. It is often found in the end (epiphysis) of long bones. It is where the red blood cells are made. The shaft (diaphysis) of a long bone is made up of compact bone and filled with yellow marrow. The entire bone is covered with a thick protective covering called the periosteum. Nerves and blood vessels weave into the diaphysis through holes (foramen) and run along grooves called fossa.

Injuries to bones generally involve fractures. Table 5.7 lists the nomenclature used to describe fractures, and provides brief descriptions of each type.

Type of Break	Description
Open/Compound	Breaks through the skin, will be high risk for osteomyelitis, a severe bone infection
Closed/Simple	Bone is broken but does not break skin
Greenstick	Splinters, bends, or cracks
Impacted/Compacted	One piece of bone jammed into another
Spiral	Bone twisted with a tortuous break
Comminuted	Bone breaks into multiple pieces
Pathological	Caused by disease process

Table 5.7—Fractures

More than 650 muscles in the body make up approximately 40 percent of the body's weight. Muscles require glucose and oxygen to make energy (ATP) for movement. Glucose is stored in the body as glycogen and oxygen is stored as myoglobin. Skeletal muscle is a striated (banded) tissue that is composed of two proteins. One protein is thin, light, and called actin. The other is a dark, heavy protein called myosin. In the presence of calcium, sticky points on the actin are uncovered and oar-like attachments from the myosin are drawn to the points with the assistance of ATP, causing the muscle to contract. We need muscles to move and maintain body temperature.

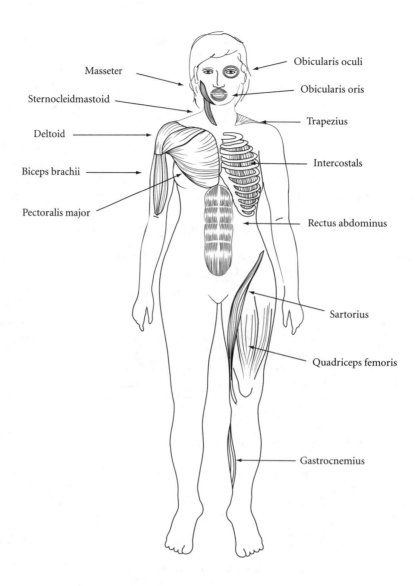

Masseter

Sternocleidmastoid

Deltoid

Biceps brachii

Pectoralis major

Obicularis oculi

Obicularis oris

Trapezius

Intercostals

Rectus abdominus

Sartorius

Quadriceps femoris

Gastrocnemius

Figure 5.9—Anterior Muscles

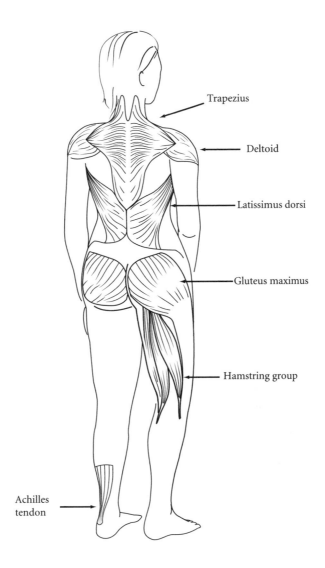

Trapezius

Deltoid

Latissimus dorsi

Gluteus maximus

Hamstring group

Achilles tendon

Figure 5.10—Dorsal Muscles

Table 5.8 lists a variety of common diseases of the musculoskeletal system, along with a description of the pathology that the diseases create. In addition, common forms of treatment for these diseases are listed.

Disease	Description	Treatment
Osteoporosis	Decreased bone mass that often occurs in middle-aged women	Hormone replacement therapy, increased calcium, weight-bearing exercise, weight loss
Scoliosis	Deviation of spine to side	Brace, surgery
Lordosis	Excessive curvature of lumbar spine (swayback)	Surgery may be used
Kyphosis	Excessive curvature of thoracic spine (hunchback)	Bracing
Osteoarthritis	Wear and tear on joints causing pain, stiffness, swelling	Medical treatment with anti-inflammatory drugs, assistive devices, exercise, joint replacement
Rheumatoid arthritis	Stiffness, swelling, and pain in joint due to autoimmune disorder	Medical treatment and drug therapy, acupuncture
Bursitis	Swelling of the fluid sac cushioning joint	Avoiding pressure on joint, medication, aspiration
Gout	Collection of uric acid crystals in joint causing pain and swelling	Low-purine diet, Allopurinol
Muscular dystrophy	Hereditary; poorly developed muscles	Physical therapy, braces
Torticollis (wry neck)	Spasm of the sternocleidomastoid muscle	Heat, antispasmodic drugs, physical therapy
Atrophy	Wasting of muscle	Exercise or range of motion exercise
Cleft palate	Congenital deformity in roof of mouth due to failure of maxillary bones to fuse	Surgery

Table 5.8—Musculoskeletal System Diseases

Nervous System

The nervous system is divided into the peripheral and central nervous system. The brain and spinal cord make up the central nervous system, which is divided into the voluntary system and the autonomic or involuntary system. The autonomic nervous system provides a rapid response to a threat where we may need to be able to run or defend ourselves. The autonomic system is made up of the sympathetic and parasympathetic systems. The sympathetic nervous system is responsible for a release of glucose from the liver, increased heart rate, increased blood pressure, increased respiration, and decreased genitourinary action. These physiological changes help humans to "fight or flight" in a dangerous situation. The parasympathetic nervous system creates the reverse responses to help slow the body down.

The brain is the command center of the body. It receives information from the world, processes it, and sends out a response. It is composed of two hemispheres of convoluted tissue. The right hemisphere controls the left side of the body and the left hemisphere controls the right side of the body. The two hemispheres are joined by tissue called the corpus callosum. There are four main parts to the brain: the cerebrum, cerebellum, brainstem, and diencephalon. The cerebrum is primarily for thinking and emotion. Both the right and left side can be broken down into frontal lobe, temporal lobe, occipital lobe, and parietal lobe. Each lobe manages special functions as listed in Table 5.9.

Lobes	Special Functions
Frontal	Emotions and personality
Parietal	Math and logic
Temporal	Processing spoken word
Occipital	Processing visual information

Table 5.9—Lobes of the Brain

When the brain is injured by illness or trauma, the result is dependent on which lobe is damaged and the extent of the damage. The cerebellum is responsible for balance and movement. The brainstem is made up of the pons and medulla oblongata. These structures are responsible for basic life functions such as respiration, heartbeat, and blood pressure. Injury to this area is often incompatible with life. The diencephalon contains structures responsible for alertness (reticular formation), body temperature (hypothalamus), long-term memory (hippocampus), and survival/animal brain (limbic system).

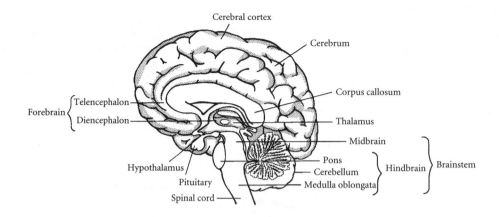

Figure 5.11—Human Brain

The brain communicates with the rest of the nervous system via the spinal cord. Both the brain and spinal cord are covered with three layers of tissue called the meninges. Table 5.10 identifies and describes some common nervous system diseases and their symptoms.

Disease	Description	Symptoms
Meningitis	Inflammation of meninges, membranes covering brain and spinal cord	Nuchal rigidity, fever, headache, vomiting
Hemiplegia	Result of stroke	Paralysis on one side of body
Paraplegia	Result of severing of spinal cord in lower back or sacrum	Inability to move legs, may have bowel and bladder dysfunction
Quadriplegia	Result of severing of spinal cord in the upper thoracic or cervical area	Inability to move arms and legs, may have respiratory dysfunction
Encephalitis	Inflammation of brain	Headache, fever, confusion
Cerebral vascular accident (stroke)	Blockage of a vessel or bleeding into brain prevents oxygen getting to brain tissue	Malfunction in the portion of the brain that is deprived of circulation
Herniated disc	Protrusion of nucleus pulposis against spinal cord	Pain that radiates down leg

Table 5.10—Nervous System Diseases

The peripheral nervous system involves the nerves that pick up information from the environment and cause a response. Input from the environment travels via nervous tissue to the spinal cord and on to the brain. An action potential is sent back via the spinal cord to nerves that trigger the muscle to move. At times, this pathway is altered. Information that is needed quickly may be processed in the spinal cord, forming what is called a reflex arc. Nerve impulses pass from one neuron to another. Impulses are picked up by dendrites and pass through the cell body (soma) and out the tail of the neuron (axon). Neurons do not touch one another. The impulse must cross the synapse (the junction between neurons) via neurotransmitters. Impulses pass more rapidly as learning takes place. That is the basic concept behind learning to ride a bike or dance. If the impulse cannot quickly pass along the axon because the coating on the axon (neurilema) is patchy, the patient would be diagnosed with multiple sclerosis.

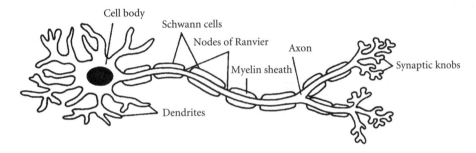

Figure 5.12—Neuron

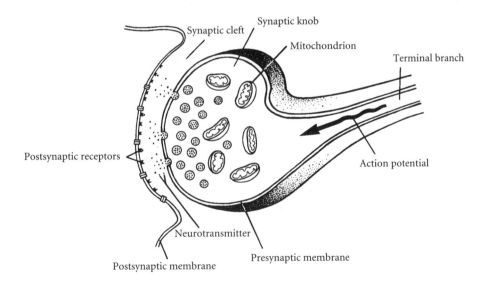

Figure 5.13—Synapse

Disease	Description
Amyotrophic lateral sclerosis	Deterioration of motor neurons
Poliomyelitis	Viral infection that leads to weakened muscles
Transient ischemic attack	Brief interludes of confusion that often precede CVA
Hydrocephalus	Enlargement of head due to accumulated fluid in ventricles of brain
Expressive aphasia	Inability to form words
Receptive aphasia	Inability to understand what is being said
Epilepsy	Abnormal electrical activity of brain
Cerebral palsy	Damage to brain that causes motor or balance problems
Intracerebral hematoma	Accumulation of blood within the brain tissue due to trauma to head or spontaneous rupture of blood vessel
Subdural hematoma	Accumulation of blood due to tear in meningeal layer
Concussion	Headache, vomiting, damage to brain tissue due to closed head trauma
Alzheimer's disease	Progressive degeneration thought to be due to plaque and tangles of brain tissue leading to regression of ability to think
Parkinson's disease	Progressive neurological disease with resulting tremors, shuffling gait, and rigidity
Multi-infarct dementia	Brain damage from chronic ischemia
Encephalitis	Inflammation of brain caused by virus, bacteria, or toxin
Bell's palsy	Temporary facial paralysis caused by virus damaging the VII cranial nerve (facial)
Trigeminal neuralgia	Severe spasm of V cranial nerve (trigeminal)

Table 5.11—Additional Nervous System Diseases

The sensory system is actually part of the nervous system and comprises touch, sight, hearing, smell, and taste. The input from the senses is conducted via the cranial nerves to the brain. The various cranial nerves and their function are listed in Table 5.12.

Nerve	Name	Function
Olfactory	I	Carries impulses for smell
Optic	II	Carries impulses for sight
Oculomotor	III	Controls eye movement
Trochlear	IV	Controls eye movement
Trigeminal	V	Carries sensation from eye, upper and lower jaw; movement of jaw
Abducens	VI	Controls facial expression, controls salivary and tear glands, carries taste
Facial	VII	Carries taste, controls facial expression
Vestibulocochlear	VIII	Carries hearing and controls equilibrium
Glossopharyngeal	IX	Carries taste, controls swallowing and gag
Vagus	X	Controls voice box, throat, and digestive juices; longest nerve; goes to abdominal cavity
Spinal accessory	XI	Controls muscles in neck and larynx
Hypoglossal	XII	Controls muscles of tongue

Table 5.12—Cranial Nerves and Functions

KAPLAN

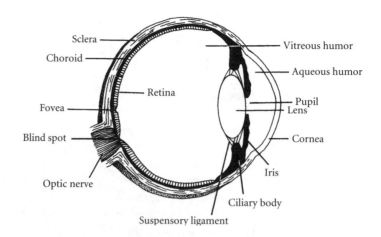

Figure 5.14—Human Eye

The eye is an orb covered with tough white tissue called sclera. In the front of the orb, a clear window in the sclera allows light to enter the eye. This is called the cornea. Light travels through the cornea and through a lens, which focuses light on the fovea centralis. Rods are specialized receptors that are sensitive to night, shades of gray, and peripheral vision. Cones are specialized receptors that are stimulated by color and daylight. Stimulation from these receptors in the retina is carried by the optic nerve to the brain. An irregularly shaped lens will cause light to focus elsewhere and result in the need for corrective lenses.

Eyes are examined as a manner of assessing the nervous system. PERRLA is a notation made when the pupils of the eye are equal in size, round, and either eye responds to a light being shined in it by contracting and the other pupil responds likewise (light accommodation). The iris is the colored portion of the eye that dilates or constricts the pupil in response to light. In conducting an eye exam, each of these items should be assessed. Some common eye disorders are noted in Table 5.13.

Eye Disease	Description
Myopia	Nearsighted; cannot see objects in the distance
Hyperopia	Farsighted; cannot see up close
Presbyopia	"Old eye," lens loses elasticity
Astigmatism	Irregular curvature of lens

Table 5.13—Eye Diseases *(continued on next page)*

Eye Disease	Description
Cataracts	Cloudy lens
Conjunctivitis	Redness and itching of conjunctiva; "pink eye"
Glaucoma	Accumulation of fluid pressure and poor drainage of aqueous humor
Macular degeneration	Abnormal blood vessel growth causing loss of central vision
Strabismus	"Crossed eyes," unable to focus independently of one another
Nystagmus	Repetitive and involuntary movement of eye
Blepharitis	Eyelid and eyelash infection
Diplopia	Double vision
Ambylopia	Lazy eye causing other eye to lose some portions of vision
Chalazion	Small, painless, localized swelling of eyelid
Hordeolum	Purulent staph infection of hair follicle of eyelid
Enucleation	Removal of eye
Keratitis	Inflammation of cornea
Nyctalopia	Inability to see at night
Pterygium	Triangular thickening of conjunctiva

Table 5.13—Eye Diseases *(continued from previous page)*

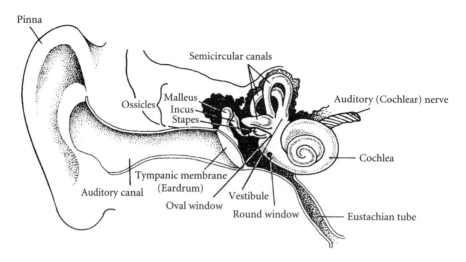

Figure 5.15—Human Ear

Hearing is a result of sound in the form of vibration of air. The outer ear (pinna) catches sound waves and directs them down the ear canal toward the tympanic membrane (ear drum). The vibration of the eardrum is passed on to the three bones of the middle ear (the ossicles). The incus (anvil), malleus (hammer), and stapes (stirrup) pass the vibration on to the inner ear. Within the cochlea, small receptors called organ of corti are stimulated by the disturbance of vibration. The cochlear nerve is triggered to send an impulse to the brain to be interpreted as sound.

Hearing may be interrupted by obstructions such as impacted ear wax or defective parts such as otosclerosis. This is called conduction deafness because of interference with the passage of sound waves or vibrations. If the deafness is caused by the cochlear nerve or failure of the brain to properly interpret sounds, it is termed sensineural deafness.

Ear Disease	Description
Otitis media	Middle ear infection, often caused by URI
Otitis externa	Outer ear infection, "swimmer's ear," caused by exposure to pathogens
Impacted cerumen	Buildup of earwax until auditory canal is occluded
Otosclerosis	Buildup of spongy bone and stiffening of stapes
Presbycusis	Decrease in hearing receptors due to aging or abuse
Meniere's	Vertigo, dizziness, and hearing loss related to inner ear
Tinnitus	Buzzing or ringing in ear/ears

Table 5.14—Ear Diseases

Olfactory stimulation is the sense of smell. Asnomia (no sense of smell) may occur because of severe chemical trauma by caustic fumes or blockage of receptor cells by a thick coating of mucus. Smell and taste combine to make flavors.

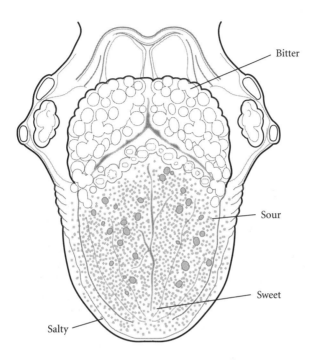

Figure 5.16—Human Tongue

Gustatory sensation, or taste, is limited to sour, salty, sweet, and bitter. The receptors for sweet are located on the tip of the tongue and helpful in teaching infants to feed from a spoon. As patients age, taste sensations diminish. The sweet receptors diminish less than the others do, so it may be helpful to administer medications to the elderly by crushing them and mixing them with sweet foods such as applesauce or pudding.

Heart and Circulatory System

The body has an extensive "highway system" of arteries, capillaries, and veins. Collectively, they are called vessels. It is necessary for many items to be circulated throughout the body. Hormones, nutrients, and oxygen are three major products that must be delivered to various distant sites via the circulatory system. Arteries are thick and elastic. They carry blood away from the heart and are buried deep in the body's tissue. Veins return blood to the heart. They are fragile and very superficially located. It is easy to rupture a vein by bumping against something.

Veins can suffer engorgement and fill with blood if blood flow in the venous system slows (e.g., varicose veins or hemorrhoids). Veins and arteries join together at capillaries, which are only one cell thick. It is in the capillary beds that tissue perfusion takes place. Oxygen, nutrients, and hormones move into the surrounding tissue and carbon dioxide and other waste is picked up and carried away. Remember, the principle of osmosis is that substances move from areas of high concentration to areas of low concentration.

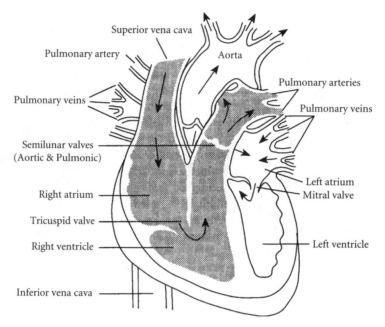

Figure 5.17—Human Heart

Blood is pumped through the circulatory system by the contractions of a double pump, the heart. The upper chambers of the heart are called the atria (left atrium and right atrium). The lower chambers are the left and right ventricles. Deoxygenated blood is returned to the right side of the heart by the two largest veins of the body, the inferior and superior vena cava. The blood that collects in the right atrium travels through the tricuspid valve and fills the right ventricle. Valves keep blood from flowing backward. The blood then goes through the pulmonary valve and out the pulmonary artery to the lungs. Oxygen is picked up in the lungs in the alveoli, where the walls of the capillaries are one cell thick. The blood then carries the oxygen back to the heart through the pulmonary vein and into the left atrium. After going through the bicuspid valve, the blood fills the left ventricle. The myocardium (heart muscle) is the thickest around the left ventricle because it must push the oxygenated blood around the entire body. The blood is finally squeezed through the aortic valve and out the aorta toward all portions of the body. Arterial branches from the aorta take blood to the head (carotid artery), arms (subclavian artery), and heart (coronary artery). The blood from the coronary artery supplies needed blood to the heart muscle so it can contract 60 to 100 times every minute. Exercise, fever, and stress increase the heart rate.

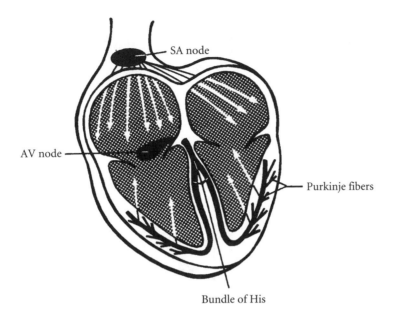

SA node

AV node

Purkinje fibers

Bundle of His

Figure 5.18—Electroconductivity of the Heart

Contractions of the heart are triggered by an electrical stimulation in the heart muscle. The electric impulse begins in the sinoatrial node (SA node) or pacemaker. The impulse spreads out through the heart and is slowed down in the atrioventricular node (AV node). The Bundle of His separates the impulse so it can travel down the septum of the heart via either the right or left bundle branches. Finally, the Purkinje fibers carry the impulse into the myocardium where it causes the myocardium to contract. This is the stimulation for the ventricles to contract. Common diseases of the heart and circulatory system are listed in Table 5.15.

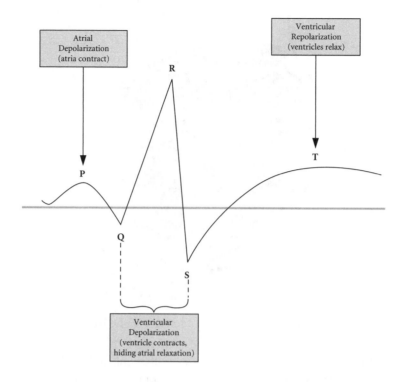

Figure 5.19—Atrial Depolarization/Ventricular Repolarization

Cardiac Disease	Description	Treatment
Myocardial infarction (heart attack)	Ischemia (lack of blood) to area of heart causes tissue death	Bypass graft around blockage or angioplasty with stent to keep coronary arteries open
Coronary artery disease	Multiple areas with start of vessel disease (narrowing and strictures)	Stop smoking; increase exercise; low-fat, high-fiber diet
Angina	Ischemia during stress or exercise, unstable angina during rest	Nitroglycerin, stop activity, stop smoking
Arrhythmia	Irregular heartbeat	Medication, surgery, pacemaker, cardioversion
Hypercholesterolemia	Total cholesterol greater than 200 mg	Diet and medication

Table 5.15—Cardiac Diseases and Disorders (continued on next page)

Cardiac Disease	Description	Treatment
Hypertension	Blood pressure elevated greater than 140/90	DASH diet, exercise, diet, medication, weight loss, stress reduction
Peripheral vascular disease	Narrowing or occlusion of vessels in legs and feet	Bypass graft or medication
Thrombus	Blood clot	Prevent clot from moving until dissolved
Thrombophlebitis	Blood clot and inflammation of veins	Heparin, antibiotics, blood thinners, exercise, avoid immobility or constriction of veins
Arteriosclerosis	Calcium and fibrous deposits inside vessels	Aspirin or blood thinners; surgery
Atherosclerosis	Fatty deposits inside vessels	Change to low-fat, high-fiber diet and increase exercise
Murmurs	Valvular disorder	Valve replacement in serious cases
Congestive heart failure	Weak ventricle (either side); allows blood to back up; left side = SOB, frothy sputum, coughing; right side = edema and cyanosis	Medication (Lasix and Lanoxin)
Aneurysm	Bulging weak spot in vessel	Graft inserted into area and sutured above and below weak point

Table 5.15—Cardiac Diseases and Disorders (*continued from previous page*)

The blood is composed of 55 percent plasma (liquid) and 45 percent formed elements (corpuscles). The plasma is made of 90 percent water, protein such as hormones, antibodies, and clotting factors and nutrients such as fats, glucose, vitamins, and minerals. Formed elements are red blood cells (erythrocytes), white blood cells (leukocytes), or platelets (thrombocytes).

Erythrocytes are disc-like without a nucleus. There are 4 to 5 million erythrocytes per cubic centimeter of blood. They live for 120 days and carry oxygen as well as the blood type protein. We are able to use the erythrocyte's four-month lifespan to look for sugar residue when we perform a glycosolated hemoglobin test on a diabetic. Leukocytes are outnumbered by red blood cells 700 to 1 and usually live from 6 to 24 hours. Their function is to fight invaders and protect against infection. They are identified through staining as granulocytes or agranulocytes. By staining the granulocytes, the lab can identify the white blood cell as a neutrophil, eosinophil, or basophil. Each can be prolific under certain circumstances, such as allergy or parasitic infestation.

Thrombocytes are part of the clotting process. These cell fragments have no nucleus and live only 10 days, but are part of the chain of events to prevent blood loss when a vessel is injured. Hemostasis begins with the release of thromboplastin by the injured tissue, followed by conversion to prothrombin and thrombin. In the presence of calcium, thrombin converts to insoluble fibrin and eventually into a clot. Despite the long chain of events, each clotting factor plays a role and when any is missing, the entire process can fail. An example of this failure would be the genetic disease hemophilia. Table 5.16 shows common blood disorders.

Name	Description	Symptoms
Thrombocytopenia	Decreased number of platelets	Bruising, easy bleeding
Leukemia	Unrestrained growth in white blood cells	Pale, weak, low-grade fever, malaise, weight loss
Anemia	Not enough red blood cells	Shortness of breath, fatigue, weakness, pale
Iron deficiency anemia	Not enough heme for oxygen to bind to on red blood cells	Shortness of breath, fatigue, weakness, pale
Pernicious anemia	Lack of intrinsic factor in gastric juice	Mental changes, weak, stiff extremities
Sickle-cell anemia	Abnormal hemoglobin; red blood cell changes into sickle shape and gets tangled up, causing blockage and pain	Pain and swelling in joints of African American children
Polycythemia vera	Red blood cell count is elevated because of living in high altitude or genetics	Phlebotomy is done at regular intervals

Table 5.16—Blood Disorders

Blood types are important in transfusions. There are four types in the ABO group:

- Type A has A antigens on the red blood cells and anti-B antibodies in plasma
- Type B has B antigens on the red blood cells and anti-A antibodies in plasma
- Type AB has A and B antigens on the red blood cells and no antibodies in plasma
- Type O has no antigens on the red blood cells and both A and B antibodies in plasma

This makes Type AB the universal recipient and Type O the universal donor.

Rh is an issue when the mother is Rh-negative and the baby is Rh-positive. The mother can be sensitized to the Rh factor if exposed to the baby's blood. Her body would treat an Rh-positive fetus as a foreign invader. An injection of Rhogam prevents problems in the Rh-negative mother's pregnancy. This usually occurs only in second and subsequent pregnancies and only if the baby has Rh-positive blood.

Lymph System

The primary function of the lymph system is to protect the body from foreign invaders. Paired with the veins, the lymph vessels contract with skeletal muscle movement. The lymph vessels help collect excess tissue fluid. The four accessory organs of the lymph system are the lymph nodes, tonsils, thymus, and spleen. The lymph nodes trap bacteria and foreign bodies and destroy them. The two main lymph nodes are under the armpits and in the inguinal area. When doing this job, a node may become enlarged and tender (lymphadenopathy). There are three sets of tonsils: the palatine tonsils, the nasopharyngeal tonsils (adenoids), and lingual tonsils (back of tongue). These tissues assist with the development of speech and are a protective barrier against infection.

The thymus lies under the sternum and is the source of immunity in the first two years of life. After the age of two years, the thymus secretes thymosin to mature T-lymphocytes that fight invaders. The thymus gland begins to shrink as a person gets older. The spleen lies in the left hypochondriac area and completes many duties. The spleen filters bacteria out of the blood, destroys old red blood cells, stores iron, provides a reservoir of blood for an emergency, and produces phagocytes to fight foreign invaders. Splenomegaly occurs in syphilis, scarlet fever, typhoid, and typhus fever.

Respiratory System

The respiratory system serves to convey oxygen into the body and remove carbon dioxide. The major organs include the trachea, the bronchi, and the lungs.

Respiration takes place in two phases: inspiration and exhalation. Movement of the diaphragm changes the air pressure in the thoracic cavity and allows air to rush into the lung via the trachea. The trachea consists of C-shaped rings of cartilage. The trachea bifurcates into the two bronchi leading to the lungs. The right lung has three lobes and the left lung has two lobes. The air travels through the lungs via the bronchi and bronchioles, and terminates in the balloonlike alveoli. It is in the alveoli that oxygen molecules move into the bloodstream and are returned to the left side of the heart. At the same time, carbon dioxide leaves the bloodstream, crosses through the capillary and alveoli membranes, and begins the pathway back up the respiratory tract to be exhaled.

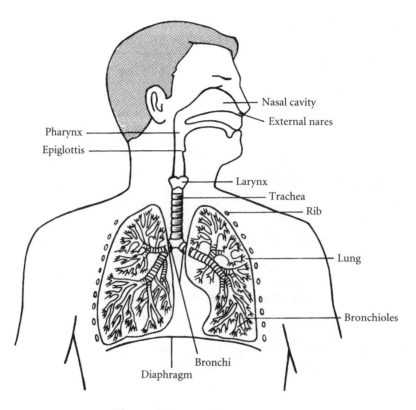

Figure 5.20—Respiratory System

Table 5.17 shows common respiratory diseases.

Disease	Description
Sinusitis	Infection of the epithelial tissue of sinus cavities
Epistaxis	Nose bleed
Coryza	Nasal discharge, rhinorrhea
Influenza	Inflammation of trachea, aches, pains, coughing, fever
Pneumonia	Air spaces filled with fluid due to viral, bacterial, chemical, or aspiration irritation
Tuberculosis	Caused by mycobacterium bacilli, night sweats, cough with bloody sputum
Atelectasis	Incomplete expansion of lung due to injury, mucous plug, cancer, or foreign body

Table 5.17—Respiratory System Diseases (*continued on next page*)

Disease	Description
Asthma	Spasm of bronchus and bronchioles due to allergy
Hayfever	Watery eyes, sneezing, runny nose
URI (upper respiratory infection)	Viral or bacterial infection of eyes, ears, nose, and throat; coughing, sneezing, and sore throat.
Pneumothorax	Collapse of lung due to nonpatent lung (bleb) or trauma
Hemothorax	Collapse of lung due to pressure from bleeding or trauma
Lung Cancer	Ten times more likely with smoking, 15% 5-year survival rate

Table 5.17—Respiratory System Diseases (*continued from previous page*)

Endocrine System

Endocrine glands secrete chemicals (hormones) that deliver messages through the bloodstream to distant tissue. The message directs the tissue to respond or perform and the endocrine gland monitors the response to determine whether additional stimulus is needed.

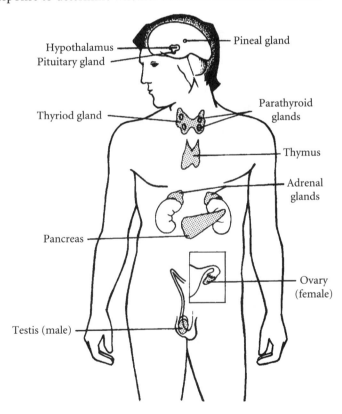

Figure 5.21—Endocrine System

Gland	Location	Hormone	Purpose
Anterior pituitary	Base of brain	Growth hormone (GH)	Stimulates growth of long bones
		Follicle stimulating hormone (FSH)	Stimulates growth of egg in ovary or sperm in testes
		Melanocyte stimulating hormone (MSH)	Regulates skin pigment
		Leutinizing hormone (LH)	Stimulates ovulation
		Thyroid stimulating hormone (TSH)	Stimulates thyroid to produce thyroxine
		Prolactin	Stimulates production of breast milk
Posterior pituitary	Base of brain	ADH	Facilitates reabsorption of water in nephron of kidney
		Oxytocin	Stimulates milk ejection and uterine contraction
Pineal	Center of brain	Melatonin	Conrols sleep/wake cycles
Thymus	Behind sternum	Thymosine	Facilitates immunity by stimulating the growth of T-cells
Thyroid	Neck	Thyroxine	Stimulates metabolism
Pancreas	Abdomen	Insulin	Assists sugar to go from bloodstream into tissue
Adrenal glands	Top of kidney	Aldosterone	Regulates sodium and potassium
		Cortisol	Regulates fat metabolism and blood pressure
Ovaries/testes	Lower abdomen/scrotum	Estrogen/testosterone	Facilitates secondary sex characteristics
Kidney	Lower back	Erythropoietin	Monitors blood for oxygen level
Parathyroids	Imbedded in thyroid	Parathyroid hormone	Facilitates calcium into bloodstream

Table 5.18—Components of the Endocrine System

Digestive System

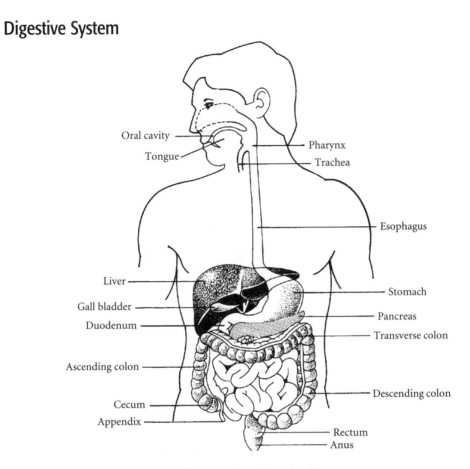

Figure 5.22—Digestive Tract

Food is ingested into the mouth, where it is mechanically broken down by 32 permanent teeth and the tongue. Mixed with the salivary enzyme amylase, starch digestion begins. Leaving the mouth, the bolus of food moves into the pharynx where reflex swallowing (deglutition) forces it into the esophagus. In the esophagus, food moves by peristalsis to the entry of the stomach, the cardiac sphincter. Sometimes this valve allows stomach tissue to slide through into the esophagus (hiatal hernia). Other times, the valve is not patent and digestive enzymes leak back up into the esophagus (gastroesophageal reflux disease or GERD).

In the stomach, gastric glands secrete hydrochloric acid and pepsin to break down connective tissue in food. The stomach stores food and releases it in small amounts as a substance called chyme. Chyme passes into the small intestine through the pyloric sphincter. Almost all digestion and absorption of food occurs in the small intestine. In the first third of the small intestine (duodenum), the chyme is neutralized by alkaline secretions from the liver, gallbladder, and pancreas. Bile from the gallbladder begins the breakdown of fats. In the second two parts of the small intestine, the jejunum and ileum, absorption of nutrients occurs through the villi of the small intestine. Amino acids (digested proteins), simple sugars, and some fat components are absorbed directly into the blood capillaries located in the villi. The liver has a variety of important functions in addition to the production of bile.

- Storage of sugar as glycogen
- Formation of blood plasma proteins
- Formation of urea from the metabolism of proteins
- Modification of fats to promote their usefulness in the body
- Detoxification of harmful substances such as alcohol and certain drugs
- Storage of some vitamins and iron

The large intestine reabsorbs water and stores and compacts waste. Elimination of solid waste is called defecation. Stool is often called feces. Gaseous waste that is expelled through the rectum is called flatulence and the gas that escapes through the mouth is eructation.

Disease	Description
Cirrhosis of liver	Chronic scarring of the liver
Hemorrhoids	Engorged and enlarged rectal veins due to increased intra-abdominal pressure
Constipation	Hard, dry stools that are difficult to pass
Diarrhea	Loose, watery stools
Peptic ulcer	Erosion of the mucous membrane of the esophagus, stomach, or duodenum due to smoking, NSAIDS, alcohol, aspirin, or helicobacter pylori
Irritable bowel syndrome	Bowel is overly sensitive to stress; pain, diarrhea, weight loss, and rectal bleeding
Leukoplakia	Thickened white patches in the mouth
Cholelithiasis	Stones formed from the substances in bile that have potential to block common bile duct and cause pain
Hepatitis A, B, C	Inflammation of the liver that may be life threatening; Hepatitis A caused by fecal-food contamination Hepatitis B and Hepatitis C caused by blood and body secretions
Pyloric stenosis	Hardened, narrow lumen of the pyloric sphincter prohibits food from entering small intestine; symptoms include projectile vomiting, poor feeding, and weight loss
Gingivitis	Inflamed, bleeding pink tissue around teeth

Table 5.19—Digestive System Diseases

Urinary System

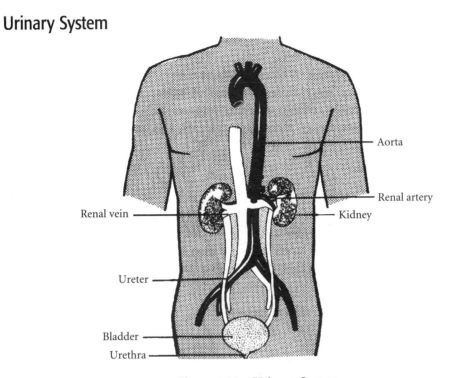

Figure 5.23—Urinary System

The urinary system eliminates metabolic waste from the body; maintains appropriate levels of water; regulates the acid-base balance (pH), blood pressure, and red blood cell production. It is assisted by other systems having excretory functions such as the digestive, respiratory, and integumentary systems. The urinary system consists of only four organs: kidneys, ureters, urinary bladder, and the urethra. The organs are the same in both male and female.

Urine is formed by millions of nephrons located in the kidneys. The nephron has a portion shaped like a "C" (called the Bowman's capsule) where the water and waste is filtered from the blood. Molecules small enough to pass through the glomerulus and the cells of the Bowman's capsule leave the blood and enter the renal tubule. Before its elimination as urine, the glomerular filtrate must be concentrated or too much water would be lost, resulting in dehydration. The pituitary hormone ADH causes the proximal convoluted tubule, distal convoluted tubule, and loop of Henle to become more permeable so that more water is reabsorbed. The kidneys process up to 180 liters of filtrate each day to create about 1 to 1.5 liters of urine. The ureters drain the urine from the kidney to the holding area—the bladder. The urethra carries the urine to the urinary meatus for excretion. Urination (micturition, voiding) is controlled by an involuntary internal sphincter muscle and a voluntary external urethral sphincter.

Urinary tract infections or UTIs affect women 10 times more often than men. This is because the urethra is approximately three inches long for women and eight inches for men—but more so because of the proximity of the female urethra to the anus. Other urinary disorders include glomerulonephritis, which may result from an inadequately treated strep infection and presents with abnormal constituents in urine such as albumin (albuminuria), pus (pyuria), glucose (glycosuria), or blood (hematuria). Kidney stones are formed from excessive calcium or oxylates. They may cause painful blockages in the ureters. The process to destroy kidney stones is called lithotripsy. When the penis has an additional opening, it is called hypospadius. It is not a common defect but can be very upsetting to a new parent.

Reproductive System

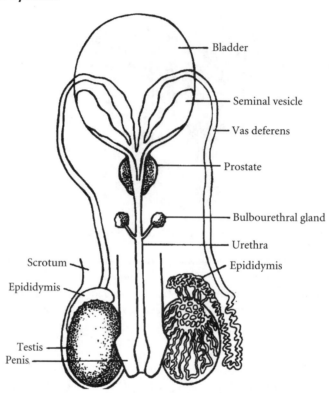

Figure 5.24—Male Reproductive System

Human reproduction requires the union of specialized male and female sex cells: the sperm and the egg. Sperm develop within the seminiferous tubules of the testes. Testosterone influences sperm cell development and also produces the male secondary sex characteristics: lower voice, male hair patterns, and the development of broader shoulders than hips. Sperm travel out of the body through a series of ducts that includes the epididymis, ductus deferens (vas deferens), ejaculatory duct, and urethra. They are transported in semen, which is composed of secretions from the seminal vesicles, prostate gland, and bulbourethral glands. Semen nourishes the sperm, neutralizes the acidity encountered in the male urethra and female vagina, and serves as a lubricant to the reproductive tract during sexual intercourse. Circumcision reduces the risk of human papilloma virus and phimosis (overly tight foreskin). Undescended testicles are called cryptorchidism and may cause sterility unless corrected by school age. Testicular cancer is common in young men aged 15–25 years. It is detected through testicular self-exam. Surgery to remove one testicle does not significantly affect fertility. Prostate cancer is common in older men age 50 years and older. It is detected by digital rectal exam or PSA exam. The PSA (prostatic specific antigen) is a blood test and fairly reliable.

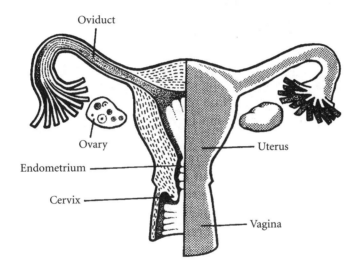

Figure 5.25—Female Reproductive System

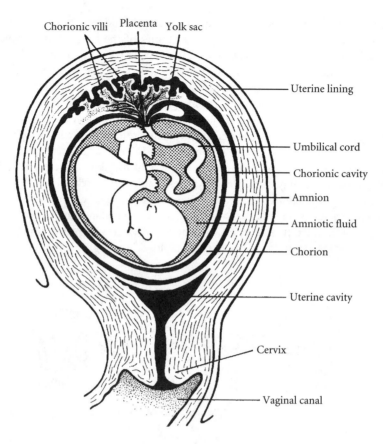

Figure 5.26—Human Fetus

In the female, the ovary forms the egg. Each month, under the effects of follicle stimulating hormone (FSH), at least one ovum matures within the follicle of the ovary. The mature egg travels down the fallopian tube. If fertilization occurs, it most often occurs in the outer third of the fallopian tube. Until implantation, the developing tissue is called a zygote. The estrogen produced by the cells of the follicle's membranous wall causes the endometrium of the uterus to begin preparation for pregnancy. The conversion of the ovarian follicle into the corpus luteum produces a large amount of progesterone for 11 to 12 weeks. Under the influence of progesterone, a fertilized egg implants in the uterus. From this point until about 8 weeks, this will be called an embryo. Eventually the placenta forms and provides oxygen and nutrients from the mother to the fetus. Pregnancy lasts for 280 days. When one fertilized egg divides into two identical eggs, identical twins are formed. When a woman ovulates two eggs that are fertilized, fraternal twins are formed. Identical twins are always the same sex. From three months until birth, the developing tissue is called a fetus. Common disorders of pregnancy include the following.

- Hypertension and spilling of protein is called preeclampsia and may lead to maternal seizures (eclampsia)

- Placenta previa is bleeding that occurs as the cervix dilates because the placenta is implanted low near the cervix
- Abruptio placenta is the sudden, violent separation of the placenta that places both fetus and mother at risk for complication from hemorrhage

Tests done during pregnancy watch for spilling of protein in the urine, ultrasonography for fetal growth and size and position in the uterus, and amniocentesis to evaluate for genetic abnormalities.

When fertilization does not occur, the corpus luteum gradually atrophies, hormone levels decline, and menses begins. The length of the menstrual cycle varies from woman to woman, but is typically 28 days.

The beginning of menstruation is menarche. The average age for menarche continues to get younger and younger. Today, the average age is 12 years old. Menopause is the cessation of menstrual cycles. Some of the adverse changes that sometimes accompany menopause are treated with hormone replacement therapy (HRT). Recently, however, there are some challenges to HRT.

Common disorders of the reproductive systems include infertility, infections, tumors, and menstrual irregularities. Sexually transmitted diseases, including HIV, are usually prevented by using a condom. Cancer of the cervix is detected thru the pap smear done annually on sexually active women.

Contraception is the use of artificial means to prevent fertilization or implantation. Surgical, chemical, and barrier methods are all in use, but vary in their effectiveness.

REVIEW QUESTIONS

1. Which of the following diseases involves incomplete expansion of the lung?
   (A) Atelectasis
   (B) Pneumonia
   (C) Tuberculosis
   (D) Epistaxis
   (E) Asthma

2. Which hormone is NOT secreted by the anterior pituitary?
   (A) Follicle stimulating hormone (FSH)
   (B) Leutinizing hormone (LH)
   (C) Thyroid stimulating hormone (TSH)
   (D) Prolactin
   (E) Melatonin

3. Which of the following is NOT a function of the liver?
   (A) Formation of bile
   (B) Formation of insulin
   (C) Formation of urea
   (D) Storage of sugar as glycogen
   (E) Detoxification of harmful substances

4. A major function of the large intestine is to
   (A) reabsorb water
   (B) break down fats
   (C) absorb nutrients
   (D) excrete water and waste
   (E) break down carbohydrates

5. Which of the following describes where the blood is filtered in the kidney?
   (A) Bowman's capsule
   (B) Distal convoluted tubule
   (C) Proximal convoluted tubule
   (D) Loop of Henle
   (E) Renal tubule

6. Urine that contains blood is called

    (A) uremia

    (B) albuminuria

    (C) hematuria

    (D) pyuria

    (E) glycosuria

7. Sperm are produced in the

    (A) epididymis

    (B) seminiferous tubules

    (C) vas deferens

    (D) prostate

    (E) seminal vesicles

8. The structure responsible for the production of progesterone to maintain the pregnancy until the placenta forms is the

    (A) ovary

    (B) corpus callosum

    (C) corpus luteum

    (D) tinea corporis

    (E) fallopian tube

9. The body system primarily responsible for protection from foreign invaders is the

    (A) circulatory

    (B) lymphatic

    (C) endocrine

    (D) digestive

    (E) integumentary

10. Which of the following would NOT be found on the ventral side of the body?

    (A) Nose

    (B) Knuckles of hand

    (C) Navel

    (D) Patella

    (E) Palm of hand

Read the following medical note to answer questions 11–14:

A patient presents to the ED complaining of lower back pain radiating to the right flank area. The patient has a history of a herniated disc at L4–L5. He also has a history of kidney stones but states that this is not the same type of pain. The doctor has ordered an MRI and an IVP to assist with the diagnosis.

11. What does ED stand for in this note?

   (A) Educational deficiency

   (B) Erectile dysfunction

   (C) Emergency department

   (D) Every day

   (E) Examining doctor

12. L4–L5 refers to the fourth and fifth lumbar vertebrae. How many each of cervical, thoracic, and lumbar vertebrae compose the spinal column?

   (A) 5 cervical, 12 thoracic, 7 lumbar

   (B) 7 cervical, 5 thoracic, 12 lumbar

   (C) 7 cervical, 12 thoracic, 5 lumbar

   (D) 12 cervical, 5 thoracic, 7 lumbar

   (E) 12 cervical, 7 thoracic, 5 lumbar

13. What does the term *herniated* mean?

   (A) Compressed

   (B) Protruding

   (C) Ruptured

   (D) Compressed and protruding

   (E) Ruptured and protruding

14. The patient is getting an MRI and an IVP. Which of the following statements regarding these tests is TRUE?

   (A) MRI stands for magnetic resonance imaging; IVP stands for inverted pyelogram.

   (B) Both MRI and IVP use radiation to produce images.

   (C) In an IVP, the patient takes an oral medication that is used as a contrast medium.

   (D) The dye used in an IVP may cause a reaction in patient who is allergic to shellfish.

   (E) There is no risk involved in taking an MRI.

15. A patient's chart has the following information: "Patient presents with a history of GERD and colitis." Which body system is being discussed?

    (A) Circulatory

    (B) Respiratory

    (C) Nervous

    (D) Gastrointestinal

    (E) Immune

ANSWERS AND EXPLANATIONS

1. **A**

   Atelectasis (A) is incomplete expansion of the lung. Pneumonia (B) is the accumulation of fluid in the lung. Tuberculosis (C) is a bacterial infection that causes coughing, night sweats, and destruction of lung tissue. Epistaxis (D) is a nosebleed. Asthma (E) is spasm of the airway in response to stress or allergens.

2. **E**

   Melatonin is secreted by the pineal gland.

3. **B**

   Insulin is formed in the pancreas.

4. **A**

   One function of the large intestine is to reabsorb water. Fats are broken down (B) in the first third of the small intestine (duodenum). Nutrients are absorbed (C) in the last two-thirds of the small intestine (jejunum and ileum). The urinary system excretes waste in water as urine (D). Breakdown of carbohydrates (E) begins in the mouth.

5. **A**

   Blood enters the glomerulus and is surrounded by the Bowman's capsule. The blood is filtered by the movement of waste from the bloodstream through the membrane on the Bowman's capsule. The distal convoluted tubule (B), proximal convoluted tubule (C), and loop of Henle (D) are part of the renal tubule.

6. **C**

   Hematuria is blood in the urine. Uremia (A) is waste in the blood. Albuminuria (B) is albumin in the urine. Pyuria (D) is pus in the urine. Glycosuria (E) is sugar in the urine.

7. **B**

   Sperm are made in the seminiferous tubules, stored in the epididymis (A), and travel through the vas deferens (C) after ejaculation. The prostate (D) and seminal vesicles (E) add nutrient fluids.

8. **C**

   The corpus luteum secretes progesterone to support the embryo until the placenta is functioning. The ovary (A) makes and ripens the egg and after ovulation, it travels down the fallopian tube (E) toward the uterus. Tinea corporis (D) is ringworm of the body. The corpus callosum (B) is the fibrous band between the hemispheres of the brain.

9. **B**

    The lymphatic system is primarily responsible for protection from foreign invaders and immunity. The circulatory system (A) is responsible for transporting oxygen, hormones, and nutrients. The endocrine system (C) secretes chemical messengers that affect target tissue. The digestive system (D) breaks down nutrients and absorbs them. The integumentary system (E) covers the body.

10. **B**

    The knuckles are on the dorsal side of the body when standing in anatomical position.

11. **C**

    When reading a medical record, one has to consider the context in which the abbreviation is being used. Although ED can mean erectile dysfunction, in this context it stands for emergency department. "Emergency department" and "emergency room" refer to the same thing.

12. **C**

    Recall that *cervical* means "neck," *thoracic* means "chest," and *lumbar* means "lower back." It is easy to remember how many vertebrae are in the spinal column if you associate it with something familiar. For instance, typical eating times are breakfast at 7 (there are 7 cervical vertebrae), lunch at 12 (there are 12 thoracic vertebrae), and dinner at 5 (there are 5 lumbar vertebrae).

13. **D**

    A hernia is a protrusion through a rupture. A herniated structure is moved or protruded from its original position. For example, in an inguinal area or umbilical hernia part of the intestines have protruded out of their normal position. In the current patient's case, the spongy disc of cartilage between the spinal vertebrae has protruded and may be putting pressure on a nerve, causing pain.

14. **D**

    Because iodine occurs in both shellfish and the contrast medium used in used in the IVP, a patient who is allergic to iodine may have an adverse reaction to an IVP. MRI is correctly identified, but IVP stands for intravenous pyelogram, not inverted pyelogram (A). The MRI produces images using magnetic waves, not x-rays (B). In an IVP, the contrast media is administered intravenously, not by mouth (C). There is always a risk to any procedure, including MRI (E). For example, patient who is claustrophobic may experience a panic attack in the MRI machine, while a patient who has a metal screw implanted in a bone may experience pain or complications if the screw moves during the MRI scan.

15. **D**

    GERD is gastroesophogeal reflux disease, in which there is regurgitation from the stomach to the esophagus. Colitis is inflammation of the colon or large intestines. All of these structures are associated with the gastrointestinal system (D).

Chapter 6: **Nutrition**

The food we consume is very important to our health because it provides our nutrients. The major nutrients include fats, proteins, carbohydrates, vitamins, minerals, electrolytes, water, and fiber. Fats, proteins, water, and carbohydrates, which are needed in large quantities in the body, are referred to as macronutrients. Vitamins, minerals, and electrolytes are needed in smaller quantities and are therefore referred to as micronutrients.

The Center for Nutrition Policy and Promotion offers guidelines for a healthy daily intake of nutrients via the program MyPlate, which guides consumers to make good food choices. It is also a visual tool for teaching young children healthy eating habits and appropriate portion sizes. Serving sizes are typically one of an item, such as one egg or one piece of fruit; 1–3 ounces of a meat or cheese; $\frac{1}{2}$–1 cup of a vegetable, sliced fruit, or cereal; or 1 cup of milk.

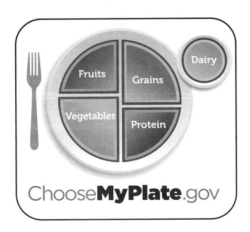

Figure 6.1—ChooseMyPlate.gov

FATS

Fats should provide approximately 20–35 percent of the average daily caloric intake. Fats serve three important functions:

1. They are essential nutrients important for the absorption of vitamins D, E, A, and K, which are fat-soluble vitamins.

2. They are necessary to provide the body's energy.

3. They assist in maintaining the core body temperature.

Fats are classified as saturated or unsaturated. Saturated fats tend to be solid at room temperature, and unsaturated fats tend to be in liquid form. Saturated fats can have an adverse effect on the body, increasing the risk for disease and cardiac damage; they are mainly found in meat and dairy products. Unsaturated fats tend to benefit health and support cardiac function; they are found mainly in foods derived from plants and fish.

PROTEINS

Protein is an essential nutrient for growth, development, and repair of skin, muscles, and other body tissues. Proteins are also necessary for the production of enzymes and hormones within the body. As proteins are digested, they break down into amino acids, which are essential for the body to build muscle and tissue.

The body is not capable of storing protein for use at a later time; therefore, a person's protein intake should constitute 10–35 percent of calories consumed daily. Practitioners typically increase protein in the diets of patients who have suffered wounds because it aids in restoring the health of tissues. The best sources of protein are plant or animal sources such as legumes, nuts, beans, soy, eggs, lean meats, fish, and dairy products.

CARBOHYDRATES

Carbohydrates provide the bulk of the caloric needs per day and should account for 45–65 percent of daily intake. They occur as sugars, starches, and dietary fiber and serve two main purposes: digestion and provision of energy. Sugar and starch break down into glucose, which is the simplest form of carbohydrate. Fiber does not break down into glucose, but it is important in digestion. Fiber also assists in weight loss by producing a feeling of satiety, or fullness.

Processed foods are typically high in carbohydrates but low in fiber. They are also high in calories and low in nutrients. Simple carbohydrates, such as those in fruit, break down very quickly in the body and produce a burst of energy. More complex carbohydrates, such as starches from potatoes, whole grains, and peas, take longer for the body to process and provide a more sustained level of energy.

VITAMINS

Vitamins are categorized as either fat soluble or water soluble. Water-soluble vitamins taken in excess are excreted and pose no threat to the body's health. Fat-soluble vitamins are stored in the body and, if taken in excess, can lead to toxicity referred to as hypervitaminosis. If fat intake is too low, or if fat absorption is compromised by a disease such as cystic fibrosis or through the use of certain drugs, the absorption of fat-soluble vitamins is inhibited. The following tables provide an overview of the vitamins and their functions.

Vitamin	Source	Function
B12 (cobalamin)	Meat, fish, seafood, eggs, milk, dairy products	Cell development, nerve function
B1 (thiamine)	Pork, whole grains, breads and cereals, legumes, seeds, nuts	Energy and nerve function
B2 (riboflavin)	Milk and dairy products, green leafy vegetables, whole grains	Metabolism, vision, skin health
B3 (niacin)	Meat, poultry, fish, breads, cereals, peanut butter, green leafy vegetables	Metabolism, digestive and nervous system function and health
B6 (pyridoxine)	Meat, fish, poultry, fruits, vegetables	Protein metabolism and red cell production
C (ascorbic acid)	Citrus fruits, vegetables in the cabbage family	Immunity, iron absorption, protein metabolism, antioxidant
Folic acid	Green leafy vegetables, orange juice, seeds, legumes	Red blood cell production, liver health

Table 6.1—Water-Soluble Vitamins

Vitamin	Source	Function
A	Animal sources, dairy products, liver, dark orange vegetables and fruits	Vision, bone, mucous membrane, and tooth health; immunity
D	Egg yolks, fortified milk, liver, fatty fish, sun exposure	Calcium absorption
E	Plant oils, green leafy vegetables, whole grains, nuts, seeds	Antioxidant, cell health
K	Green leafy vegetables, with smaller amounts in fish, liver, eggs, and cereals	Blood clotting

Table 6.2—Fat-Soluble Vitamins

Vitamins can behave in different ways in different bodies:

- Alcoholics are prone to a secondary vitamin B6 deficiency.
- Individuals with a vitamin B12 deficiency are likely lacking an intrinsic factor in the stomach. If pernicious anemia is diagnosed, these patients require an injection of B12 on a monthly basis.
- Infants are born with a low level of vitamin K. An injection of this vitamin is administered shortly after delivery to enhance clotting and deter intracranial bleeding associated with the trauma of delivery.

MINERALS

Minerals are a necessary part of the body's chemistry:

- Potassium is essential for muscle contraction, and any deviation from the normal amount may result in cardiac problems or death.
- Calcium is needed for strong bones and teeth, as well as muscle contraction.
- Iron is important as a precursor to red blood cells' ability to carry oxygen.
- Fluoride is important to prevent cavities (dental decay).
- Sodium needs are easily exceeded. Salty foods like potato chips, pretzels, ham, pickles, and table salt are easily recognized as sources of excess sodium, but significant sodium intake also comes from less obvious sources. Processed foods, for example, such as canned vegetables and frozen dinners contain high levels of sodium.

Mineral	Source
Potassium	Oranges, bananas, broccoli, potatoes, tomatoes
Calcium	Milk, sardine and salmon bones, fortified orange juice or bread
Iron	Red meat, liver, raisins, tomato juice, dried fruit
Fluoride	Fluoridated water, toothpaste
Iodine	Seafood, iodized salt

Table 6.3—Sources of Minerals

ELECTROLYTES

As the name implies, electrolytes are substances that dissolve to produce a solution that conducts electrical impulses. Electrolytes include sodium, potassium, calcium, magnesium, chloride, bicarbonate, and hydrogen phosphate.

Important points to remember about electrolytes include:

- The body needs electrolytes to sustain life.
- Electrolytes are found in fruits and vegetables.
- Electrolyte imbalance or deficiency results in symptoms of confusion, irregular heart rate, blood pressure changes, numbness, muscular twitching, weakness, and, in severe cases, seizures.
- The elderly are susceptible to electrolyte imbalances.
- Various diseases, conditions, and medications affect electrolyte levels:
  ° Kidney disease affects all electrolytes.
  ° Heart failure causes a low sodium level.
  ° Diabetes is associated with low sodium levels.
  ° Cancer is associated with high calcium levels.
  ° Certain diuretics cause loss of potassium through the kidneys.
  ° Vomiting, diarrhea, and dehydration cause electrolyte imbalances.
  ° Anorexia and bulimia affect electrolyte levels.

Electrolyte replacement may be necessary in patients presenting with these symptoms. Oral replacement solutions, such as Gatorade or Pedialyte, may need to be diluted for use in infants or an elderly patients due to their high electrolyte concentration. It is always better to err on the side of caution and consult the patient's provider prior to instituting electrolyte replacement therapy.

WATER

The human body is 60 percent water, and maintaining a healthy level of water is important in preserving life and maintaining homeostasis. Hydration is important for the transport of nutrients, the moisture of tissues, and the removal of waste products. Essentially, water regulates most activities in the body, including the activity in lymph, blood, glands, tissues, and cells. Water is lost through perspiration, respiration, and elimination.

The amount of water consumption required per day depends on a variety of individual circumstances, including a person's age, activity level, geographic location, and general health. The Institute of Medicine recommends that men consume about 3 liters (13 cups) of water per day and women consume 2.2 liters (9 cups). Although the rule of thumb of drinking eight 8-ounce glasses of water per day is still valid, water needs really do depend on the individual situation.

FIBER

Fiber is found in most fruits and vegetables. Dietary supplements of fiber are available, as are foods that are fortified with fiber such as some cereals, yogurt, and granola bars. However, supplements and fortified foods do not supply the vitamins and nutrients that whole foods provide. Unlike other nutrients, fiber is not digested or absorbed; it passes directly through the gastrointestinal tract. Soluble fiber dissolves and forms a gelatinlike substance. This type of fiber is found in oats, barley, carrots, peas, beans, apples, and citrus fruits. Insoluble fiber increases stool bulk and is found in whole wheat flour, nuts, beans, and vegetables such as cauliflower, potatoes, and green beans.

Most people associate fiber intake with the goal of preventing or relieving constipation, but its value goes beyond this function. Benefits of fiber include:

- Lowering cholesterol
- Normalizing bowel movements and maintaining bowel health
- Contributing to the prevention of colorectal cancer
- Controlling weight by producing a lasting feeling of fullness
- Helping control blood sugar levels

Fiber does tend to produce additional gas, bloating, and cramping if implemented too quickly into the diet. Adjust the body's fiber intake gradually, increasing it over several weeks until it reaches approximately 25–35 grams per day. Additional water also aids in absorbing fiber and facilitating elimination.

DIETS

Patients with specific health conditions will have special dietary needs. For example, gluten-free diets are necessary in patients with celiac disease. Patients who are unable to tolerate milk or dairy products are likely lactose intolerant and may need to use different products such as soy milk. Glucose-controlled diets are necessary for diabetic patients; these patients will also need to have regularly scheduled mealtimes.

Patients often need dietary modifications to meet their special needs. Most diets can be modified for consistency, spices, fiber, caffeine, and caloric level. The following table reviews the most common therapeutic diets.

Diet	Use	Description
DASH	Lowers blood pressure	Fresh fruits and vegetables, no alcohol, low salt, high fiber
BRAT	Controls diarrhea	Bananas, rice, applesauce, and tea
Soft diet	Decreases strain on GI tract	No fresh or raw fruits and vegetables, no strong spices, no gas-forming vegetables
Bland diet	Decreases GI irritation	No caffeine, no alcohol, no pepper, no chili, no nutmeg, no fried foods, no concentrated sweets
Low salt	Decreases blood pressure or water retention	Avoid processed foods (canned and frozen); no added table salt; no cured meats like ham, bacon, or sausage; minimal dairy products; avoid pickled items; avoid salty snacks
Low fat	Promotes heart health	Avoid saturated fats, pastries, icings, butter and whole milk products, and fatty cuts of meat; remove poultry skins
Low cholesterol	Promotes heart health	Avoid egg yolk, shrimp, organ meats, coconut and palm oils, and lard; increase foods that elevate HDL (avocados, nuts, legumes, canola oils)
Antioxidant	Prevents cancer	Dark green and yellow vegetables, green tea, red wine, oregano, sesame, rosemary, thyme, and cloves
Vegan	Lifestyle	No animal products, all nutrients from plant sources
Lacto-vegetarian	Lifestyle	Plant sources of nutrition supplemented by dairy products
Lacto-ovo-vegetarian	Lifestyle	Plant sources of nutrition supplemented by dairy products and eggs

Table 6.5—Special Diets

Metabolism is the production of energy from food; the body's internal temperature is related to metabolism. Caloric intake requirements are dependent on many factors, including health status, age, activity level, and male or female sex. Women's recommended caloric intake is usually 1,600–1,800 calories per day, and pregnancy requires approximately 300 calories more per day. Lactation requires approximately 800 calories more per day. Men's recommended caloric intake is usually 1,800–2,000 calories per day.

REVIEW QUESTIONS

1. Which vitamin plays an important role in the body's absorption of calcium?

    (A) Vitamin A
    (B) Vitamin B12
    (C) Vitamin C
    (D) Vitamin D
    (E) Vitamin K

2. Water intake is valuable for all of the following EXCEPT

    (A) replenishing body fluids
    (B) increasing the bulk of stool
    (C) treating congestive heart failure
    (D) aiding in nutrient absorption
    (E) facilitating removal of waste products

3. Which of the following fat soluble vitamins is important for vision?

    (A) Vitamin A
    (B) Vitamin B12
    (C) Vitamin D
    (D) Vitamin K
    (E) Riboflavin

4. Which of the following patients would most likely be linked to an electrolyte imbalance?

    (A) An adult patient who eats three meals per day that incorporate all the food groups
    (B) An adult patient with a history of anorexia as a teen that lasted five years
    (C) An infant who is breastfed and refuses to take the bottle when being weaned
    (D) A diabetic who has adjusted insulin intake to accommodate for additional exercise
    (E) A cancer patient undergoing chemotherapy

5. The main nutrients consumed each day are

    (A) carbohydrates
    (B) fats
    (C) proteins
    (D) fiber
    (E) vitamins

6. Which of these is a danger of fat-soluble vitamin intake?

    (A) They interfere with other nutrients being absorbed into the body.

    (B) They can accumulate and lead to toxicity.

    (C) They cause unnecessary expense because they will be excreted if taken in excess.

    (D) They reduce the appetite, causing a decrease in consumption of other important nutrients.

    (E) They cause constipation.

7. A patient who has diarrhea may benefit from which diet?

    (A) Soft-food

    (B) DASH

    (C) BRAT

    (D) Lactose-free

    (E) Vegan

8. Which mineral is important for normal cardiac function?

    (A) Potassium

    (B) Sodium

    (C) Chloride

    (D) Fluoride

    (E) Iodine

9. Which combination of nutrients is MOST beneficial for wound healing?

    (A) Carbohydrates and iron

    (B) Fiber and water

    (C) Fats and vitamin D

    (D) Protein and vitamin C

    (E) Calcium and protein

10. An average of 3–5 servings per day should be consumed from which category?

    (A) Dairy and cheese

    (B) Meats

    (C) Cereals

    (D) Vegetables

    (E) Fruits

ANSWERS AND EXPLANATIONS

1. **D**

   Vitamin D promotes calcium absorption. The human body obtains vitamin D from forti-fied foods such as milk or synthesizes it when the skin is exposed to sunlight. Vitamin A (A) is important in forming and maintaining healthy skin, teeth, and mucous mem-branes; it is also important for eye health and is also known as retinol because it produces the pigments in the retina for the eye. Vitamin B12 (B) is essential for brain and nervous system functioning. A person who is deficient in vitamin B12 is subject to pernicious ane-mia and needs a monthly injection of the vitamin. Vitamin C (C), also known as ascorbic acid, is important for wound healing and for normal growth and development. Common sources of vitamin C are citrus fruits and leafy green vegetables. Since it is water soluble, vitamin C requires constant replacement in the body. Vitamin K (E) is a fat-soluble vita-min stored in the body that is important for normal blood clotting. Leafy green vegetables are a good source of vitamin K.

2. **C**

   Patients with congestive heart failure (C) may need liquids restricted due to the fluid buildup in the system.

3. **A**

   Vitamin B2 (B) aids in vision but is water soluble. Vitamin A (A) is a fat-soluble vitamin found in dairy products, orange fruits, and vegetables such as yams and carrots; it is ben-eficial for eyesight.

4. **E**

   Any condition that is not managed can lead to electrolyte imbalances, but a cancer patient (E) is the most likely of the patients listed to develop an imbalance. All the other patients' diets are monitored or controlled.

5. **A**

   Carbohydrates (A) constitute 45–65 percent of the average daily intake of calories. Fats and proteins follow next in the macronutrient category.

6. **B**

   Fat-soluble vitamins are stored in the body and therefore should be taken in smaller quantities to avoid hypervitaminosis or toxicity (B).

7. **C**

   A BRAT diet (C) consists of bananas, rice, applesauce, and tea. These items are very mild on the gut and easy to digest. They contain nutrients and assist in hydration until the diarrhea is resolved.

8. **A**

   Potassium (A) is important for muscle contraction. Abnormally low levels of potassium can lead to poor cardiac muscular contraction.

9. **D**

   Protein and vitamin C (D) are both important in cellular regeneration and tissue health, aiding in wound healing.

10. **D**

    After the bread and cereal group, for which 6–11 servings per day are recommended, vegetables (D) are the category with highest number of recommended servings per day, with 3–5.

KAPLAN

Chapter 7: **Psychology**

Medical assistants routinely interact with patients during a wide range of encounters from routine appointments to emergency treatment, and from acute care to chronic illness. Patient responses to the care and treatment provided are heavily influenced by their developmental stage, cognitive abilities, intellect, and general state of psychological well-being. The interplay between factors that affect both the body and mind in health and illness are interwoven. It is important to understand and apply key information from the study of psychology in daily work with patients. This chapter includes a brief review of the field of psychology, a summary of the major theorists, and the developmental stages that you are likely to encounter.

Psychology refers to the study of the mind. Human psychology includes the thoughts, behaviors, and emotions of individuals across age groups, genders, and cultures. Over the course of time, major schools of psychological study have emerged as scientists continue to explore the wide variability of the human mind from both normal and abnormal perspectives. As a field of science, psychologists conduct research and apply the scientific method to the study of human behavior. A common example is the effort to determine the relative importance of nature (genetic and biological influences) versus nurture (social and cultural influences) on behavior.

SIGMUND FREUD (1856–1939)

One of the earliest theorists to examine and describe the human mind was the Austrian physician Sigmund Freud. Freud was the first to label what he considered the hidden area of the mind, the unconscious. The area was believed to contain thoughts, emotions, and memories of which people are largely unaware. In psychoanalytic therapy, Freud used a technique he named *free association of ideas* to allow patients to recognize and recall unconscious memories and deal with them in the conscious mind. Freud's work, referred to as psychoanalysis, is based on his belief that psychological problems are the result of repressed impulses and conflicts stemming from childhood. The goal of psychoanalysis is to bring these issues into conscious awareness so patients can deal with them in the present.

In addition, Freud viewed the structure of the human mind as containing distinct parts that shaped the personality and thus the behaviors of all human beings. He coined the terms *ego, id,* and *superego* as the areas of the mind that govern unique processes. The ego is the conscious state that directs the personality and works to deal with the state of reality. The id contains the unconscious memories and impulses, that Freud believed were based on sexual and aggressive drives. The id drives the personality to seek pleasure and instant gratification of unconscious desires. Finally, the superego represents the judgment center of the mind where internalized ideals and values are held. Problems in human behavior and psychological pain occurred as a result of the struggle and interplay of the id, the ego, and the superego. The goal of therapy was to bring repressed information to the conscious mind and allow the patient to handle the conflict.

Freud felt that personality development occurred during the early years of a child's life. Later problems were rooted in unresolved conflicts from childhood. Freud viewed the developmental stages as psychosexual in nature. During these stages, the id sought pleasure through stimulation of erogenous zones of the body. First, the infant experienced the oral stage where pleasure was sought through sucking, chewing, and biting. Next, from age 18 months to age 3, the child experienced the anal stage when control over bowel and bladder elimination dominated the id. During the phallic stage, from about 3 to 6 years of age, the id focused on the genital area of the body, and the child developed sexual desires. It was during this stage that Freud believed that boys went through an Oedipal complex of loving their mothers and desiring them sexually, while feeling threatened by and fearful of their fathers. Freud felt that eventually children repress these feelings and learn to cope with them by a process of identification with the same sex parent and the values held in the superego. Though much of Freud's work has been dismissed by modern psychologists, his fundamental contributions to the field remain intact.

JEAN PIAGET (1896–1980)

Piaget, a Swiss psychologist, studied the basis for learning and development of the mind. He is considered to be the founder of cognitive psychology. Cognitive psychology is the study of thinking, logical reasoning, and the ability of the human mind to understand abstract and symbolic ideas. Piaget studied the development of children and their progressive stages of motor development. He believed that motor activity stimulated mental development. For example, an infant beginning to experience her environment may shake a rattle, which produces a noise. Over time and with repetition, the infant learns that this motor activity produces a sound. Piaget theorized that cognitive development is based on the child's interaction with her environment. The following table summarizes Piaget's developmental learning stages.

Developmental Period	Age Group	Description
Sensorimotor	Birth to 2 years	Children learn about the world through their senses and motor skills

Table 7.1—Piaget's Developmental Learning Stages *(continued on next page)*

Developmental Period	Age Group	Description
Preoperational	2–6 years	Children begin to think symbolically and form language skills; they pretend and fantasize during play; thinking is self-centered
Concrete operations	7–11 years	Children perceive differences and begin to reason; they can classify and attend to multiple situations
Formal operations	12–adulthood	Children and adults can grasp abstract concepts, more formal notion of time, and long-term goal setting develops; learning takes place by relating new material to past material

Table 7.1—Piaget's Developmental Learning Stages *(continued from previous page)*

ERIK ERIKSON (1902–1994)

Erikson based his theories in psychology on social development across the human lifespan. His work was conducted in the late 1960s, and it has formed the basis for the field of developmental psychology. He believed that people in each stage of life faced age-specific, competing psychosocial tasks that manifest as crises that had to be resolved before the person could move successfully into the next stage of psychological development. According to Erikson, there are eight stages of development. The stages are listed in the following table, along with the competing tasks associated with each stage, and a brief description of each stage. Erikson believed that resolution of the crises in each stage led to the formation of an individual's identity as a person. You will apply your knowledge of the tasks of each stage of development in working with patients. The unmet developmental tasks often become apparent during medical treatment or life crises.

Age of Developmental Stage	Developmental Issues	Tasks Associated with Developmental Stage
Infancy up to 1 year	Trust vs. mistrust	If basic needs are met, the child learns to trust
Toddler 1–2 years	Autonomy vs. shame and doubt	Child learns to exercise free will and accomplish tasks or doubt his abilities
Preschool 3–5 years	Initiative vs. guilt	Child learns to initiate activities and plans or feels guilty about his inabilities
Elementary school (6 years up to puberty)	Competence vs. inferiority	Child gains pleasure from accomplishments or he feels inferior

Table 7.2—Erikson's Developmental Tasks *(continued on next page)*

Age of Developmental Stage	Developmental Issues	Tasks Associated with Developmental Stage
Adolescence (teens into 20s)	Identity vs. role confusion	Teens refine their identities and try different roles or they lose their sense of who they are and what they will become
Young adults (20s to early 40s)	Intimacy vs. isolation	Young adults seek to develop close and intimate social relationships or remain socially isolated
Middle-aged adults (40s to 60s)	Generativity vs. stagnation	Adults develop a sense of well-being through contributions to work and family or they feel a lack of purpose
Later adults (late 60s and beyond)	Integrity vs. despair	In reflecting on their lives, seniors sense satisfaction or failure

Table 7.2—Erikson's Developmental Tasks *(continued from previous page)*

ABRAHAM MASLOW (1908–1970)

Maslow, an American psychologist, is considered the founder of humanist psychology. Maslow followed Freud's psychoanalytic model and viewed his work as an extension rather than a replacement for other theory. Maslow is best known for his hierarchy of human needs. Maslow believed that human behavior was motivated by a series of hierarchical needs ranging from basic physiological survival to self-actualization.

The following chart displays a graphic of the levels of human need in Maslow's hierarchy. Maslow believed that having basic survival and physiologic needs unmet prevented individuals from addressing safety needs and issues. In turn, safety needs for security, stability, and protection must be met before people can deal with love and belonging needs in social relationships. Once social relationship needs are met, the person can focus on developing self-esteem through achievements and accomplishments. Once all of the levels of need are met, the individual seeks self-actualization, which is attainment of peak performance living. This person has met and accomplished what he is best suited for in life, and is reaping the rewards of living.

Maslow recognized that life circumstances create situations that move people between stages. You will need to recognize what life realities and needs your patients face as you assist in your office practice. It will be important to assist patients who are struggling with basic physical needs or safety needs by referring them to social service agencies or other human service organizations in your community. Being aware of where a patient is on this hierarchy will help guide your interventions and communication to be more effective.

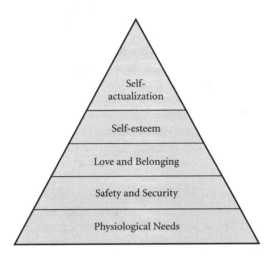

Figure 7.1—Maslow's Hierarchy of Human Needs

LAWRENCE KOHLBERG (1927–1987)

Kohlberg, a Harvard University developmental psychologist, studied the field of moral development beginning in the 1970s. Kohlberg believed that moral development and ethical behavior, like cognitive development, depended on the age and problem-solving ability of the individual. His work built upon that of Piaget and other developmental psychologists. According to Kohlberg, children and adults move through three major stages of developing a sense of justice and moral beliefs. These beliefs formed the basis for ethical behaviors. The first stage of moral development is termed preconditional. In this stage, young children learn to behave based on rewards and punishments. Essentially, they learn that by doing what is "good" they will avoid punishments and gain rewards from their parents and other adults. The next stage of moral development was referred to as the conventional level. At this stage, right and wrong is determined by others and is approved behavior. Later in this stage, law and order and fixed rules and regulations are recognized. Moral behavior consists of following the rules of society, authority, or religion. The highest stage of moral development was termed the postconventional or principled level. In this stage, rights are part of a greater social contract, such as the U.S. Constitution. At this level, individuals hold to universal good and ethical principles. Kohlberg believed that individual moral development depended on a person's cognitive or thinking capacity and exposure to different ideas and human experiences.

ELISABETH KÜBLER-ROSS (1926–2004)

Dr. Elisabeth Kübler-Ross is famous for her work with patients who were experiencing death and grieving during the final stages of life. Through her observations and interviews with patients, she identified five stages that are typically observed by individuals going through the dying experience. The stages are denial, anger, bargaining, depression, and acceptance.

In working with terminally ill patients, she noted that newly diagnosed patients frequently face shock and disbelief in dealing with the information. They may feel invincible even in the face of major signs and symptoms. During this stage, patients may reject treatment or seek multiple providers to avoid facing their disease. Once they move through denial, many become angry. It is typical for patients to feel anger that despite following prescribed treatments, healthy life-styles, or other actions, they are the victims of illness. The outward anger may be directed at health care providers, family members, or others deemed to be responsible. The next stage of grieving is bargaining. In this stage, people may bargain with "if-then" thinking. For example, "If I pray and attend church regularly, then God will save me." Once bargaining has been completed, it is common for depression to set in. Facing multiple losses of family, friends, functional status, appearance, and often livelihood may lead to sadness and isolation. The final stage of grieving is acceptance. In this stage, people facing terminal illness come to terms with this reality. They say their good-byes and may develop an appreciation for what they are leaving behind. Often patients in this stage will seek to leave a legacy in writing or in pictures for their loved ones. They may begin to assist in planning for their own funerals and actively put their affairs in order.

Kübler-Ross noted that not every patient or family member experienced each of the five stages. In addition, patients may move back and forth in the stages. She was one of the first scientists to explore not only the stages of the grieving process, but also the lack of understanding and appreciation by the majority of the health care professionals for these experiences. Her book, *On Death and Dying*, was instrumental in directing the movement of hospice and end-of-life care in the United States.

DEFENSE MECHANISMS AND COMMUNICATION

People often have emotional reactions to their experiences, and this of course includes patients. When events arouse difficult feelings in a patient—such as guilt, fear, or shame, among others—he or she may react defensively. Defense mechanisms are a person's conscious or unconscious effort to protect the ego and self-esteem. However, they can create a barrier to communication. Furthermore, defense mechanisms that last for excessive periods of time, or that do not resolve, can raise mental health concerns.

As a medical assistant, you must be able to recognize defense mechanisms. You must also learn to navigate them by incorporating therapeutic communication into your daily activities. Following are some common defense mechanisms that you may encounter in the health care setting.

Denial is a refusal to accept something that may be painful, and it often follows a traumatic event such as a death in the family or a diagnosis of cancer. A patient in denial will not be able to focus on the news you are conveying.

Regression is a means of retreating from unpleasant situations. The regressive patient may retreat to a happier, more secure time in their life. An example of this defense mechanism is a child who has been toilet trained but begins bed-wetting again when a new sibling is born.

Rationalization is labeling as acceptable a behavior that may not be healthy. In essence, the individual is making excuses—rationalization is the mind's way of avoiding guilt or embarrassment. For example, a driver may rationalize that it is acceptable not to wear a seatbelt because he travels only a few miles to work.

Undoing is meant to make amends for unacceptable behavior. For instance, an abusive spouse might shower excessive gifts upon the victim in a bid to "undo" or negate the abuse.

Sublimation is a means of channeling something socially unacceptable into an acceptable form. It would not be acceptable to be aggressive toward a medical assistant, for example, but someone who has aggressive tendencies might exhibit those behaviors through a sport such as football.

Projection is blaming others or attributing one's own thoughts to others in order to avoid accepting accountability. For instance, a parent who abuses her child may lash out at a medical assistant for being too rough during a pediatric exam preparation.

In **compensation**, a person substitutes a strength for a weakness to avoid embarrassment or acknowledgement of deficiencies. For example, an oversized child who is not very intelligent might use his size to compensate, by exhibiting some power over other children.

PUTTING THEORY INTO PRACTICE

As a medical assistant, you will be working closely with patients and coworkers from a variety of age groups and backgrounds. Understanding basic principles of human behavior and development will be fundamental to your practice. As you work to communicate effectively, consider the age and developmental stages of your patients. When designing an effective teaching plan, you will need to consider the ability of the patient to learn. Health behavior of patients will be influenced by their basic stage in the hierarchy of needs. If they are seeking safety and security, they are not going to be open to higher-level health behaviors and actions. In working with problems or conflicts, try to determine if what you are observing may relate to the person's psychosocial tasks and moral development. Psychological theory and basic knowledge from the major theorists in the field can be an important resource to draw on throughout your years in practice.

REVIEW QUESTIONS

1. The social worker at a clinic has arranged for a safe and secure apartment for a young single parent and her children. According to Maslow's hierarchy of needs theory, which of the following is the next level of need for her to meet?

    (A) Food and water

    (B) Love and belonging

    (C) Self-actualization

    (D) Sexual needs

    (E) Esteem and recognition

2. Freud was the first person to discuss which of the following concepts in psychology?

    (A) The developmental stages

    (B) Dreaming

    (C) The hierarchy of needs

    (D) The unconscious mind

    (E) Human sexuality

3. According to Kohlberg, many people

    (A) never develop a sense of right or wrong

    (B) do not follow laws

    (C) do not reach the highest level of moral development

    (D) are afraid of their parents

    (E) never develop a sense of morality

4. According to Kohlberg's theory of moral development, young children who obey their parents do so because of their

    (A) sense of right and wrong

    (B) awareness of law and order

    (C) awareness that family harmony is the ultimate good

    (D) desire to avoid punishment

    (E) older sibling's behavior

5. According to Piaget, the following behaviors would be shown by children in the sensorimotor stage of development, EXCEPT

    (A) placing objects into their mouths

    (B) drawing a picture of an apple

    (C) watching a pinwheel turn

    (D) playing peek-a-boo

    (E) rubbing their faces on a soft blanket

6. A patient continues to smoke despite repeated instruction and information that the medical assistant provides at appointments. She says that she smokes because her friends all smoke. Which of the following age groups is she likely to be in?

    (A) Senior citizen

    (B) Middle-aged adult

    (C) Adolescent

    (D) School-age child

    (E) Late 20s adult

7. By the age of 18–24 months, children may cry or become frightened at the sight of a medical assistant wearing a lab coat. Which psychological theory is this an example of?

    (A) Conditioning

    (B) Cognitive therapy

    (C) Grief and loss

    (D) Hierarchy of needs

    (E) Play therapy

8. Providing an obese child with a gold star sticker at each appointment at which they experience a weight loss is an example of

    (A) role playing

    (B) patient education

    (C) behavior reinforcement

    (D) patient-centered care

    (E) cognitive therapy

9. A four-year-old child who has been potty-trained for almost a year begins wetting the bed. No medical basis is identified, and the parents state that the bed-wetting began soon after the birth of a sibling. The toddler probably is exhibiting what defense mechanism?

    (A) Repression

    (B) Projection

    (C) Denial

    (D) Compensation

    (E) Regression

10. A physician recommends surgery for a female patient who is found to have a mass in her breast. The patient refuses surgery, stating that she will decrease her caffeine intake and the mass will go away. What defense mechanism is the patient displaying?

    (A) Denial

    (B) Undoing

    (C) Regression

    (D) Sublimation

    (E) Rationalization

ANSWERS AND EXPLANATIONS

1. **B**

   Love and belonging is a need that can only be met after the basic human survival needs for food and water (A), oxygen, excretion, and sex (D) are met, as well as the need for safety and security. The need for love and belonging is followed by the need for esteem and recognition (E). Maslow believed that self-actualization (C) could only be achieved if all the preceding human needs had been met. In Maslow's hierarchy, self-actualization is the highest level of need.

2. **D**

   Freud was the first person to use the term "unconscious mind" to discuss an area of the mind that functioned outside of our day-to-day awareness. Though Freud interpreted dreams (B) as part of his process with patients, he viewed dreams as a component of the unconscious mind.

3. **C**

   Kohlberg felt that many adults never reach the state of altruism that represents the highest stage of moral development. Instead, they obey laws and do what is deemed right in the eyes of society.

4. **D**

   Kohlberg observed that school-age children learn to obey rules based on what they are told by parents, teachers, and other authority figures. Their moral development at this stage is based on avoiding punishment. Items A through C reflect higher levels of moral development. Sibling behavior (E) was not considered in Kohlberg's theory as an element of moral development.

5. **B**

   Drawing a picture of an apple requires that the child has the perception of the use of symbols and symbolic reasoning. Sensorimotor is Piaget's developmental stage for infants and toddlers who experience their environment through their senses of touch, taste, smell, vision, and movement. The other answer choices are all sensory activities.

6. **C**

   A common characteristic of adolescent behavior is the influence of peer pressure. The fact that her friends smoke will be a strong motivator for the patient to begin and continue smoking despite knowledge of the hazards of this habit. Peer pressure is less likely to influence the patients in the other age groups in this example.

7. **A**

    This exemplifies conditioning, where a known stimulus comes to be associated with another stimulus that accompanies it. In this case, the child may have received a shot at the medical office and now associates office personnel with that pain and fear. Cognitive therapy (B) is a form of psychological counseling. Grief and loss (C) are experiences in response to illness, death, and changes in function. Hierarchy of needs (D) was used by Maslow to explain a progression in the stages of human needs from simple survival to self actualization.

8. **C**

    Behavior reinforcement is providing a reward for a desired patient behavior, in this case weight control. If the child interprets the gold star as a reward for staying on his diet plan, then the medical assistant is reinforcing this behavior. None of the other items are a fit with this activity. Role playing (A) involves asking the patient to pretend to assume a new identify, patient-centered care (D) is a strategy to focus medical interventions specifically on the needs of a particular patient. Cognitive therapy (E) is a form of psychology that relies on a patient's conscious thoughts.

9. **E**

    When faced with a stressful situation, a person may regress, or retreat to an earlier, more secure time in life.

10. **A**

    Denial is a frequent first response to a traumatic event. It may also be used to avoid any painful situation. Denial is often a barrier to effective communication.

KAPLAN

Chapter 8: **Patient Communication**

An important component of medical assisting is ensuring effective communication. You will need to convey information and converse with patients, families, and a host of other health care providers. Much of your job will involve communication skills. You will communicate both verbally and in writing via face-to-face encounters, telephone messages, email messages, and patient documentation and reports. You must also be able to communicate nonverbally. This chapter will assist you by reviewing the critical elements of therapeutic communication and addressing communication with special-needs populations. In addition, a variety of typical clinical communication encounters such as patient interviewing, telephone calls, and writing will be covered.

OVERVIEW OF BASIC COMMUNICATION PATTERNS

Communication is defined as the sending and receiving of messages. Critical components of any communication include four elements. First, the *sender* begins the exchange by forming and conveying a clear thought or piece of information. The sender transforms the information into speech or actions (symbols), which are organized according to a certain syntax and grammar. This process is called encoding. The second element is the *message* itself, which is the information being sent. The third component in communication is the *receiver*, who takes in (decodes) the message. The most common forms of receiving messages are listening and reading. Finally, every communication includes *feedback*, which is the response of the receiver verifying the exchange of information.

The Communication Process

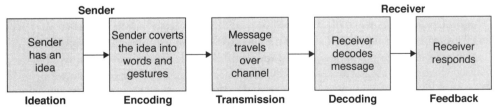

Sender			Receiver	
Sender has an idea	Sender coverts the idea into words and gestures	Message travels over channel	Receiver decodes message	Receiver responds
Ideation	**Encoding**	**Transmission**	**Decoding**	**Feedback**

Figure 8.1—The Communication Process

Many factors can influence or distort the basic communication cycle described above. Noise is anything that gets in the way of effective communication. Individual interpretation of words, facial expression, and the setting of the communication are just a few of the potential influences.

THERAPEUTIC COMMUNICATION

In our day-to-day lives we communicate on a social level in many different situations. This communication requires no special set of skills or knowledge. However, in the professional world of health care, you as a medical assistant will be called on to use therapeutic communication with patients, families, and other professionals. Therapeutic communication occurs when patients who have particular concerns or needs seek your help to resolve or alleviate their problem. This specialized form of communication requires that you be open to others, be respectful of cultural and ethnic diversity, be a good listener, be aware of your own biases, and be truly interested in helping others. In a therapeutic encounter, you will also need to avoid becoming overly involved in a patient's emotional and physical distress. Such a level of involvement may cause you to lose objectivity or become codependent and be unable to provide the necessary assistance.

Effective Therapeutic Communication Strategies

The best communication occurs when the entire exchange of information adheres to the "five C's." This means that the communication is complete, concise, concrete, clear, and considerate. Therapeutic communication can be most effective when you pay attention to the message that you are sending. A message must be empathetic to the patient and must involve reflexive communication skills. You will need to pay attention to your nonverbal communication patterns as well as those of your patient. You should be aware of the impact that environmental and cultural differences may have on your therapeutic communication.

Empathy

Empathy means that you are in touch with and aware of the feelings your patient is experiencing. It implies that you are able to "walk in her shoes" and that you appreciate and accept her feelings. Empathy is often compared to and contrasted with sympathy, which is responding to the emotional state of another person with your own emotional reaction. During a time of stress or illness, patients are best served by professionals who can empathize with their situation. An excellent strategy for conveying empathy in a sincere and honest way is through reflective communication. Remember that you cannot always say, "I know how you feel," because it is likely that you have not been in that situation, so you really do not know. An empathetic response would be, "I understand how that must make you feel."

Reflective Communication

The techniques and talent of reflective communication may seem simple; however, they will require a great deal of practice and attention to be used well on the job. Reflective communication involves listening to the patient closely and carefully while observing their nonverbal cues such as facial expressions, gestures, and body language. During reflective communication, you are not only taking in the message, but its meaning to the patient and how the message seems to be influencing the patient's emotional state. Your sincere interest is conveyed by head nodding, direct eye contact, and paraphrasing what the patient said. In paraphrasing, you state back to the patient in your own words what you heard him say. You may also comment on the feelings that seem to be conveyed in the message. For example, if an elderly patient tells you that she is being urged by her family to give up her home and move into an assisted-living facility, you may reflect by stating, "Your daughter feels that you would be safer in an assisted-living facility." Restating the patient's words, tying the words together with their emotional meaning, and reflecting this back to the patient is a core skill for medical assistants. To be good at reflective communication you need to listen actively, pay attention to the spoken word, and observe the patient carefully.

Nonverbal Communication

You may be familiar with the saying, "Actions speak louder than words." This saying underscores the meaning and importance of all forms of nonverbal communication. As a medical assistant, you will need to attend to both your own nonverbal cues and to those of your patients and coworkers. Nonverbal communication includes appearance and style, facial expressions, hand gestures, body position, and movements. Often gestures and stance send more meaning than the spoken message in a conversation.

Dress and appearance convey a great deal of information and, like it or not, we all tend to form our first and lasting impression of people based on their physical appearance. Grooming, appropriateness of dress, accessories, and ornamentation will influence your impression of the patient and his impression of you. As a medical assistant, you will need to be well groomed and neat. Avoid extremes in jewelry, nail length, hair styles, and ornaments in the workplace. In today's world, men and women are freer in expressing their individual styles through body piercing, tattoos, hair color, and fashion. It is likely that you will see a wide variety of states of personal grooming, dress, and appearance. Many people make judgments and interpretations of others based on their appearance. You need to be aware of what your own biases are in regard to style and appearance and take care to act professionally with all patients.

Body language includes posture, stance, gesturing, eye contact, and movement. During therapeutic communication you will want to sit on the same level as the patient, facing the patient, making direct eye contact, and respecting the patient's personal space. You need to observe how congruent the patient's words are with her facial expression and body stance. Arms folded across the chest may indicate a closed or defensive posture. Downcast eyes may be a sign of embarrassment or discomfort. Sitting with arms and legs crossed may be a sign of avoidance. If a patient tells you that she is okay during a procedure but you observe that her fists are clenched, you may want to ask if she is uncomfortable or in pain.

There are no hard and fast rules in interpreting nonverbal communication. If you do not see consistency between a patient's words and gestures or expressions, ask a question before you assume that there is a meaning behind the message you are getting. You will want to validate your observations and give feedback about the communication from your sender.

Environmental and Cultural Influences on Communication

The Environment of Care

To enhance communication in the medical office, you want to create an environment that supports interaction. Some environmental factors that will contribute to open and free communication include a professional office space, privacy, secure storage of documentation and medical records, and avoidance of noise, distractions, and interruptions during patient contacts. Patients should be interviewed and examined in private. You should knock, announce yourself, and wait for the patient to acknowledge you before entering the exam room. If at all possible, arrange seating so that the patient is directly across from you and at eye level during your conversation. You want to convey your full attention, and even in a hectic office practice, the habit of sitting down and making eye contact will convey your attention to the patient. If possible, avoid interruptions during a patient visit. If you are documenting information in a patient file during the interview, make sure that you look up regularly and make eye contact with the patient. To protect patient confidentiality, you should give the patient instructions, test schedules, and other information in a private location.

Cultural Considerations in Communication

Major demographic changes in the U.S. population have occurred, producing a wide diversity of cultural and ethnic groups. It is likely that you will be treating a mix of patients from different countries, speaking different languages, and engaging in different social behaviors and practices from those of your own family. It is important that you take time to learn some basics about the culture and belief systems of the patients in your workplace. While there are no hard and fast rules, you need to appreciate that people from around the world will not always think and act as you do. This information will assist you in gaining the trust and confidence of those you serve.

Many individuals new to the United States will need time to translate your words and their meaning into their own language and then translate their response into English. This is a complex process and there may be phrases or figures of speech that do not translate. For some, English as a second language means that they do not think in English and must decode your words and meaning into their own language. It is important that you ensure that you are being understood clearly. Speaking slowly may help with the decoding; speaking louder will not.

In some cultures, issues as fundamental as time and its meaning are less precise. In Native American or Mexican cultures, arriving at the office for an appointment at a specific time may not be valued and will need to be explained to patients. This will prevent confusion and help them understand the office's expectations. Facial expressions and conversational etiquette are also a cultural variation. For example, in some Asian countries such as Cambodia and Laos, making prolonged direct eye contact is interpreted as a sign of disrespect and is impolite. As this example demonstrates, effective communication across cultures will require that you take the time to understand and appreciate the cultural aspects and diversity in the patients you treat on a regular basis.

COMMUNICATING WITH SPECIAL-NEEDS PATIENTS

As a health care professional, you will be working with a broad group of patients who have unique diseases and disabilities that affect their functional status and communication capabilities. In this section, you will review some basic strategies to enhance your ability to effectively communicate with these individuals.

Blind or Visually Impaired Patients

Patients with low vision or blindness will need some accommodations to support effective treatment and communication in the medical office setting. You should be aware of the cause of the visual impairment and the level of functional eyesight of your patient. Blind patients may be accompanied by another person or a guide dog. You will need to remember that the guide dog is at work while in your setting, and although it is tempting to pet and play with the dog, this is a distraction that the working dog has been trained to avoid. In addition, the dog is trained only to respond to commands from its owner. Some blind and low-sighted individuals use a cane to navigate their environment. You should ask such patients what assistance they need from you to get to the exam room, to change clothing, and to complete any procedures. You should avoid reaching out and touching these patients without prior verbal cues to avoid startling or invoking a sense of intrusion. You will need to provide detailed instructions and step-by-step explanations of your actions. For example, if you need to leave the exam room to get equipment or supplies, let the patient know that you are leaving and when you will return. As with any patient, knock on the door to signal your return and wait for the patient's acknowledgment. If you work in a specialty practice, you may have patient teaching materials in Braille; however, not all visually impaired children and adults are able to read Braille. You may need to audiotape complex patient information or instructions for these patients.

Deaf and Hearing-Impaired Patients

Caring for deaf or hearing-impaired individuals requires some adaptations and accommodations to your communication practices. Not all deaf or hearing-impaired patients communicate in the same way. For some, lip reading is used to communicate in the hearing world. Lip readers need to have unencumbered access to your face while you are speaking. It helps to speak slowly and deliberately. Some deaf individuals are trained to speak, but their voices and speech patterns may be garbled or difficult to understand. You may need to ask for an interpreter if the communication is complex. Some deaf people communicate using American Sign Language and will need a sign language interpreter to be available at their office visits. When speaking through a sign language interpreter, it is still proper to direct your comments and communication to the patient. When working with deaf patients, you can use demonstrations, written material, and gestures to communicate.

Elderly Patients

Communicating effectively with older adults will sometimes require that you use the full gamut of communication techniques. You should be familiar with your patient's functional abilities and note any impairment in concentration, memory, or recall. If the patient has memory impairments, you will need to make sure the caregivers, spouse, or significant other is involved in health teaching or patient instruction. You may need to break complex procedures into simple step-by-step instructions with both written and verbal review. Patients should be asked, when possible, to give return demonstrations or to review your directions with you in their own words. If the elderly patient does not drive or leave the home independently, you should find out how he will obtain any needed supplies, equipment, or medication. You may need to assist the patient by making referrals for home health nursing, medical equipment, dial-a-ride, or other community resources. In most communities, you can obtain a directory of resources for seniors through the National Association of Area Agencies on Aging. More information is available at www.n4a.org.

Children

It is important that you integrate your understanding of childhood growth and development stages and apply this information as you work with children of various ages. All individuals fear the unknown and unfamiliar. These fears are even stronger for children who may not understand what is happening or why a medical office visit is occurring. As a health care professional, you can help lessen children's fears and anxiety by giving them your attention and respect, and providing clear and accurate information about treatments or procedures. Children should be given a chance to see and, if possible, touch your instruments and equipment. Never tell a child that a procedure will not hurt if that is likely to occur. You should observe the interaction between the parent and child and reinforce how a parent can and should assist you in an interview, exam, or procedure. Do not assume that parents readily know what to expect and what you need from them during an office visit.

A few special considerations will assist you in working and communicating with younger children in your office. The environment should be bright, cheerful, and childproofed. It is helpful to have toys and books that can be easily cleaned and stored in the office. You should avoid prolonged waiting periods for young children who will become anxious and potentially uncooperative. Having separate reception areas for sick children and well children is an effective concept.

It is helpful to speak directly with the child at eye level. Usually it is not a good idea to pick children up. Use a friendly and open approach, but avoid talking down to children or using terms or language that is too complex for them to understand. Give children encouragement for positive behavior during the exam or treatment. It is helpful to wait until the end of the appointment to complete any invasive or painful procedures as these may elicit crying or anger. Allow children to express their feelings and fears before and after their treatment. Acknowledge their hurt, and try to provide a simple reward or reinforcement for good behavior. It will also help if you listen both to the concerns of the child and of the parent.

Seriously Ill Patients

When patients are seriously ill, their energy levels, cognition, and ability to communicate may be distorted or limited. Health care providers should respect the reality that lengthy interactions, polite small talk, or social conversation can become a drain. The patient's appointment should be scheduled accordingly to avoid waiting time and to allow extra time for accommodating limited mobility or the need for special devices and equipment. You should also pay attention to family and other caregivers. Keep the appointment focused and be prepared for any procedures by having equipment and supplies handy. Pay attention to the patient's level of physical and mental comfort while she is in the office. Often a trip to the physician's office is a major undertaking for the patient and the family that requires advance special transportation, painful movement and manipulation into mobility devices, and extra work for families and caregivers. Try to make the visit as comfortable, timely, and supportive for the patient as possible.

Non-English-Speaking Patients

As discussed earlier, the diversity of the U.S. population is on the rise. When working with non-English-speaking patients, you should have an available and reliable interpreter. In many health care settings, a listing and access to foreign language interpreters is available. In addition, there are prepaid phone translator services that can provide real-time simultaneous interpreting services for a wide variety of languages. You have an obligation to ensure that medical and health information is provided accurately to your patient and that she understands all instructions, treatments, and medication regimens. If a patient's family member is available to translate, spend a few minutes talking to this person and make a decision as to his fluency and comfort with English, rather than assuming that your messages will be accurately sent and received. You may want to have common patient education materials translated into the most common languages of your local patient population.

Illiterate Patients

Special accommodations need to be made when communicating with patients with little or no ability to read and write. Perhaps the most difficult aspect is recognizing the problem. Many people feel guilt and embarrassment about being unable to read and go out of their way to hide the problem of illiteracy. Take the time to review and discuss any written forms and materials that are used during the course of medical care. In particular, you will want to review the patient rights and responsibilities used in your setting, and make sure that you review the notice of privacy statements. Assist the patient or delegate others in the office to assist the patient in completing any health- or history-related forms. When it comes time to provide patient education, you may use symbols or graphics to assist the patient. For example, you may draw a picture of the sun on a sheet of paper and tape it on the pills that the patient needs to take for her morning dose as a teaching aid. Review instructions in simple language and ask the patient to relate the instructions back to you to make sure that she correctly understands you. You must realize that this accommodation may take more time in the daily schedule of your patient visits.

Angry and Anxious Patients

A reality of all helping professions is that you will encounter people who are undergoing stress. Each person has a unique response to stress; however, a frequent response is anxiety or some level of anger. As a medical assistant who understands human behavior, you will recognize that the anger is not personally directed at you, although you may be the target or trigger for a patient's anxious or angry behavior. A few tips can guide you in communicating with anxious and angry individuals. The angry person wants to be recognized and listened to. You will get nowhere by interrupting someone who is upset and expressing his anger. If possible, give the person your full attention and take him to a place where you can have a private conversation. Listen and let the person tell you his story. It helps to speak in low voice tones, as this behavior alone may defuse his anger. If some unfortunate set of circumstances has occurred, such as a misscheduled appointment or a prolonged wait, apologize to the patient.

This apology can be worded simply: "I am very sorry. We do not like for our patients to wait for more than 15 to 30 minutes to see the physician. Today we had an emergency. I understand that this delay is inconvenient for you." This response to the angry patient acknowledges the source of his anger and the disruption that it may have caused. It demonstrates that you have listened and reflected back his concerns.

When communicating with an angry person, you should avoid getting into a dispute over the facts of the situation. This is likely to result in an escalation of the patient's anger. Sometimes it is helpful to get a third party or coworker to take over if you do not feel that you can calmly and objectively manage the communication. If the other person becomes insulting or uses inappropriate language or threats, end the conversation. You do not want the safety and security of your office, your patients, or yourself to be at risk.

Seeking medical attention, even for routine treatment, is often a source of anxiety for many people. You can assist the anxious person by giving clear and simple instructions and information. You may need to repeat the information and confirm that your instructions are understood. If possible, sit down and speak directly with the anxious patient. Give the person time to take in new information and to ask questions. If any follow-up instructions are needed, provide them in writing as anxiety may interfere with the person's ability to listen carefully.

GIVING INSTRUCTIONS TO PATIENTS

An important role of medical assisting is providing information and instructions to patients. Providing timely and accurate information regarding medications, health maintenance, medical equipment, and supplies is essential. You will also be responsible for interpreting your office policies and practices to patients. This section of your review material will focus on patient education and instruction.

In the hectic medical office, you may find that your time for providing effective instructions and health education to patients is limited. You can resolve this problem by using every encounter and discussion with a patient as a chance to provide health information. During the initial health interview, you are likely to hear about the patient's health history and the nature of her unique health problems. These health problems, along with your knowledge of age-specific health risks and occupational risks, will give you a starting point for patient instruction. Remember that individual patient instruction will need to be based on the person's learning style, age and developmental stage, motivation to learn, emotional state, and any barriers to communication. Effective education must also consider the time limitations for your instructions, the teaching environment, and the availability and level of teaching materials.

A systematic approach to patient instruction begins with assessing the information needs of the patient, determining the existing knowledge of his state of health or illness, and determining his learning style. Some patients prefer to read written articles, pamphlets, or brochures. Others respond to verbal instruction or teaching audio or videotapes. For important information, you may reinforce instruction by providing information in more than one format. Having a well-stocked set of patient instruction materials that feature colorful charts, illustrations, and simple explanations will support your patient-instruction efforts. Drug companies, health-related organizations such as the American Heart Association, and medical equipment providers are often able to give you patient-teaching materials for the office and to distribute to patients. In working with printed material, you will want to review it for timeliness and accuracy. It should be easy to read and avoid technical language or information that is too detailed for patients to understand. The level of content that is most effective is written to the eighth-grade reading level, which will be a fit for all but highly educated patients who may indeed seek information from medical texts and references. You want to make sure that you review any supplemental patient instruction information with the patients or their caregivers and avoid simply handing the material over and feeling that your instructions are over.

In addition to determining the patient's learning style and learning needs, you will want to set priorities for your patient teaching. If a patient has multiple health issues or a complex treatment regime, you will need to prepare a teaching plan and provide the information in reasonable amounts based on consideration of your time, the patient's ability to comprehend, and the amount of information that needs to be presented. Creating a teaching checklist for patients of different ages and common disease and health states will help you organize your teaching sessions and materials. A checklist will ensure that you have covered the major areas that the patient will need to take care of her health needs between appointments.

As a medical assistant, you will want to reinforce any instructions provided by the physician in your office. You also will want to encourage the patient to understand his disease state, health risks, and health behaviors, and participate actively in his own health. You will need to adapt your patient instruction to overcome any disability or limits to communication that the patient is experiencing. Also remember that teaching requires repetition and review for reinforcement.

Instruction on Health Maintenance

Healthy living and health maintenance is a fundamental goal of health care providers. Providing patients with information about nutrition, healthy diets, food choices, and therapeutic diets are one aspect of health maintenance instruction. Patients can benefit from information about exercise and physical activity designed to maintain fitness and manage weight. Some patients will need to be instructed on progressive activity-upgrading schedules following surgery or hospitalization. Do not assume that your patient will understand the meaning of vague or general instructions such as "take it easy." If any limits in activity are needed, be specific about the exact nature of the activity to avoid, for what duration, and when it can be resumed. Discussing the need for sleep and rest is another aspect of health teaching. Determining the patient's normal sleeping patterns may be covered at the initial interview, and it can be discussed again at follow-up appointments. You may want to use a healthy lifestyle patient log and include the patient in being responsible for recording data such as her weight, physical activity, pertinent health signs and symptoms, and medication schedules. Having the patient record this information between office visits will reinforce your health maintenance teaching. Remember to include age, gender, and health risk factors in your teaching. Provide instruction about any specific health-screening tests that are appropriate, such as mammograms, colonoscopies, or TB testing. Assist the physicians in your office by reminding them of patient-specific health maintenance activities and interventions so they are completed according to recommended schedules.

Medical Equipment Instructions

As medical technology advances, more and more medical devices and equipment are being used by patients in their homes. Equipment can range from standard wheelchairs and hospital beds to complex home infusion pumps and dialysis machines. Be aware of the medical equipment providers in your community, what they can provide, and what level of customer service and support they offer to patients. You need to know and explain associated costs of the equipment and the payment options available to the patient.

Instructing Patients on General Office Policies

It will be important for you to provide your patients with clear and concise information about your standard office policies. These are likely to include your office hours, as well as the methods of reaching a provider in an emergency or when the office is closed. You will want to make sure that patients are informed of their responsibilities for payment and what forms of payment are accepted in your office. Patients should be able to understand and interpret their bill and know who to contact with questions or concerns regarding payment or insurance coverage. You should review your expectations for cancelled and no-show appointments and any limitations on walk-in or last-minute appointments. Many practices provide a patient brochure or handout that clearly lists these policies. Having this material ready and available to patients will help ensure that policies are followed and that the office runs smoothly. You may design a set of frequently asked questions (FAQs) if you find that you are routinely asked about a certain item or issue.

CONDUCTING PATIENT INTERVIEWS

Medical assistants regularly conduct the patient interview, and take and record both new and established patient health histories. They may conduct certain components of the physical examination to support physicians. It is important that you be organized in your approach to patient interviews. You will need to use all of your listening and observation skills to accurately and thoroughly gather patient information during the interview. You must become proficient in documenting your findings and observations in the patient's medical record. In this section, you will review the basic structure and elements included in a patient interview. Follow all policies and format requirements that are unique to your practice setting. Many offices have standard forms or formats for patient interviews that may be manual or computer based. You will need to adapt the general interview strategies to your work setting.

Setting the Stage for Effective Interviews

If this interview is the patient's first visit to your office, make sure you greet him and explain your role and functions as a medical assistant. Let the patient know what to expect during the interview and health examination and approximately how long the process may take. It would be a good idea to discuss this and any laboratory tests or procedures that are generally included in the first visit on the phone before the visit is conducted. Patients can help by bringing in information such as health records or medication records to the appointment.

Make sure that the examination room is clean and comfortable and that all equipment and supplies that you or the physician may need are assembled and prepared for use. Make sure that the patient needs for privacy are protected during the interview. Arrange for any accommodation that the patient may need for an effective two-way communication. You will want to have a gown, draping cloths, and examination gloves handy. In some practices, a health history form is sent to the patients in advance so they can self-record their family health history, personal health history, and complete a review of body systems or signs and symptoms that they are currently experiencing or have experienced. Some forms contain questions regarding lifestyle and behaviors such as smoking, drinking, and use of medications. If the form has been brought in to the visit, it is important to review it completely with the patient and validate any significant items or concerns noted in the self-report. If your office does not provide this self-report, you will want to obtain a health history as part of the interview. See Chapter 12 for information on the standard components of a health history.

Health information is recorded in the patient's medical record along with pertinent quotes from the patient when possible. After the interview, you will review the information with the patient and instruct him to change into a gown for a physical examination. You may be participating in the exam by taking the patient's vital signs. If you are examining a child, you will want to record the height and weight on a growth chart. For infants up to one year of age, you will also record the head circumference.

For routine office visits or follow-up appointments, your interview should begin with the patient's chief complaint, history of present illness, and any updates to the past medical history since her last appointment. Many offices use a problem-oriented medical record that allows the physician, nurses, and medical assistants to document subsequent treatment into the categories of health problems and health interventions noted in the patient problem list.

TELEPHONE COMMUNICATION

As a medical assistant, you may conduct a great deal of your daily work activities over the telephone. It is important to remember that your patients, other providers, and members of your community will be judging the level of service and quality of your office based on the way that phone contacts are managed. As the medical assistant, your voice and level of customer service over the phone set the tone for how the quality of care is perceived. Some of the most common phone work will include scheduling patient appointments for new or existing patients, handling calls from patients who are experiencing health problems or who have questions, receiving laboratory results, taking calls from consultants and other physician offices, and handling calls from insurance companies and salespeople. You should not act as if phone calls are irritations or interruptions in your day. You should treat each caller with respect, and use the techniques of therapeutic listening just as if the patient or caller were having a face-to-face encounter with you.

Maintaining confidentiality and divulging information only to authorized individuals is imperative. Therefore, it is paramount that you confirm the identity of the caller. You can do so by asking demographic questions on the caller's birth date, telephone number, address, and last four digits of a Social Security number. Each medical office may its own standard policies and procedures that you will need to follow when communicating by telephone.

General Screening and Referrals

An organized medical office should develop a systematic approach to triaging phone calls. Telephone triage means that your office has a pre-established method of determining the nature and urgency of patient problems and providing directions for the level of care required. It is helpful to have a patient triage list organized by category of problem with the physician-specific guidelines for the practice. In addition, a list of local ambulance services, pharmacies, hospital directories, and other frequently used referral agencies should be available and kept up to date by the office staff. Your patient-care policies should include standard processes that should be taken when a patient is sent to the emergency room. Having these materials ready and available will help you respond in a more timely and efficient manner.

Messages and Call Logs

In a medical office, patient calls and subsequent instructions are considered a form of treatment. It is therefore critical that detailed logs of these interactions be recorded in writing and kept according to the state-regulated statutes for medical records.

Taking a message may seem simple, but it is helpful to review the elements of an effective telephone record.

Make sure that messages are recorded on a logbook that is designed for this purpose. It will be difficult to trace and track random pieces of paper or notes scribbled on the back of other documents. Have a central logbook that everyone in the office is familiar with and uses on a regular basis.

When a caller contacts you, it is important that you provide prompt and courteous service. Answer the phone with a greeting that is acceptable to the physician, and state your name to the caller. It is unacceptable to immediately place the caller on hold or to leave callers on hold for a prolonged period. You may need to ask if you can make a return call back if required.

Be ready to record the name of the caller, spelled correctly and written legibly. Indicate the time of the call and the reason given for the call. List any specific directions or actions that you recommended to the patient. Note the caller's phone numbers and the best times and methods for call-backs. It is helpful after getting this information to read it back for verification. Having all of this information will assist both you and other office staff who need to reconnect with the patient. If you tell the patient that you or the physician will call back, estimate a time in order to avoid phone tag.

Information about clinically related calls should be placed in the patient record. This would include instructions regarding medications, laboratory tests, doctor's orders, or health care recommendations. Prescription refills should be approved only by the physician, who may then direct you to contact the patient's pharmacy. Although telephone contact does not substitute for face-to-face treatment, your responses and responsibilities are just as crucial. Phone records and information provided to patients is considered a component of medical treatment from a legal perspective. Documentation is necessary.

Emergency Calls

Handling emergency calls from patients effectively is based on the particulars of your practice and the preferences of your physician or employers. It is best to have written protocols established for the most prevalent and common emergency issues that you may treat. The first step in triaging an emergency call is to determine if the matter is truly urgent. Next, you will want to have a clear idea of what steps you should recommend to patients in this situation. It is good to obtain some key baseline information to provide to the physician. Get the phone number where the patient can be reached in case the call is disconnected. Find out what specific symptoms are occurring and when they started. You should ask if this type of problem has occurred in the past. If the patient is alone and does not have transportation, you may need to arrange for emergency transport. All of this information should be conveyed to the physician as soon as possible and documented in the patient's chart.

Problem Calls

Problem calls can include calls from angry patients, complaint calls, and people seeking private health information. It is important to remember the skills involved in therapeutic communication. Let the person tell their story uninterrupted. Remain calm and avoid taking the complaints personally. Get the facts of the situation and provide reassurance that you will try to get the matter or need resolved. If patients or others call you to obtain lab results or other health information, you should have a system to verify that they are in fact the patient or the patient's legal representative. Some offices now use a call-back system and verify that the person on the line is correctly identified. For example, you may request two patient identifiers, such as date of birth or social security number to validate that you are speaking with the approved individuals. You must not provide patient health information to unauthorized parties at any time.

WRITTEN COMMUNICATION

You will be working with the physicians and others in your practice on a wide range of letters, reports, medical forms, and other written materials. Medical writing is a form of technical writing using scientific and clinical terms along with Standard English words and phrases. In many documents, physicians and others use myriad abbreviations, symbols, and grammatical shortcuts. You will need to interpret this information and convey it accurately and clearly in your writing. This review will cover some fundamentals of effective writing, including sentence structure, punctuation, and spelling tips. Written work completed by you and the other members of your medical office are a reflection of the quality of care that you provide. In addition, it is likely that the bulk of your written work will be related to patient health information and, therefore, will be a part of the legal record.

Sentence Structure

A sentence conveys a thought or idea in writing. There are many types of sentences, but all have two basic elements: a subject (noun) and a predicate (verb), along with the words that describe the verb. The subject conveys the *who* in the sentence and the predicate conveys the *what*, or the action or activity that is happening. If a sentence does not have both, it is considered a sentence fragment, and it does not convey a meaningful thought. Sentences can be *simple* and contain only one subject and one predicate, or *complex* and contain more than one of each. However, in writing complex sentences, it is important to make sure that you do not convey too many thoughts or you will create a *run-on sentence*. If you write a letter or a document, you should begin with a topic sentence that introduces the purpose and scope of the document. Next, you want to convey important ideas or findings in subsequent sentences.

For sentences to be clear, some general rules to follow are to tighten up wordy sentences. Avoid redundancies such as *basic essentials* when writing. If you have time, you may want to prepare a rough draft and have someone else review it for clarity and accuracy. Make sure that the verb tenses agree throughout the document. In addition, the sentences should have the same point of view. A more casual approach may be in the first person such as, "*you* will need to take the medicine daily." A more formal point of view may be in the third person and state, "*patients* will need to take the medication daily." The purpose of the document should guide your use of style in sentences.

Punctuation

In this section, you will review the most common forms of punctuation and their correct usage. If in doubt, refer to a style manual or grammar usage text as a reference. Correct use of punctuation will increase the effectiveness of your written communication.

Periods and End-of-Sentence Punctuation

End-of-sentence punctuation includes periods, question marks, and exclamation points. Each tells your reader that the thought is ending and a new one will begin. In addition, periods are used after many abbreviations such as *M.D.* or *Ph.D.* When abbreviating names of states or two or more initials using all capital letters, like *USA,* periods may or may not be used. You should be consistent in using periods for these and other abbreviations within a document.

Commas

Commas are the most common punctuation form used in writing. They are used for a variety of reasons, including those in the following list.

1. To separate clauses in a sentence

   Example: *The infant was delivered vaginally, but high forceps were used.*

2. To set off introductory words in a sentence

   Example: *First, the patient went to the emergency room.*

3. To set off nonessential phrases or asides in a sentence

   Example: *Secondary smoke, though not bothersome to all, is associated with lung cancer.*

4. To separate a list of items or words in a series within a sentence

   Example: *The physician reviewed the symptoms, measured the weight, and palpated the abdomen.*

Colons and Semicolons

A colon (:) is inserted after an independent clause in a sentence. It is used to alert the reader to the information that is listed or quoted following the clause. A colon should be used as in the following example: *A routine exam includes the following: a health history, a physical examination, and a series of laboratory tests.* A colon is also used in a formal business letter after the salutation (for example, *Dear Sir/Madam:*).

Semicolons (;) are used between items in a series that are joined together in a sentence. They are also used between independent clauses that are not joined by a conjunction. Most often, clauses are joined by conjunctions such as *and, but, or, nor,* or *so.* If you do not include these terms to link clauses in a sentence, then a semicolon can be used to separate the clauses. In the following sentence, the semicolon is used instead of the word *and: The patient filled out the form; the physician read it.*

Apostrophes

Apostrophes (') are used to indicate possession and contractions. Possessive nouns generally indicate ownership, as in the doctor's office or the assistant's desk. If the noun is plural and ends in the letter s, the apostrophe should follow the word.

In contractions, the apostrophe takes the place of the missing letters. For example, in the phrase, *don't \do not\ eat or drink before the test*, the apostrophe takes the place of the letter *o* in the word *not*.

Apostrophes are also commonly used to abbreviate the first two digits in a year or decade. For example, *she graduated in the class of '59*, or *she is from the '60s*.

Spelling

It is likely that you will be preparing many documents on a computer, using word processing software. Speli-checking and grammar-checking tools are embedded in these products and should be used routinely. However, spell-checkers do not flag improper use of common words like *its and it's*, nor do they note incorrect use of words like *do* and *due*. You must take care in proofreading your documents for accuracy. Make use of a medical dictionary to look up terms and to ensure that correct spelling is used. It is a good idea to have a list of common medical terms that are unique to your practice available as a reference.

Ensure that your writing is concise, precise, and clear to the reader. Spell out medical symbols and abbreviated words. The medical community has recently been challenged to avoid excessive use of some abbreviations, as they can be linked to serious medical errors in medications and treatments. Your job will be to translate abbreviations and symbols into sentences for reports and other clinical documents. Your office should have a list of accepted abbreviations that are frequently used. If the document you are preparing is handwritten, make sure your handwriting is legible and signed and dated with your name and title. It is a good idea to have a style manual and a medical dictionary available as reference tools.

PATIENT PORTALS

Patient portals enable patients to take a more proactive stance in their health care and serve as an effective means of communication between the provider and the patient. Patient portals were included in the meaningful use requirements of the Centers for Medicare and Medicaid.

Portals are secure websites that are accessible to the patient 24 hours per day, 7 days per week. In addition to being able to view test results, immunizations, reports of medical visits, and other health data, patients can use a portal also to request medication refills, ask questions, schedule appointments, and view educational materials. The use of patient portals is sure to expand in the future as patients assume more responsibility for their health.

REVIEW QUESTIONS

1. Which of the following actions, if performed by the medical assistant, does NOT promote effective therapeutic communication?

   (A) Making direct eye contact with the patient

   (B) Siting down and taking notes during a patient interview

   (C) Looking at watch while the patient answers a question

   (D) Rephrasing the patient's statements and restating them

   (E) Noding head in agreement with a patient's statement

2. A mother brings her three-year-old into the office for a checkup and immunization. To assist the child and improve communication, the medical assistant should

   (A) ask the mother to wait in the waiting room while the child is given the immunization

   (B) offer the child a lollipop when he arrives to keep the child distracted

   (C) tell the child that the shot won't hurt and to be brave

   (D) give the child information on immunizations and risks of childhood diseases

   (E) let the child hold your stethoscope and listen to his own heartbeat so he understands what you are going to do

3. A new patient from the Middle East comes to the office for her first exam. Her husband fills out all of the health forms and comes into the exam room during the medical assistant's interview. The patient sits calmly while her husband answers all of the medical assistant's questions. This is likely an example of

   (A) domestic violence

   (B) cultural diversity

   (C) a deaf patient

   (D) male domination

   (E) stereotyping

4. On his way home, a medical assistant sees a blind woman walking with a guide dog. The guide dog is walking toward a puddle. Which of the following actions should the assistant take?

   (A) Take the woman by the arm at the elbow and direct her.

   (B) Reach down and gently move the dog away from the puddle.

   (C) In a loud voice say, "Hey, you are about to step in a puddle!"

   (D) No action is needed; the dog is trained to handle this situation.

   (E) Tell the woman that he will help her cross the street to avoid the puddle.

5. Which of the following is the best way to explain the concept of empathy?

(A) Feeling the same feelings as the patient

(B) Observing a patient's gestures

(C) Acknowledging a patient's emotional state and the meaning this has to her

(D) Being nice to your patients

(E) Paraphrasing the patient's statements and reflecting them back during an interview

Answers and Explanations can be found on the following page.

ANSWERS AND EXPLANATIONS

1. **C**

   Looking at his watch while the patient is being interviewed does not exhibit interest, concern, or respect for the patient. All of the other items are appropriate behaviors during a therapeutic communication session with a patient.

2. **E**

   Letting the child hold your stethoscope is the appropriate step in this situation. This action will allow the child to feel included in the procedure, reduce anxiety, and promote communication. Leaving the mother in the waiting room (A) would likely cause fear in a young child and you may need the mother to assist you with the exam and immunization. Giving a lollipop (B) should come as a reward for being brave and holding still during the immunization. Telling the child the shot will not hurt (C) is not true; the shot is likely to hurt and it will break down trust between you and the child. Giving health information (D) is not age-appropriate for this patient.

3. **B**

   Cultural diversity is likely the source of the behavior of the husband and wife in this encounter. In their country of origin, it is likely that women do not speak with strangers or conduct business outside of their homes. None of the other items is appropriate; however, if an American family conducted the visit in this manner, the concern for spousal abuse or intimidation may be raised.

4. **D**

   The medical assistant does not need to do anything; the guide dog is trained to effectively lead and guide the path of the blind woman. You would not want to reach out and touch a blind person without prior verbal cues (A), nor would you touch a guide dog while he is working (B), as it may be a distraction. Items (C) and (E) are not necessary.

5. **C**

   Empathy means being able to acknowledge and understand the emotions of another, and being able to interpret the meaning that the emotional state has on the patient. Empathy is often compared and contrasted with sympathy, which is described in (A). Observing the patient's gestures (B) and being nice (D) are elements of therapeutic communication, but do not define empathy.

Chapter 9: **Professional and Legal Knowledge**

As a medical assistant, you must be familiar with the regulatory and legal aspects of medical practice. You are not expected to be a lawyer, but in a general way, you should know the key legal issues that medical assistants encounter in their work. Medical assistants are employed in medical offices, hospitals, clinics, and insurance companies performing a variety of clinical and administrative tasks including billing, collections, coding, accounting, EKGs, phlebotomy, and giving injections (in some settings). The variety of work depends on the setting and state laws.

Laws relating to the practice of medicine are found in each state's constitution under medical practice acts. Licensure is the strongest form of professional regulation. Mandatory licensure proves a minimal level of competence. Physicians and nurses are licensed. Often, states have agreements to allow a person licensed in one state to practice in another state. This is called reciprocity. Licensure allows the state to control the behavior of professionals. Licensed health care workers who engage in criminal behavior, unprofessional conduct, or are incapacitated can have their license revoked. Licensing boards determine the renewal requirements, which may include continuing education and renewal fees, enforcement of statutes related to the profession, and the approval and supervision of training institutions.

Medical assistants can either be certified or registered. Programs accredited by the Commission for Accreditation of Allied Health Education Programs (CAAHEP) prepare their graduates to sit for a voluntary national certification exam. Programs accredited by the Accrediting Bureau of Health Education Schools (ABHES) prepare students to take the Registered Medical Assisting exam. Students attaining a CMA or RMA status are attaining a level of recognition that showcases their knowledge.

MEDICAL LAW AND MALPRACTICE

When a person makes a mistake that breaks the law in health care, it falls under civil law. Civil laws are different from criminal laws. There are two types of civil crimes: torts and breach of contract.

Torts can be intentional or unintentional. Intentional torts are always crimes committed against a person or property and are punished with fines. It is essential that a health professional know what situations can lead to an intentional tort. A patient can recover monetary damages in situations where an intentional tort has been committed. The following are examples of torts:

1. Assault: the threat and perceived ability to touch a person without permission

2. Battery: the intentional act of touching someone without his consent

3. False imprisonment: constraining a person against her will

4. Defamation of character: *slander* is false information spoken to a third party with the intent of harming a person; *libel* is false information written with the intent of inflicting harm

5. Invasion of privacy: divulging or sharing information without patient consent

6. Infliction of mental distress: causing a patient serious emotional suffering

7. Malicious betrayal of professional secrets: unauthorized disclosure of privileged information

8. Fraud in the fiduciary relationship: intentional misrepresentation of information

9. Abandonment: improper termination of patient care by physician

Unintentional torts are those commissions or omissions by the health professional that a reasonable or prudent person would not do under similar circumstances. This is called negligence and may result in a charge of malpractice. Unintentional torts are just as illegal as intentional torts. Negligence is punished with fines, but in order for a plaintiff to recover damages, all four "D's of negligence" must be present.

1. The defendant must have an established *duty* toward the plaintiff.

2. The defendant must be *derelict* in performing the duty.

3. The action must be the *direct cause* of injury.

4. *Damages* or injury must have occurred as a result of the action.

Based on the action, malpractice can be categorized as misfeasance, malfeasance, or nonfeasance. Misfeasance is the incorrect performance of a legal act. Caring for a patient includes accepting the responsibility to deliver a prevailing standard of care. This means delivering care similar to what a reasonably prudent person would do acting under similar circumstance. The legal standard defining "reasonable action" takes into consideration the person's age, sex, physical condition, education, knowledge, training, and mental capacity. For that reason, it is important to never represent oneself improperly. The medical assistant must be careful not to refer to herself as "the nurse" lest she be held to different standards. An example of misfeasance would be not using a clean needle to give an injection.

Malfeasance is the performance of an illegal act. In most states, giving intravenous drugs would be malfeasance. Nonfeasance is failure to perform when a duty exists. Forgetting to apply a dressing ordered by the physician would be nonfeasance.

There are several types of defense against malpractice; however, there is no defense in ignorance of the law. A defense of denial places the burden of proof on the plaintiff to prove that the four D's of negligence exist. One type of affirmative defense is contributory defense. In it, the plaintiff is found to be at least partially responsibility for injury and, therefore, the health care provider is not held liable for negligence. In a comparative defense, damages are awarded based on a percentage of negligence for both plaintiff and defendant. With intervening cause, an independent factor affected the outcome. Assumption of risk means that the patient voluntarily accepted the risks. A technical defense is decided by a judge as a point of law. When the evidence is so overwhelmingly against the health practitioner that the burden of proof shifts to the defendant, we call it *res ipsa loquitur* (the thing speaks for itself). An example of this would be a patient who complains of pain in the abdomen after surgery and is then found to have a towel clamp in the abdomen. Obviously, the surgeon left the foreign object there and is responsible. The burden to prove otherwise is incumbent on the surgeon. Criminal negligence is outrageous carelessness or disregard for patient safety.

CONTRACTS

The trusting relationship between a highly trained service-oriented person and a client seeking services is considered a fiduciary relationship. In health care, an agreement for treatment is a contract. There are three parts to the legal contract. A product or service is communicated for consideration and acceptance is offered. A consideration would be payment or an exchange of something of value. For example, the physician will perform a physical exam for $175 and you agree. The physical exam is the service and the consideration is the $175. In offering a patient an appointment, the medical office makes a contract between the patient and physician. The contract must be made by competent parties. Persons who are confused are still allowed to make binding contracts, unless that person has a guardian, power of attorney, or is declared incompetent. Minors, persons under 18 years of age, are unable to make any contracts. However, persons under the age of 18 years who support themselves, are married, have children, or are active military are considered emancipated minors and as such, can make their own decisions and engage in contracts. Persons under the age of 18 who are considered "emancipated minors" and may make their own decisions to seek substance abuse or psychiatric treatment or reproductive health care.

Some patients will need to be reminded that the contract requires them to be responsible for the "consideration" or bill. Any arrangement with a third party to pay the bill is a contract between the patient and the third party. The physician has a right to hold the patient accountable for payment.

Terminating the physician-patient relationship must be done properly or it can be considered the breaking of a legal contract. Abandoning a patient is a serious charge and could lead to charges of an intentional tort. The patient can choose to terminate the relationship with a physician at any time. The physician, however, must properly terminate a physician-patient relationship and only if there is just cause. The patient must have been noncompliant with treatment recommendations, repeatedly missing appointments, or refusing to pay for services. A policy for termination of patient care must be established and followed each time it is required. The patient must be notified in writing by certified mail, return receipt requested when care will no longer be provided. The patient needs to be given a reasonable length of time to find alternative medical care. There is no set time limit for a "reasonable length of time," but most experts agree that 6–8 weeks is sufficient. The return receipt and a copy of the letter must be filed in the patient's chart. A patient may terminate the relationship at any time.

The relationship between medical assistant, physician, and patient all include trust, honesty, and caring. Many offices give out a sheet detailing the rights and responsibilities of both parties to make sure certain expectations are clear and consistent. In some states, the Patient's Bill of Rights must be posted in all health care facilities.

The patient/physician contract should not guarantee a cure or specific treatment outcome. It merely promises a treatment plan and personalized care that will be documented completely and accurately. It is understood that the physician will provide alternative coverage on days off and request consultations when indicated and referrals when needed. In exchange, the physician will select working hours, location of practice, and the type of patients to treat. She should expect timely payment of bills and personal time off. The patient has a right to honesty and complete information about his diagnosis, treatment, and prognosis. The patient has a right to confidentiality and a standard of treatment that does not reflect discrimination based on race, gender, age, sexual orientation, ability to pay, religion, color, or nationality. The patient has a right to decline to participate in teaching or research projects. The patient is responsible for disclosing all information relevant to his medical condition, being compliant with appointment and treatment plans, and accepting the consequences for refusing treatment. The medical assistant's duty is to respect all patients without regard to race, religion, sexual orientation, national origin, age, or gender, and to skillfully perform duties designated by the physician employer with concern for the dignity of the patient.

LEGAL PROCEEDINGS

Legal issues are decided in court by a jury (other citizens) or bench trial (judge). Sometimes the lengthy and expensive costs of a trial can be avoided by arbitration and mediation. In mediation, a third party attempts to bring a settlement between two parties. When parties agree to submit their differences for judgment by an impartial mediator or panel, they can agree to make the decision "binding." This process is called arbitration. It is often used to screen and evaluate malpractice cases.

The person who has a complaint is the plaintiff. The person who has been accused of wrongdoing is the defendant. An indictment means that there is enough evidence for a trial. Evidence is the proof submitted supporting the plaintiff. A verdict is the final decision based on evidence. A subpoena is an official demand to come to court to testify. A deposition is giving sworn testimony outside of court. With the exception of *res ipsa loquitur*, it is incumbent on the plaintiff to prove an injustice has occurred and that the defendant is responsible. In public law and in criminal cases, evidence must prove beyond a reasonable doubt that the defendant is guilty. However, in civil cases, there must only be a preponderance of evidence. A medical assistant working for a physician is an agent representing the physician in making contracts or promises to a patient. The physician is vicariously responsible for the medical assistant's actions as the employer. The legal term is *respondeat superior*, which means "let the master answer."

MEDICAL RECORDS

There are four purposes to a medical record. It is a legal record, a record of health treatment, a communication tool between members of the health care team, and a research tool. Falsification of records is a criminal offense. A medical record will contain personal information such as names of patient, addresses, phone numbers, parents, spouses, children, insurance, and social security numbers. If the patient has a living will or power of attorney for health care, it should be in the chart. A living will authorizes the continuation or withdrawal of life support when a patient is too sick to voice an opinion. Many persons want to designate another party to make all decisions for them in the event they are unable to speak for themselves. This is called a durable power of attorney for health care. Copies of this document should be placed in the chart as well. The Uniform Anatomical Gift Act allows those over the age of 18 years to provide their bodies or body parts for medical education, research, or transplantation. It is important that the physician be aware of the wishes of a patient; this communication is often kept in the medical record.

It is important for you to remember that the patient history and physical examination and entire medical record are legal documents. As such, you need to ensure that your documentation is accurate, objective, and legible. Avoid abbreviations that are not approved in your setting. Do not leave components of the form blank or incomplete. If the patient was unwilling or unable to provide information for whatever reason, note this in the record. Identify the source of interview information whether from the patient, relatives, prior health records, or other sources. Make sure that your entries are made in blue or black ink and are signed and dated. Do not use correction fluid or tape in a clinical record. If you make an error, draw one line through the error and insert the correct word or information neatly in the space available and initial your entry. It is important that health records be safely and securely stored to protect the confidentiality of health information. If the records are stored electronically, they should be password protected and accessible only to individuals who need them for care, treatment, and business use.

Psychosocial history including occupational or marital issues, sexual behavior, birth control, alcohol and drug history will be in the chart. Health and social histories contain information on relationships, vaccinations, past illnesses, laboratory, treatments, complaints, and medications. It may be discussed in great detail and this intimate information belongs to the patient. It has been shared in a trusting manner with the physician, but cannot be disclosed to anyone without the patient's express permission. In simple terms, the patient owns all information inside the medical record and that includes the right of allowing others to know what is in the chart. The only exclusion is mental health records where the patient or staff might be harmed by allowing the patient to see records. Ownership of the actual paper upon which the information is written belongs to the facility in which treatment was provided.

Strictly speaking, the physician who prepares a patient's medical record owns that record, while the patient has a right to the information within it. Patients have the right to request copies of their health records and your office should have a policy on the correct procedures for releasing medical records and health information to patients and to other providers. Normally these requests are required in writing and should be spelled out clearly in your patient notice of privacy practice and office procedure manual. The legal issues mentioned are but highlights of an entire set of patient privacy requirements under federal law. Please consult your office Health Insurance Portability and Accountability Act (HIPAA) information polices and procedures for more detailed information that is beyond the scope of this review.

When faced with a lawsuit, good medical records will help refresh the memory and prove if there is a deviation from a standard of care. Standard of care means someone providing the same quality of care as any other person with the same level of training in an equivalent area. Keeping medical records (retention of records) is quite important. In reality, the legal time that they must be saved varies from state to state and depends on the patient's age. With modern health information storage techniques, however, it is reasonable to retain records indefinitely. As minors reach majority age (21), they can initiate lawsuits and many injuries are not recognized until several years after occurrence. Records for a deceased patient should be retained for insurance and liability issues. The statute of limitations or time during which a person can file a lawsuit differs from state to state. If records are not retained, they must be burned or shredded. Be very careful in disposal of computer information.

Charting should be done in black or blue ink, dated, timed, and signed. Always use abbreviations approved by the Joint Commission on Accreditation of Hospital Organizations. Corrections should never obliterate the original writing or be erased even with correction fluid. Drawing a single line through the error, then writing the date and person's initials with the word "error" is the proper way to correct a mistake. Never skip lines between entries. Always sign entries with a full name and title. The chart should contain every visit, every record of physical examination, laboratory results, diagnostic procedures, hospital discharge summaries, and consultations. No judgments or opinions should be charted, just facts. Missed appointments and any action taken with abnormal lab results should be charted. Phone calls, advice given to the patient, safety instructions, a patient's ability to return a demonstration, and presence of family members who received instructions need to be included in the chart. In court, if something is not charted, it was not done.

Information documentation is a major source of controversy in today's world. Computer storage allows information to be accessed in an emergency situation when displaced persons need access to their health records and paper charts are no longer available. With computer records comes the risk of information theft if those records are illegally accessed. Consider, for example, the personal information disclosed between 2010 and 2013 alone, when data breaches compromised over 29 million U.S. health records (Liu V, Musen MA, Chou T, "Data Breaches of Protected Health Information in the United States," *Journal of the American Medical Association*, April 14, 2015).

When responsible for transferring records, make certain to send only photocopies of original material. There must be permission from the patient to transfer records. Records cannot be withheld for nonpayment of a bill, but a reasonable charge to photocopy can be charged. On occasion, the court will ask for records. This is called *subpeona duces tecum*. Never take the original chart. Make certified copies of the requested information and nothing more. Copy and number the pages and place them in a folder. Place a prepared table of contents in the front of the file. Lock the original document in the office safe. Obtain a notarized statement that the chart is reproduction of the original made by the physician's staff. Take it all to court on the appointed day and time. Do not give it to anyone other than the judge. Obtain an official receipt and be prepared to testify if necessary.

CONFIDENTIALITY

The Hippocratic oath is the historical basis for the laws of confidentiality. If a patient is damaged by information that is disclosed, it may be construed to be a breach of confidence. Even a physician needs permission to disclose, unless one of the following occurs:

1. A subpoena has been issued by the court

2. The physician is being sued by a patient

3. The doctor believes he must disclose information to protect the welfare of a patient or third party (includes information such as births, deaths, child or elderly abuse, criminal acts such as stabbing, gunshot wounds, or assault, as well as infectious, contagious, or communicable diseases)

If a patient requests a release of information, that release must include:

1. The name of the physician who is asked to disclose information

2. The name of person to whom the information is disclosed

3. The dates of service that can be discussed in disclosure (dates can be limited)

4. A signature of the patient asking for disclosure and the date of signature

5. Signature of a witness

The decision to disclose information is the patient's choice. If the patient requests disclosure of information to another party, the doctor cannot refuse. However, each party to whom a physician can disclose requires new authorization. The patient has the right to rescind an authorization to release information. This is best accomplished through a written and dated request to disclose no further information.

Confidentiality policies should be reviewed each year by every employee. As agents of the physician, all employees are responsible for keeping information secure in the office and maintaining confidentiality. Reporters, insurance companies, pharmaceutical companies, and well-meaning friends and family members may work to trap you into disclosing confidential information. Information must not be overheard from phone calls or conversations in the office nor seen on computer screens. Fax machines should not be used to share medical information except in a life or death emergency. Access to records should be limited by storage under double locks. Charts must never leave the office. Even a patient's name should be confidential. Discuss patient information with only those who have a need to know. Never discuss patients outside of the office or in front of other patients. Speak in a modulated, soft voice. Be aware of sounds passing through walls and windows. Do not allow persons to wait in office hallways. Close doors to discuss health issues, lab results, finances, refills, or personal issues. Stay current with state laws and regulations regarding HIV confidentiality.

CONSENT

Consent is not always written. Consent can be implied by offering an arm to check blood pressure or opening the mouth for a throat culture. When there are many risks, consequences, and alternatives to a proposed procedure, express consent can be obtained orally or in writing. The Patient Self Determination Act of 1990 protects patient rights including the right to agree to or refuse medical treatment. To enable the patient to decide, the physician has the duty to explain to the patient all the information necessary to clearly evaluate the proposed treatment. This is called the Doctrine of Informed Consent. Informed consent requires making the patient aware of the nature of their condition and the purpose of a proposed procedure. Benefits, risks, and consequences associated with the procedure, alternative treatment, and accompanying benefits and risks must be given to the patient. Lastly, the benefits, risks, and consequences of no treatment must be understood by the patient. It is the physician's responsibility to ascertain that language barriers do not interfere with providing informed consent.

If this information is upsetting to the patient, it is her right to decline the information. Many times, however, family members and patients have additional questions to ask the physician. When all concerns have been answered by the physician, the patient must sign and date the informed consent. The physician and a witness must sign the consent. Confused patients who are not incompetent have the right to sign consent, but many prudent physicians will want a family member to sign the consent as well. Patients always have the right to rescind any permission or consent given. The medical assistant's role in informed consent is to witness the signature.

Do not confuse consent issues with offering emergency care to an injured person. Emergencies can occur where a patient requires immediate medical attention. Often health care persons are afraid to perform first aid because of the Doctrine of Informed Consent. The Good Samaritan Act protects the actions performed by health care persons who act in an emergency situation outside of the health care facility, as long as they act within the scope of their training. Make sure that your state carries a Good Samaritan law.

HEALTH CARE DUTIES AND OBLIGATIONS

Medical assistants are key agents in the chain of custody of specimens and evidence. When there is a crime such as rape or battery that requires a physical exam or laboratory specimen, the medical assistant needs to be aware of the importance of verifying that any potential evidence is safeguarded against tampering. That means each person who touches the evidence must record his or her name. Potential evidence is never out of direct sight unless locked in a secure place where those who have access must record their names. This may include routine drug testing as well.

All drug and alcohol treatment information is under federal jurisdiction and must never be disclosed without patient permission. According to the Public Service Act, anyone disclosing this type of information is subject to criminal fines.

Patients receiving mental health treatment require a high degree of confidentiality. Treatment of the mentally ill may be involuntary if the patient is in imminent danger. Laws vary from state to state, but usually involve a petition for involuntary admission by someone who has no direct interest in the case but has observed dangerous behavior. Additionally, two certificates within 24 hours are usually required to keep a patient against his or her will. A formal, legal hearing is usually held within five days. The patient must have legal counsel, if desired. Like any other patient, mentally ill patients have rights to adequate humane care, timely discharge, to be free of mechanical and chemical restraints, to handle their own business and money, to communicate in private, to send and receive mail, and to vote in any election. Depending on the nature of the illness, mentally ill persons may lose a gun permit or not be able to obtain one.

Medical assistants have access to Schedules II through V substances and are responsible for maintaining all regulations required by the Drug Enforcement Agency (DEA). All physicians prescribing these substances must register for a DEA number using form DEA 224. Controlled substances are those with the potential for addiction. The medical assistant may be responsible for making certain the DEA number that identifies the physician is renewed every three years. The office is responsible for having policies established for dispensing, handling, and storing scheduled drugs and keeping current and up-to-date records. See Chapter 14, Medications, for additional information.

Hiring and firing of staff may be a responsibility of the medical assistant. It is essential that no laws are broken in the hiring process. There are strict guidelines designated by the Equal Employment Opportunity Commission (EEOC) to ensure hiring practices remain fair. Questions about age, race, religion, nationality, handicaps, and children are illegal. It is not legal to ask about arrests, but it is acceptable to ask about convictions. Asking about marriage is not illegal, but might be construed as discriminatory and is not advised. Hiring based on ability, training, and certification is the best practice. All new employees should have a clear job description and an employee handbook clearly stating the expectations and disciplinary procedures. Employee records and evaluations should be stored in a secure, locked area. The hiring process includes completion of a W-4 for the Internal Revenue Service (IRS) and I-9 for the U.S. Citizenship and Immigration Services (USCIS). Other business forms that the medical assistant may be responsible for include the W-2 Wage and Tax Statement sent at the end of the year itemizing annual wages and taxes withheld, Form 941 Employer's Quarterly Federal Tax return, and Form 940 Employer's Quarterly Federal Unemployment Tax return.

Medical assistants are mandated to report abuse and neglect of children or elderly persons. Abuse to the elderly can be neglect, financial, emotional, physical, or sexual abuse. Child abuse is neglect and abandonment as well as sexual, physical, or psychological abuse. It can manifest itself in physical or emotional ways. Most states have hotlines that can be used for reporting suspected abuse.

A medical assistant may be the person appointed to report communicable illnesses and vital statistics to the public health department. This is one of the public duties performed by physicians. Diseases such as measles, mumps, polio, syphilis, gonorrhea, tuberculosis, and HIV are tracked for trends and epidemics. Births, stillbirths, deaths, rapes, gunshots, knife wounds, and animal bites may be part of the vital statistics recorded in a state. Most counties require the filing of birth and death certificates at the county clerk's office as well. The medical assistant must know the regulations of the state in order to comply with making certain all information is provided in a timely manner.

Many medical assistants are responsible for billing third-party payers such as insurance, Blue Cross/Blue Shield, Medicaid, and Medicare. Medicare is a federally administrated program in which all persons over a certain age or those who are disabled are entitled to health benefits. Medicaid is a need-based program for health benefits administrated by individual states. It is important to know the correct billing procedures, guidelines, and laws so as to avoid fraud.

Medical assistants help protect patients and the environment by properly disposing of medical waste and biohazardous materials. Medical assistants make sure sharps in puncture proof containers and the items disposed of in biohazard bags are uniformly packaged, labeled, and taken to incinerators by biohazardous waste companies. It is important to conform to federal standards that have been developed by the Occupational Safety and Health Administration (OSHA) and the Environmental Protection Agency (EPA) to protect health care workers. Failure to comply can lead to large fines.

EMPLOYMENT SAFETY AND LAWS

The health and safety of health care employees is guarded by the federal agency called the Occupational Safety and Health Administration (OSHA). This watchdog agency provides for the physical safety of employees regarding training, equipment, exposure, and disposal of waste. Material safety data sheets help medical personnel use and dispose of chemicals that are known to be harmful. Medical offices are required to keep a record of harmful products and supplies on the premise as a reference for all staff. OSHA has mandated safety by requiring employers to provide personal protective equipment (PPE) such as gloves, safety needles, sharps containers, eye wash stations, an exposure plan, and biohazardous warning labels. OSHA regulations are laws. Compliance with OSHA means protecting patients and staff from exposure to unsafe conditions. Breaking OSHA guidelines can lead to employee injury, fines, or penalty for the employer.

The Civil Rights Act of 1964 makes it illegal to discriminate against anyone on the basis of race, color, religion, nationality, or ethnic origin. The Age Discrimination Act protects the employment of persons in the age range of 45–60 against unlawful discharge or termination.

The Americans with Disabilities Act allows access to jobs and facilities for the physically challenged that are qualified to do a job. No employer is required to hire a disabled person if the candidate is not qualified for a reason other than the disability. However, an employer is required to make physical accommodations for a qualified individual with a disability. These benefits accommodate disabled patients and also promote hiring a diverse population of persons.

The Fair Labor Standards Act regulates the minimum wage and standardizes the number of hours an employee is allowed to work. Fair labor practices require overtime pay for some categories of employees.

The Social Security Act provides for disability and retirement compensation, survivor benefits, and Medicare for those over 65 years of age.

ERISA stands for Employee Retirement Income Security Act and protects pensions.

The Family and Medical Leave Act allows workers to take unpaid time off from their jobs to deal with serious family and health issues without jeopardy to their job. There are limitations to the amount of unpaid leave.

Health Information Portability and Accountability Act (HIPAA) of 1996 provides national standards to protect the privacy of personal health information and standards for electronic health care transactions. This act has provided tools and funding dedicated to the investigation and prosecution of health care fraud. In excess of $700 million has been refunded to state and federal governments as a result of this act.

COBRA insures that persons changing jobs do not lose insurance.

The Fair Credit Reporting Act of 1977 allows patients to see their credit reports.

The Equal Credit Opportunity Act prohibits discrimination against extending credit based on race, sex, gender, religion, or marital status.

The Consumer Protection Act of 1960 or "Regulation Z" requires that if more than four extended payments will be made, the contract must be in writing.

Fair Debt Collection Practice Act requires that collectors must contact debtors between 8:00 AM and 9:00 PM, Monday through Friday. Privacy must be protected by not leaving messages or calling people at work. Threats or vulgar language cannot be used.

Workers' compensation is coverage for the bills incurred because of an injury on the job. This is the only case in which the medical information does not belong to the patient. Information specific to the claim belongs to the company that is covering the injury.

FACILITIES

To protect the office, the physician should have malpractice insurance on himself and his employees. If a lawsuit is filed against an employee, the employer is usually listed as well under the doctrine of *respondeat superior*. However, all medical assistants may want to consider a malpractice policy through their accrediting body because many employers' policies have a "right of recovery" for expenses caused by the person named. Employers should also have an insurance policy covering the facility for injury sustained on the premises. Employees who handle money may need to be bonded.

Medical facilities are regulated by both the state and federal government. A certificate of need (CON) is the process required for approval of any new hospital, facility, or service based on need. The federal government's Clinical Laboratory Improvement Act (CLIA 88) outlines lab standards of quality assurance, quality control, and test-specific procedures for any facility doing outpatient lab tests in the physician office laboratory (POL). The U.S. Department of Health and Human Services (HHS) maintains regulatory standards for those laboratories that perform tests beyond the simple CLIA-waived tests and expect reimbursement from Medicare or Medicaid. Ambulatory Surgical Centers (ASC) are regulated as to which surgical procedures can be done safely as outpatient services.

ETHICS AND BIOETHICS

Laws must evolve to meet a changing environment. Hippocrates lived in ancient times and managed to write a code of ethics for physicians that is still recited today (the Hippocratic oath). The AMA and the AAMA have codes of ethics for the modern physician and medical assistants. Both codes address human dignity, death, honesty, confidentiality, the responsibility of the physician to improve society and the doctor-patient relationship as a sacred trust.

As you might imagine, the American Medical Association's *Code of Medical Ethics* is extremely detailed. It would be impossible to paraphrase even a small part of it; however, just because the code is lengthy, does not mean you are not responsible for being aware of its major tenets. The Council on Ethical and Judicial Affairs (CEJA) keeps this code, created in 1847, updated so that it remains relevant to current practices. A copy of the *Code of Medical Ethics* can be purchased online at the AMA website or you may also download a copy.

The *Code of Medical Ethics* is not to be confused with the nine Principles of Medical Ethics, which were adopted in June 2001. To summarize, the principles require that physicians:

1. Provide quality care while upholding human rights

2. Embody the highest level of professionalism and to expect the same of colleagues

3. Adhere to the law

4. Place a high importance on patients' rights and the rights of others

5. Continue to learn, study, and research so as to provide the best care

6. Maintain the right to choose where and with whom to work (emergency situations excepted)

7. Attempt to improve general public health

8. Consider the care of the patient their most important task

9. Promote medical care for every person

The AAMA has its own code of ethics. This, of course, relates specifically to the profession of medical assistants. In general, the medical assistants' code of ethics requires that medical assistant pledge to:

1. Provide quality service while preserving human dignity

2. Adhere strictly to confidentiality laws except when it becomes legally or otherwise necessary to disseminate information

3. Maintain honor and professionalism

4. Continue to study and increase knowledge for the benefit of patients and coworkers

5. Act at all times, even outside of work, to improve the health of the general public

From reading the codes of ethics, it should be obvious that ethical behavior and maintaining patient rights are of utmost importance in this field of health care. Anyone not willing or able to follow the law or to act in the best interest of the patient has no business becoming a medical assistant. As a rule, you should consider these codes carefully before entering this profession.

In health care, there has been an explosion of new procedures and options. Many times, laws have not been written to cover the cutting-edge technology (bioethics). Health care providers must turn to using their own beliefs (ethics) to decide what is right or wrong. Many health care professions have written ethical codes of behavior to help their membership to decide how to handle tough decisions. Medical assistants have an ethical code on their accrediting body's website.

Many ethical issues today are based on advances in science such as artificial insemination, transplantation, surrogacy, euthanasia, cloning, gene therapy, fetal tissue research, stem-cell research, abortion, harvesting of embryos, and in vitro fertilization. Many areas of health care have inconclusive answers to what is right or wrong. Each individual is allowed to refuse to participate in an activity that violates the individual's values (conscience clause). The conscience clause should be documented in the employee's record.

REVIEW QUESTIONS

1. The document that represents the wishes of an individual regarding end-of-life treatment is called a/an
    (A) living will
    (B) power of attorney
    (C) durable power of attorney
    (D) power of attorney for health care
    (E) advance directive

2. A state statute that outlines the requirements to practice medicine, licensure requirements, and guidelines for revocation or suspension of licensure is
    (A) OSHA
    (B) Nursing Practice Act
    (C) Patient Self-Determination Act
    (D) Medical Practice Act
    (E) HIPAA

3. The statute that protects health care givers when providing emergency care within their scope of ability is the
    (A) Medical Practice Act
    (B) Nursing Practice Act
    (C) Good Samaritan Act
    (D) Patient Self-Determination Act
    (E) Doctrine of Informed Consent

4. Which of the following is not a licensed health care worker?
    (A) Pharmacist
    (B) Social worker
    (C) Nurse
    (D) Medical assistant
    (E) Physician

5. CLIA is the abbreviation for

   (A) Criminal Law Intervention Act

   (B) Certified Lab Identification Act

   (C) Clerical Labor Interests Act

   (D) Clinical Lab Improvement Act

   (E) Common Licensure Interface Act

6. Informed consent involves understanding which of the following elements?

   (A) Benefits of treatment

   (B) Nature of the patient's condition

   (C) Purpose of treatment

   (D) Risks of treatment

   (E) All of the above

7. Medical malpractice is defined as

   (A) breach of confidentiality

   (B) deviation from the office procedures manual

   (C) fraud

   (D) personal liability

   (E) professional negligence

8. The legal term for an employer's responsibility for the acts of an employee is

   (A) chain of custody

   (B) consideration

   (C) *res ipsa loquitur*

   (D) *respondeat superior*

   (E) *subpoena duces tecum*

9. A medical assistant publicly criticizes a physician's diagnostic skills. This is an example of

   (A) breach of confidentiality

   (B) professional negligence

   (C) slander

   (D) testimony

   (E) veracity

10. Who is the legal owner of the information in a patient's medical record?

   (A) The insurance company

   (B) The patient

   (C) The physician

   (D) The patient and the physician

   (E) The U.S. state in which the patient resides

ANSWERS AND EXPLANATIONS

1. **A**

   A living will names no agent but states the desires of a person regarding how he or she would like to see their end-of-life issues handled. An advance directive (E) is a document naming an agent to speak for the patient if he or she is unable to express a choice. Durable power of attorney (C) or a power of attorney for health care (D) empowers that agent to make all property, financial, and health care decisions for the person, whereas a power of attorney (B) may only make property and financial decisions.

2. **D**

   Medical Practice Acts cover all the requirements to practice medicine including education, licensure, and guidelines for suspension and revocation of licensure for physicians. Guidelines for registered and licensed practical nurses fall under nursing practice acts (B). OSHA (A) involves the laws protecting the safety of the health workplace. The Patient Self-Determination Act (C) empowers the patient to make decisions for accepting or rejecting health care for themselves. HIPAA (E) involves privacy of health information and control of use of those records.

3. **C**

   The Good Samaritan Act protects certain health care workers from lawsuits when they offer emergency aid within the scope of their training. The Patient Self-Determination Act (D) empowers patients to decide what medical treatment to accept or reject. The Doctrine of Informed Consent (E) requires that the patient know all potential dangers from a treatment or procedure, any alternatives, and the risks of doing nothing. Medical Practice Acts (A) cover the licensure and guidelines for medical practice, whereas the Nursing Practice Act (B) covers education and licensure of nurses.

4. **D**

   The AAMA and AMT tests medical assistants. Each organization offers proof of accomplishment beyond basics. The AAMA offers certification and the AMT offers registrations to those students passing a national examination.

5. **D**

   The Clinical Lab Improvements Act offered standards for medical laboratory tests run in the physician's office lab (POL).

6. **E**

   Informed consent involves all the listed options. Patients should made be fully aware of the nature their condition (B), the purpose of the prescribed course of treatment (C), and its risks (D) and benefits (A). This information should be conveyed by the provider. The medical assistant plays the valuable role of clarifying what the provider has conveyed.

7. **E**

    Professional negligence can include actions of omission (which is nonfeasance), in which services were not rendered that should have been, or actions of commission, in which an error was made. In either case, malpractice is most often a civil tort that carries a financial penalty. In criminal negligence, often an unnecessary death has occurred, and the provider would be charged with manslaughter; fines and/or imprisonment may ensue.

8. **A**

    Respondeat superior, meaning "let the master answer," is a legal doctrine providing that the employer/provider is ultimately responsible for the actions of employees. Although the medical assistant is held to a standard of care, if the medical assistant makes an error, he/she will be held liable and so will the medical assistant's employer. Chain of custody (A) refers to safeguarding specimens that may be needed as evidence and documenting each person who handles them. Consideration (B) is another word for the bill for services rendered by the medical office to the patient. *Res ipsa loquitur* (C), meaning "the thing speaks for itself," is a legal concept that places the burden of proof on the practitioner when circumstances strongly suggest malpractice. *Subpoena duces tecum* (E) ("summons for the production of evidence") is an order for medical records to be delivered to the court.

9. **C**

    Slander is defined as using false spoken words that would harm the reputation or credibility of another. Breach of confidentiality (A) is disclosing patient information without authorization. Professional negligence (B) involves omission of appropriate medical services and/or carrying out incorrect medical actions. Testimony (D) is evidence given verbally under legal questioning. Veracity (E) means truthfulness.

10. **B**

    The patient is the owner of the information within the medical record, and it may not be released without express written permission from the patient and/or guardian. The physician, however, owns the documents and the documentation on the record. Be aware that there is a lot of controversy regarding ownership of the medical record, and the issue is often left to individual states for clarification.

Chapter 10: **Office Administration**

A key aspect of your role as a medical assistant is supporting the efficient and effective administration of the office practice. The administrative duties will vary by the size and scope of your practice setting; however, you will likely be involved in patient scheduling, managing appointments, management of medical records and reports, and assisting with office equipment. In this chapter you will review the essential elements of these duties.

SCHEDULING

Making Appointments

One of the most important administrative duties for a medical assistant is to make appointments and maintain the practice appointment book. The person responsible for scheduling the appointments plays a key role in making sure the office runs smoothly. Patients do not want to wait any longer than 15 to 20 minutes before being seen by the doctor, and the doctor wants a smooth flow of patients. Patients who are very ill or have an emergency want to be seen promptly by their primary physician whenever possible.

Patient satisfaction or dissatisfaction with the experience of making an appointment can determine whether the patient will remain with the practice or find another physician. Your demeanor on the telephone is very important. Speak clearly and do not appear rushed. Give your total attention to the person on the other end of the telephone. Repeat information back to avoid errors. Always be friendly, courteous, and interested in what the caller has to say. To avoid long wait times, schedule the correct amount of time for the type of appointment you are making.

Methods of Scheduling Appointments

Appointments are scheduled either manually using appointment books, or by computer using scheduling software. An appointment book is usually spiral-bound, so it can lie flat. It may have pages for a single day, pages that show a week when open, or pages with two or three doctors' schedules for a single day. Appointments may be set up in 10- to 15-minute intervals. Initial appointments or those requiring complete history and physical exams are generally longer, as are some medical procedures and office-based procedures. It is helpful to create a list with the preferred time frames for a variety of appointment types in your practice.

A computerized appointment schedule shows the same information as in an appointment book. The doctor has a screen for each day, which can be printed. Corrections, additions, and deletions can be done easily on the computer. The daily printout can be used at the end of the day to note cancellations and "no-shows" in the patient record.

Some basic information must be obtained when you are scheduling appointments.

- Patient's full name: obtain a correct spelling of the patient's name; date of birth should be used to confirm the correct identity for patients with common names

- Home and work telephone numbers where the patient can be reached by your office; repeat phone numbers to ensure accuracy

- Purpose of the visit (e.g., routine visit, health exam, immunizations); your office should have an estimated length for each type of visit

Tuesday

April 10, _____

Time	Patient	Phone	Insurance
9:00	Anna Miller	555-2348	
	New Patient		BlueCross/HMO
9:15	XXXXXXXXXXXXXXXXXX		
9:30	Stephen Smith	555-0000	
	follow up/flu		self pay
9:45	Patrick McCarthy	237-0110	
	second opinion		PPO-Blue Cross
10:00	XXXXXXXXXXXX		
10:15	Pharmaceutical Rep		
10:30	Sally Halper	555-0230	
	Earache		Medicare
10:45	Hector Ramirez	630-6700	
	Headaches		HMO/Unicare

Figure 10.1—Appointment List

Daily appointment lists are printed or copied for office use so that medical records can be pulled for the upcoming daily appointments. Additions or corrections are made in ink, because this list is an official legal record of patients seen on a given day.

No-shows (people who do not show up for their appointment) and those who call to cancel on the day of the appointment are marked in red on the daily schedule. This information is also noted on the patient medical record. Documentation of no-shows protects your practice if the patient later claims the office did provide care. A list of cancellations may also be kept on the computer.

Legal Status of Appointment Book

The practice appointment book is considered a legal record. Your office should have a policy on retaining old appointment books in an archive. Because the appointment book could be used as evidence in legal proceedings, entries must be clear, written in black ink, and easy to read. Never erase a name or use correction fluid to blot the name out. Instead, draw a single line through the name and beside it write "can" for canceled or "NS" for a no-show patient. Also write the date, time, and reason (if known) why the appointment was missed or canceled, and then initial the entry. This information should also be documented in the patient's chart.

Some offices permit the use of pencil to allow for changes or corrections if necessary. If pencil is used, at the end of the day you or another designated staff member should write directly over the penciled entries in ink to create a permanent document.

Appointment Systems

There are several different types of scheduling systems. The physician or the practice will choose which system is best for their practice. Open-hours, time-specified, wave, modified-wave, double-booking, cluster, advance, and combination scheduling are the different methods used when setting up your appointment book.

In an open-hours scheduling system, patients arrive at their own convenience with the understanding that they will be seen on a first-come, first-served basis, unless there is an emergency. A drawback to open-hours scheduling is a patient may have a long wait time. Open scheduling is seen in public health clinics and urgent care centers. This system increases the possibility of inefficient downtime for the physician.

Time-specified scheduling is scheduling patients at regular, specified intervals. Minor medical problems usually require 15-minute appointments. This type of scheduling leaves more time to schedule physical exams or procedures that can require 30- to 60-minute appointments. Time-specific scheduling controls the flow of the day and how the doctor's time is spent.

Wave scheduling works best in large medical facilities that have enough departments or personnel to give service to several patients at one time. With wave scheduling, the medical assistant asks the patients to all arrive at the top of the hour. This system is based on the experience that some patients will arrive late for their appointment while others may need more time for an appointment than initially expected. Patients are seen in the order of their actual arrival time. A disadvantage of wave scheduling is that patients can become annoyed or angry if they realize that several patients have an appointment at the same time.

The wave can be modified in different ways. Patients can be scheduled in 15-minute increments, regardless of appointment type. Another method of wave scheduling is to schedule four patients to arrive at planned intervals during the first half hour, leaving the second half unscheduled. Appointments that need more time should be scheduled at the beginning of the hour. Less time-consuming appointments would be scheduled in 10- to 15-minute time slots. The use of this method allows time for catching up.

When two or more patients are scheduled for the same appointment, the scheduling is called double booking. The double scheduling assumes that both patients will be seen in this time slot. If the visits are short or there are multiple practitioners available, it can make sense to double book. If both patients need the 10- to 15-minute time slot, then the office falls behind. If you work in a practice where two patients can be seen at once, this method does work. Double booking also helps when a patient calls and needs to be seen that day. As a medical assistant, you will work with the physician to prepare and treat both patients in different rooms.

Clustering scheduling is grouping similar appointments together during the day or week. This method is helpful when specialized equipment or services are available only at certain times.

Specialists often book patients weeks or months in advance. This method is advance scheduling. The physician usually leaves a few slots open every day to accommodate urgent appointments.

Practices often combine two or more scheduling styles, and more offices are using the computerized scheduling. With this method, the computer can be programmed to lock out selected appointment slots so that these times will be available for emergencies. Another advantage of computerized scheduling is that the schedule can be accessed from all the computers in the practice. It also is a great way to keep track of the patients who are late or miss appointments, and it can identify length of appointment times. In addition to patient appointments, you may be asked to schedule appointments with representatives from drug companies, medical equipment suppliers, and other vendors. Some physicians keep times available on their practice schedules for these and other administrative activities.

Managing the Physician's Schedule and Travel

Maintaining the physician's time and daily activities schedule is another duty of the medical assistant. Physicians regularly attend meetings and conferences, make hospital rounds, meet with colleagues, complete paperwork, and perform other duties. You must be careful to avoid overbooking as well as underbooking patient appointments. Underbooking occurs when the physician's schedule results in too many gaps between appointments. These gaps are inefficient and costly to the practice. Remember that maintaining the schedule requires regular attention. The physician may have an emergency in the hospital or be called away and you will have to contact the patients and reschedule appointments.

Some physicians set aside certain times and days when pharmaceutical sales representatives can be seen by the physician to talk about the latest drugs or equipment. Pharmaceutical reps often leave samples of the drug to encourage the physician to write prescriptions. Physicians do not want to fall behind with the patients, so keeping track of the pharmaceutical reps can save the physician needed time for patient care.

Other duties related to the physician's schedule include setting up meetings and possibly making travel arrangements for the out-of-town engagements. Scheduling time with the physician every week to go over the office schedule helps keep the practice running smoothly.

Referrals

There will be times when the physician needs to send a patient to a specialty practice. You may be asked to assist in the referral to the consulting physician. Keep a list of the preferred consultants used by your practice. The patient should be given the specialist's name, address, and phone number. You may be asked to schedule the appointment for the patients. Patients who have HMO insurance will also have to be given a written referral to bring with them to the specialist's office. Some HMOs have a unique list of required consulting physicians. Check with the patient or review their coverage prior to initiating a referral to a consulting physician. This will be necessary for the insurance to pay the bill for the specialist. Explain to the patient how the referral works. Ask if the patient has any questions. The patient will have to follow up with the primary physician after seeing the specialist. A referral form should include the patient's demographic information, the reason for the referral, and the follow-up action requested by your office.

Follow-up Appointments

Patients should be encouraged to follow their physician's advice and schedule follow-up appointments with the physician in a timeframe specified by the physician. Patients should schedule the follow-up appointment before leaving the physician's office if the office uses wave, time-specified, modified-wave, or advance scheduling.

RECORDS MANAGEMENT

Medical Records

When a new patient comes to the doctor's office, a medical record must be compiled. The medical record or chart is a legal document that is not removed from the doctor's office. There are different systems used to document patient information. One method is source-oriented. The information is arranged according to the professional who supplied the data. This type of record describes all problems and treatments on the same page. The record contains physician notes, nursing/assistant notes, laboratory records, radiology reports, and insurance information.

The problem-oriented medical record (POMR) is another way to document patient information. This method makes it easier for the physician to follow a patient's progress and treatment. The information in the POMR is the history and physical exam database; a detailed patient problem list; an educational, diagnostic, and treatment plan; as well as the progress notes.

The database includes a record of the patient's history, information from the initial interview with the patient, and all findings and results from examinations, any tests, and other procedures.

Each problem the patient presents is listed separately, given its own number, and dated when it was identified. The physician must be aware if the patient has personal problems or family issues, such as marital problems, that may interfere with treatment. Along with each patient problem, there should be a detailed diagnostic and treatment summary in the record. Subsequent visits are documented by listing the problem and describing the current status, new complaints or symptoms, treatment, and the patient's response to the treatment plan. You should review the problem list and make sure that age- and gender-specific health promotion and disease prevention problems are noted and tracked in the POMR.

Problem-Oriented Medical Record

Name of Patient: *Mary Smith*

DATA:

Patient: *Patient "unemployed after 30 years at the same company."*

B/P: 180/94, P: 90
X-ray of spine: Normal
Blood test: Cholesterol   300

1. *4/1/16*   *headaches*
2. *4/1/16*   *lower back pain——pain worse after sitting for long periods of time*

Family: *Patient's son unemployed also. Lives at home. Sleeps all day——not looking for work*

Signs/Symptoms: *"temple throbbing——right side" pain lasts all day waking up from sleep with headache*

Figure 10.2—Problem-Oriented Medical Record

The SOAP approach, which is used in many medical records, gives orderly steps for documentation of clinical information. SOAP is an acronym that stands for the following items:

Subjective: this information comes from the patient describing his or her signs and symptoms; it is recommended that you use direct quotes or paraphrase the patient's subjective comments about their status

Objective: this information comes from the health care provider's observations and measurements including vital signs, examination results, and laboratory test results

Assessment: this information describes the diagnosis of the patient's problem or what the provider believes is the condition facing the patient

Plan: this component of the documentation states action or steps that will be taken to address the patient's problem; this includes recommended medications, treatment, consultations, patient's education, and follow-up care. The plan should always be discussed with the patient prior to the end of the office visit. In some cases, written instructions should be provided.

SOAP Progress Note

Patient Name:	Sidney Holmes Date of Birth: 6/7/65 Chart #66738
Date:	3/31/16
Subject	Patient complaining of pain in lower right quadrant. Patient had a fever of 101.2 for the past 3 days.
Object:	BP 130/80. Temperature 102.0 F. Abdominal exam revealed rebound tenderness.
Assessment:	Appendicitis
Plan:	1. Admit to hospital 2. Surgery to remove appendix

Figure 10.3—SOAP Progress Note

It is important that medical records are neat, legible, and complete. Never use correction fluid or tape in medical records. If an error is made, cross out the word(s) using one line, make the correction above the corrected word, initial it, and date it.

Medical records should be kept up to date and filed in an organized way so that current information is available to the physician during office visits. Use a professional tone in documenting. Record information in the patient's own words when appropriate, using quotation marks. Do not record your personal opinions, comments, or speculation.

Medical records are legal documents and must be handled accordingly. Patients who see the doctor must have the chart up-to-date and patients who have not seen the doctor in a year can be placed in the inactive file cabinet. Records of patients who are deceased or have moved away should be placed in a closed file cabinet. The medical file belongs to the physician or medical group, but the information in it belongs to the patient. Patients who are changing doctors will request to have their records sent to the new physician. A signed release of records must be obtained prior to transferring the medical record. The original file is placed in the inactive file. Medical records are kept for 7 to 10 years or according to the policy in your practice. If you treat children, records should be retained until the child reaches the age of 21, plus the statute of limitations for adult records. Some physicians do not want the records destroyed and have the inactive charts placed in storage or computerized. When disposing of a medical record, it must be shredded or burned.

Outguides

An outguide is a stiff marker that is placed on a medical file when the file is removed. The outguide serves as a placeholder in the file cabinet so that any files that are removed are traceable within the office. Outguides have either a list to sign out the file or a clear pocket where a slip of paper can be inserted listing the location of the record and which office member has signed it out. When the file is returned to the file drawer, the outguide is removed. Different color outguides can be used for each physician in a medical office. Outguides are helpful for keeping track of the files.

Filing Systems

Medical records are organized using a filing system. A medical office may use any variety of filing systems, but the patient records must be stored using a system that allows for ease of access and retrieval. The most common filing system for maintaining patient files is the alphabetic system. In the alphabetic filing system, files are arranged in alphabetical order by the last name of the patient. Files are labeled with the patient's last name first, followed by the first name and middle initial. If the patient has a common name, you may include the date of birth or social security number to track specific patient files.

Another system is the numeric filing system. In this system, each patient is assigned a number. The number used for a new patient is assigned in sequential order. Only numbers are found on the outside of the folder. Some numeric file systems imbed the year or month of treatment into the ordering system. The numeric system can be expanded to indicate the location of the files. A master list with the numeric system of the patient's names with the corresponding numbers can be helpful in keeping track of the files when a numeric system is used.

Color-coding is used when there is a need to distinguish between files in a filing system. An example would be using a certain color to distinguish new patients to the practice. Color-coding may allow you to find a file quickly and easily. You can color-code the files in a variety of ways. Folders, labels, stickers, and plastic tabs all come in a variety of colors. Using a color-coded system also allows for easier identification of misfiled records.

Pulling and filing patient records will be a part of your job as a medical assistant. There will be times when you can return a file to the cabinet or medical records area immediately after use. Other times the files will be put in a holding bin until the file can be returned to the file cabinet. It is good practice to return all medical records to their proper location at the end of the business day.

There are three types of records that you will need to file: new patient records, individual documents that belong to existing patient records, and patient records that have previously been filed and now require refiling. There are five steps that should be used for filing patient records: inspecting, indexing, coding, sorting, and storing. Inspecting means making sure that the documents are ready to file. All documents should be signed, dated, and complete. Remove any paperclips or rubber bands. Removing paperclips and rubber bands will make the folder less bulky. Indexing is another word for naming the parts of a file or the area of the record in which the document should be filed. The coding method is using an identifying mark on the document to ensure that the file is placed in the correct area within the clinical record.

Patient charts should be stored in a safe and secure area in your office. Either a locked room or locked file cabinet should be used. It is important that you protect the records from view of office visitors, vendors, and others who are not directly involved in providing care and treatment to the patient. Medical records contain protected health information and failing to secure confidential information violates the privacy rights of your patients.

Filing Guidelines

There are specific guidelines that are used to file more efficiently. When you pull a file or file a patient's chart, glance at it. Make sure that the papers are in proper order. Always keep the files neat. It will be easier to locate the documents that you need. The papers should fit neatly into the folder and not be sticking out. Folders have to be able to remain closed when laid down, so make sure the files are not overstuffed. You may need to thin a patient file or set up several volumes for long-term patients. Folders have to be lifted out of the drawer when filing, so make sure that all papers are properly inserted and fixed inside of the record binder. If using a cabinet for storage, the drawers should not be crowded. Files have to be able to fit in the drawer easily.

Use a combination of uppercase letters and lowercase letters on the label of the file. An example would be: Smith, David. The letters of the first and last name stand out, which makes it easier to read. Using a different tab position when filing the folders will assist in making the folders easier to locate and pull out for use.

Lost files can have devastating consequences. If a file cannot be located in 24 to 48 hours, it should be considered lost. Try to locate lost files within the office, and make sure that the record has not been misfiled among other records. As a last resort, you may have to reconstruct the file with information that is available or computerized.

Electronic Health Records (EHRs)

Implementation of electronic health records (EHRs) was included as part of the Centers for Medicare and Medicaid Service's meaningful use requirements. The Health Information Technology for Economic and Clinical Health (HITECH) Act, enacted as part of the American Recovery and Reinvestment Act of 2009, provided $19 billion to fund the adoption of information technology into health care, thus creating financial incentives for physicians, hospitals, and other health care providers to adopt EHRs. The goal of this initiative was to improve the overall health of the U.S. population. As a result, according to the Office of the National Coordinator for Health Information Technology, 87 percent of office-based physicians had adopted EHRs as of 2015. Failure to implement EHRs results in a decrease in the reimbursement from Medicare for services performed.

Some of the barriers to full implementation of EHRs include high costs, lack of system integration, and deficiencies in staff knowledge of computer systems. As a medical assistant, you may be part of the effort to implement an EHR, assisting your practice office in the transition to this new and much-improved system of data collection, storage, and retrieval. This section will describe the benefits of using computerized records, relate some key concerns and potential limitations of their use, discuss tips for implementation, and point out some key features of EHR systems.

Benefits of EHRs

If you have ever spent time searching for a medical record or a particular report, chances are you have encountered the situation of having lost or misplaced a file or having located a record after a search and finding that it is incomplete. One of the key benefits of an electronic health record is that it maintains the entire record in a consistent location that is readily accessible to the providers in a health care facility or medical office practice. In addition to being available and intact, the electronic format is legible and easy to follow in a chronological format. The ability to trace care delivery from one encounter to the next and integrate hospitalizations, changes in prescriptions, preventive health activities, and phone contacts supports continuity of care and avoids repetition of expensive tests and treatments. Record retrieval for release of information to third party payors, patients, and other parties is simplified. In many cases the files can be transferred to these parties electronically, resulting in a savings of time and money. Generally the entries in the record are able to be date- and time-stamped as they are produced so that the integrity of the chart is maintained automatically. Alterations in the record made through error correction, late entries, or addenda can be recorded and tracked to a particular provider. Using an electronic record allows the facility to enter providers into the system at the time of hire, when they are issued proper credentials and passwords. Each member of the practice or team can be granted authorship rights for the select functions that apply to his or her position. In this way, the system supports the privacy and confidentiality rights of patients and their protected health information. In addition, when providers leave the facility, their use and access privileges can be removed to avoid record tampering and system violations.

A major benefit of electronic health records is the ability to access, aggregate and analyze health information. Most systems are designed so that information entered into the electronic record system goes into a database that can be sorted by a variety of variables. For example, if the medical assistant needs to identify all patients with a common diagnosis—such as congestive heart failure—the system can be searched on the diagnosis code, and a list of patients with this diagnosis can be prepared for review. In this way, providers are able to track key information about patients, payors, and service use. In terms of patient care delivery, this ability enables medical assistants to track key preventive health measures—such as mammograms or immunization records—for individual patients, for specific age groups, and for the practice as a whole. Information retrieval via electronic methods simplifies clinical record reviews conducted for quality improvement and other purposes.

In addition to ease of access and the ability to retrieve and report on health information, the electronic record can be formatted to comply with medical record standards established by the provider. For example, the patient admission history and physical can be standardized and sequenced to allow ease of data entry as the provider interviews and examines a patient. The key elements that are important for the particular specialty practice can be included. For example, all pediatric cases can include data fields for height, weight, and head circumference. These data points can then be automatically graphed on standardized growth charts for children. If the record system is networked with a document imaging system, copies of paper-based reports or test results can be added to the electronic record for a particular patient.

Another important benefit of electronic records is the ease of information storage. No longer will records and charts take up the costly resource of space in the office. Health records can be maintained indefinitely on electronic media such as hard drives or tapes. Off-site storage of backup copies of health and billing records will protect the integrity of what could formerly be lost, misfiled, or even destroyed in a natural disaster.

Key Concerns Related to Electronic Records

A common concern among providers is the perception that entry of information into the EHR is cumbersome and causes loss of contact with the patient. In many ambulatory practices the computerized record is contained in a desktop computer that is placed out of the direct, view of a patient. It requires the medical assistant or physician to have their back turned to the patient during the interview and this can be seen as a barrier to communication. In addition, the data entry requires a level of comfort in keyboarding and data entry. Some facilities provide basic computer training for all staff, to ensure that they can save and retrieve files and successfully manage the database and software system, prior to going live with an EHR.

In addition to the communication and skill barrier, some feel that EHRs can be violated by security breaches both from hackers and from professional staff who are not directly involved in a particular patient's care. An EHR requires a system for data administration and maintenance that can ensure that confidential information is not routinely accessed by uninvolved parties and that tight security measures are implemented. Backup copies of records should be kept in off-site storage for ease of retrieval in the event of power outages or other disruption of service.

Finally, a concern in any facility is the major change of transitioning from a familiar and comfortable clinical and business record to a new system. The process requires careful planning and decision-making about the system that is selected for use and its integration with other office systems, such as those that support business, billing, and accounting functions. Staff training and the time required to convert paper records to electronic media should be considered. In addition, decisions will need to be made about how to integrate the EHR across settings with hospitals, pharmacies, laboratories, and other providers.

Despite the concerns discussed above, the move to EHRs is definitely underway. Current incentives to foster this move include offering reimbursement to practice offices that make the switch to electronic records.

Features and Functions of EHRs

Numerous software and hardware vendors are entering the market for EHRs. A provider should take care to plan the implementation and selection process carefully, beginning by creating a list of the preferred features and characteristics of their desired EHR. Following are some specific components of the system that can be considered.

- Web-based versus software-based systems: A web-based system means that all providers access the record system via the Internet, where it is maintained and stored. The vendor regularly updates the system and is responsible for upgrades, enhancements, and changes; this relieves the need for an onsite system administrator. New users from a particular office can be added easily and given credentials that can be altered or removed as needed.

- Fully integrated systems: A fully integrated system should link demographic information, patient scheduling, health records, history information, laboratory results, communication from phone calls and emails, patient education materials, medication records, and billing and financial information. In addition, a sophisticated system may link to office and supply inventory and reports. The state-of-the-art systems that are currently in development can link the practice office to select laboratories, pharmacies and suppliers to enable real-time communication and information exchange.

- Point of care data entry: Some EHRs are designed to allow clinical staff to enter patient information via a PDA or handheld device that allows maximal interaction between the patient and the provider. Another possibility is the use of Computers on Wheels (COWs), which are mobile workstations, using notebook computers that can be moved from exam rooms to the bedside or other locations.

- Clinical record: A well-organized and systematic database for entry and retrieval of patient information is an essential element of an EHR. The database should include patient history and physical examination reports, medication lists, problem lists, contact records, test results, and consultation reports. The data should be searchable and stored in easy-to-access electronic files. It is also helpful if the flow of the record mirrors the practice workflows so that clinical staff can easily adapt to the computer conversion. Some systems automatically supply ICD and other codes when the patient diagnostic and treatment information is entered.

- Specialty information and patient information: An EHR should match the needs of the patient in the practice setting in an effective manner. Examples include disease state templates that prompt clinicians to address common patient needs and problems at various encounters. Additionally, the availability of patient instructions on treatments, medications, and disease states for downloading and printing helps save time and increases office efficiency while supporting the delivery of quality care.

Successfully Implementing EHRs

Step one in a successful implementation of an EHR is planning. The plan should include an estimate of the available funds to support the system purchase and installation. It may be helpful to hold a team meeting to get the input of all staff in the facility regarding the functions and characteristics they feel are most crucial to guide selection of a vendor or product. Once a comprehensive list is developed, staff can survey and interview vendors and request hands-on demonstrations of a select group of systems. Once a new system has been chosen, staff training and implementation can occur. One aspect to consider in implementation is how to manage existing patients. One very large national health care company decided to go back and enter all patient data from their historical paper files so that the entire facility could be electronically based. Another option is to convert patients to EHRs as they come in for regular encounters and to routinely admit new patients using the system. In either case, a major focus of the implementation will be staff training, staff support, and effective change management. Having an electronic record that is easily accessed, fully integrated, and legible is a reminder that the effort is worthwhile.

OFFICE POLICIES AND PROCEDURES

Policies are rules that tell employees the day-to-day workings of the medical office. Policies will vary from office to office, but there are several policies that are used in most medical offices. The physician and/or management staff create the policies and procedures of the office. Examples include office hours, dress code, job descriptions, duties of the staff, vacation, sick time, salary, bookkeeping, scheduling system used for appointments, and how mail is handled. An office manual of established policies and procedures should be available to all employees to review. Standard procedures would be explained in detail in this manual along with clinical procedures and quality assurance measures. An example of an office policy would be a written explanation of the format for a medical record for a new patient. The medical assistant may be asked to update and maintain the policy and procedure manual for the office. It is a good practice to review this manual and make necessary changes and additions on a yearly basis or more often if the nature of the practice changes.

DATA ENTRY

Data is made up of the raw facts, numbers, letters, or symbols that the computer processes into meaningful information. Data is also the information that is put into the computer. The type of data in a typical office database would be the name of the care provider, patient demographic information, insurance carriers, diagnosis codes, procedure codes, and transactions. Following is a more detailed list of the types of data.

Provider: name, address, phone number, tax and medical identifier numbers, and other information about the physician and the practice

Patients: each patient's medical record number and personal information

Insurance carriers: name, addresses, other data about each insurance carrier that the physician accepts

Diagnosis codes: codes from ICD-10-CM (*International Classification of Diseases, 10th Edition, Clinical Modification*) specify the diagnostic information about the illness, injury, or condition for which the patient is under treatment

Procedure codes: procedure codes from CPT (*Current Procedural Terminology*) specify the care and treatment provided in the office setting; the codes are used for billing and charges for care rendered in your practice office

Transactions: information about the patient's visit, diagnoses, procedures, and received and outstanding payments, recorded in the form of charges, payments, and adjustments

SOFTWARE APPLICATIONS

Software applications are programs available in office computers. They perform a variety of important functions for the medical office. Application software falls into the following areas:

- Word processing
- Graphics
- Database
- Spreadsheet
- Presentation
- Utility
- Communication

Word processing software is used to write doctors' notes, reports, transcripts, memos, and letters. When you need to write any type of correspondence, it has to be proofread before it is sent out. Using proofreader's marks on the document to correct errors will ensure that the corrections are made accurately.

Graphics software produces information using pictures. It can also be used to input illustrations or photos into medical reports or documents.

Most offices use medical office **database** software that provides templates for a variety of office-related activities. Databases may include progress notes, health histories, laboratory information, and medication lists for patients. Databases not only store information but many also allow the user to sort and aggregate patient information for management purposes.

A **spreadsheet** is a worksheet that performs numeric calculations on data that is entered in the worksheet. Spreadsheets are used in budgeting, financial reporting, and invoicing.

Presentation software assists in designing the layout and content for presentations, lectures, and staff training materials.

A **utility** helps maintain the function of a computer system. An example of utility software is antivirus software.

Communication software is used to communicate to others in the medical office or in the health care system. Communications applications include email and Web browsers.

OTHER COMPUTER CONCEPTS

Computer hardware refers to the physical components of computer equipment, such as the central processing unit (CPU), monitor, keyboard, and printer. The keyboard, disk drive, and scanner are input devices; that is, you use these devices to put information into the computer. Output devices include the monitor and printer; these display information from the computer.

Office computers should be password protected for security and integrity of patient information. This will ensure that unauthorized people cannot get any information about your patients. Each person working in the office should have a unique password. A monitoring system is another tool used to ensure that patients' medical records are secure. Whenever someone goes into the system to access information, the system tracks the user's name and which files have been viewed.

Backup files are used to protect information from being lost, damaged, or destroyed. Backup files need to be made regularly. Storing backup files on a Zip disk, CD, or other method of storage is the best way to protect the information. In case of a computer virus or fire, you will still have the information. Backup files are often maintained in an off-site location for protection.

Computer viruses are common and your office should protect computer systems with up-to-date antivirus software. A virus can appear on your computer by opening an infected disk or opening infected email or downloading information from the Internet. A good rule to follow is not to open an email from someone you do not know. There are computer detection and protection programs that can be purchased to fight viruses.

The Internet was developed by the U.S. government and is a global network of millions of computers. The intranet is a local network internal to a company.

OFFICE EQUIPMENT

When thinking of office machine equipment you probably think of stethoscopes, blood pressure monitors, and x-ray machines but the medical office has many other kinds of office machines to help the office run smoothly. Medical offices need to have a telephone system, fax machine, computer, photocopier, calculators, postage scale, postage meter, dictation-transcription equipment, and a paper shredder. All these pieces of equipment can help you keep running the office properly.

Computers have become a necessary part of the medical office. Computers are used to schedule appointments and keep data, including information on patients, billing information, diagnostic information, and specialist information. The size of a medical office determines how many computers are needed for the office.

Telephones

Without the telephone system it would be impossible to run a medical office. Not only do we need the telephone to communicate with patients but also with other physicians, other employees, hospitals, laboratories, and other businesses. The size of the medical practice will determine how many lines the office will need. Even in a one-physician practice the office will have more than one line so that callers will not get a busy signal. Having more than one line will make it more difficult for you and the other employees to keep track of the calls coming in.

Telephones will be in several locations in the medical office. The reception area will have more than one telephone while the other telephones will be in other areas of the office. Exam rooms often will have telephones in them so that the medical assistant can communicate with the physicians when an urgent matter arises. Telephones in the exam rooms should not, however, be used for personal calls or otherwise when a patient is present in the room.

When taking telephone calls from patients, remember to answer the telephone by the third ring and ask the caller if it is okay to hold. Wait for the caller to agree. The caller may have an emergency and be unable to hold. Each caller must be given your full attention. Assistants in medical offices with multiple lines will find it difficult at times to answer the telephone by the third ring, but by practicing this method and being courteous with each caller, they will help the medical practice to thrive. You, the medical assistant, are the first person to whom the caller speaks. By answering the telephone quickly and giving that call your full attention, you will keep the patients happy and they will continue to see that physician.

When you have to put a call on hold, remember to get back to the caller as soon as possible. Apologize for keeping her waiting. Do not act as if you are in a hurry. Speak clearly and repeat the patient's name, phone number, and appointment date and time to them. This will help prevent any errors that could cause confusion later on.

Fax Machine

A fax machine is a must in the medical office. A fax machine can be used to send information to other physicians, insurance companies, or to send referrals. Your office should design a standard fax cover sheet that clearly identifies your address and phone number, and specifies who is transmitting the fax information. Medical office faxes should contain language that specifies the confidential nature of health information and alerts the recipient of the fax to return or destroy incorrect information. This disclaimer should be clearly displayed on all fax cover sheets. Faxing protected health information should be avoided.

Calculators

Calculators are used to balance daily receipts or other office transactions. You will want to have a calculator that uses a paper tape to keep a record of these calculations. Bank deposits, for example, should be totaled each day and deposited with a copy of the daily tape record stored for accounting purposes.

Postage Scales

Postage scales are used to weigh envelopes for the correct postage, while the postage meter secures and stamps the envelope.

Shredder

When disposing of papers that are confidential, a paper shredder is used. When patient records, financial records, or other documents are no longer required or retained, the shredder ensures that no one will be able to access the information.

Photocopiers and Scanners

Photocopiers are used to make copies of documents. A patient may want a copy of a test result or a copy of the visit may be needed for billing purposes. A patient's insurance card (front and back) is copied and put in the chart so that it is available for billing purposes. Some newer photocopiers include scanners. This is used to send a scanned document to an electronic medical record or to a particular person whose email address is programmed into the machine. Once it is scanned, the document goes directly to the receiver's email address.

Dictation-Transcription Equipment

As use of electronic health records (EHRs) increases, the need for transcription of dictated information from physicians is declining. However, as a medical assistant you may be asked to prepare or transcribe memos, letters, or patient records. Dictation is when the physician records the information to be typed. Transcription is when the medical assistant types out what was dictated. The physician should speak clearly and slowly so that you can clearly understand what is said. It is helpful to ask that the dictator spell out any names or addresses that may be unfamiliar to you. Also ask the dictator to repeat anything that you cannot understand. The physician will tell you if what you are transcribing is a memo or letter. After you have completed the document, you will proofread it and make any corrections to the document. When it is 100 percent accurate, you then give the document to the physician for signature. It may be your job then to address an envelope and use the postage meter to get it ready for mailing. It is a good idea to make a copy of the document or save a copy on the computer for future reference.

A medical practice cannot run smoothly without the help of a variety of office machines. It may be your job to ensure that the machines are working properly and stocked with necessary supplies. It is also important to keep maintenance records on the equipment and assure that preventive maintenance is done on a regular basis.

OFFICE DOCUMENTS

Letters

Letters are external documents. They originate in the office and are sent to patients, associates, and other outside recipients.

Letterhead

Letterhead is the paper that the physician will use for official correspondence. It will have the office name on the top (or the doctor's name), the address, and phone number of the office. You will use the letterhead paper in all your correspondence whether to another physician, patient, or vendor. Letterhead or stationery is a higher quality paper than plain paper.

Content

There are four main elements to every letter. These are:

1. heading
2. opening
3. body
4. closing

The heading is generally something standard to office stationary, or letterhead. Since you don't have to create this yourself, the only other element you must be sure to include in the heading is the date. To avoid confusion, the month should be spelled out first, followed by the date, and then the year should be included in its entirety (e.g., April 5, 2017, as opposed to 4/5/17).

The opening is the next element of a letter. The opening starts with the recipient's name and full address. Even though this is not used for delivering the letter, the name and address should be accurate and complete. Title, name, street number, street address, city, state, and ZIP code are all required.

Below the address, the opening of some letters contain an attention line ("ATTN:" or "ATTENTION:") to direct the letter to a specific person. If this is not required for your letter, you should begin with the greeting. The greeting can be a person's title and name followed by a colon for business letters or a comma for more personal letters (e.g., "Mr. Lennon:" or "Mr. Lennon,"). If the specific recipient is unknown, the greeting should read: "To Whom It May Concern:".

As expected, the body of the letter contains the main contents of the letter. The body is followed by the closing. The closing begins with something such as "Yours" or "Best regards" or other such compliments. This is followed by the author's signature under which the author's typed name appears. Next comes the reference notation, which includes the author's initials in capital letters followed by the lower case initials of the person who actually put the letter on paper. It looks like this: SG:ab or SG/ab. This line is only required if the author of the letter is not the one who types it.

If copies of the letter are sent to others or if there are enclosures to a letter, two additional lines are needed. Enclosures are noted with one of the following: "Enc:" or "Enclosure:" or "Enclosures:".

If copies of the letter are sent to others, a copy notation is used. This is indicated by adding "cc:" along with the name of the recipient of this carbon copy. If there are multiple recipients, the recipients' names should be alphabetized. Blind carbon copies ("bcc:") might also be sent. They are indicated in the same way as carbon copies, but do not appear on the original letter.

The final element of the closing is the ever-popular postscript ("P.S.") This is for any additional information the author wants to include that has not yet been found in the letter. Typically, formal letters do not contain a postscript.

Spacing

One important aspect of each element of a letter that has not yet been discussed is placement on the page. Following is a list of each element of a letter and where each of the aforementioned elements belongs on a document.

- Letterhead (at top of page)
- Date (3 line spaces below letterhead)
- Address (4 line spaces below date)
- Attention (2 line spaces below the address)
- Greeting (2 line spaces below the attention)
- Body (2 line spaces below the greeting; the letter should be single-spaced but there should be double-spaces between paragraphs)
- Closing compliment—e.g., "Sincerely" (2 line spaces below the body)
- Signature (leave 4 or 5 blank line spaces to accommodate the signature)

- Typed name (4 to 5 blank lines below the closing compliment)
- Reference notation (2 lines below the typed name)
- Enclosure notation (1 or 2 lines below the reference)
- Copy notation (1 or 2 lines below the enclosure)
- Postscript (2 lines below the last line)

Generally, letters should have 1-inch margins. If letters are particularly short (fewer than 100 words) or slightly longer (100 to 200 words in length), then 2-inch or 1.5-inch margins, respectively, should be used.

Format

There are five main business letter formats: full block, modified block, semi-block, hanging indentation, and simplified. Following are the main characteristics of each. (Please note, since letterhead is specific to each company or organization, its location is not accounted for in these formats.)

- In **full block format**, all content is aligned on the left side of the document.
- In **modified block format**, the date and the closing compliment are centered on the page. All other content is aligned on the left side of the document.
- In **semi-block format**, the date and the closing compliment are centered on the page. The start of each new paragraph in the body is indented five spaces to the right, but all other content not already specified is aligned on the left side of the document.
- In **hanging indentation format**, the date and the closing compliment are centered on the page. The first line of every paragraph in the body and other content not already specified is aligned on the left side of the document. The subsequent lines of every paragraph in the body are indented five spaces to the right.
- In **simplified format**, all content is aligned on the left side of the document. However, this format does not include a greeting or a closing compliment.

Memoranda

Unlike letters, memos, as they are commonly known, are internal documents. They generally have four different headings:

1. TO:
2. FROM:
3. DATE:
4. SUBJECT: (you sometimes see "RE:" instead of "SUBJECT:")

For each of these headings, the relevant content should appear on the same line. For example:

TO: Joseph Angelo

The body of the memo should appear three line spaces after the subject line. Like letters, memos may have reference or copy notation. The same rules that applied to letters regarding these elements apply to memos. More often than not, specific medical offices will have a template that should be used for all memos.

Manuscripts

If your office submits manuscripts for publication, chances are the publisher will provide specific information about the style and format required of all submissions. Some general elements you should be sure that each manuscript includes are:

- title page
- acknowledgments
- summary
- text
- references
- footnotes
- bibliography
- graphic elements

Remember, it is most important that you follow the submission guidelines provided by the publisher. These guidelines take precedence over the general information found here.

MAIL PROCESSING AND SCREENING

Envelopes

It is best to use a business-size envelope to mail all correspondence. The business envelope is a No. 10 and measures $4\frac{1}{8}$ by $9\frac{1}{2}$ inches. You may also use a smaller envelope inside the correspondence for the patient to return payment. The postage meter will seal and stamp the envelope once it is ready to be mailed.

Labels

It can take a lot of time to address envelopes for bulk mailings. Address labels, which are printed from a computerized mailing list, will reduce the time needed to address the envelopes. To make your job easier, you can prepare the labels with the medical practice's name and address on the label for the return address. Labels can be used in other correspondence from the medical office such as referrals and business mail. Be sure to follow the U.S. Postal Service (USPS) guidelines for addressing envelopes.

Invoices and Statements

You may be responsible for mailing out the invoices and statements every month. Preprinted invoices are used to send an original bill. The amount that is due will be preprinted on the invoice. Preprinted statements are mailed out from the medical office as a reminder when an account is 30 days or more overdue. Computer-generated invoices and statements are automatically generated each month. You would have the responsibility to ensure that the envelopes are mailed. Superbills are another piece of mail that may have to be mailed monthly.

Preparing Outgoing Mail

The address or address label must be placed in a certain spot on the envelope. The handwritten address or label needs to be placed on the envelope with a one-inch border on the left and right side of the envelope. The address also is placed two-and-a-half inches from the bottom of the envelope to the top of the address. The USPS uses optical character recognition (OCR) to sort mail. It is important to prepare outgoing mail to meet the requirements for OCR.

Folding the letters and invoices into the envelopes needs to be done neatly. It is important that the correspondence fits in the right-sized envelope. When using a small envelope, fold the letter in half lengthwise before inserting it. While using a business-size envelope, fold the letter in thirds. The best way to fold a business-size letter is to fold the bottom third up first, then the top third down. When using envelopes with a window, the mailing address must be clearly seen through the window. Fold the bottom third up, and then fold the top third back so that the address appears in the window.

Different Postal Delivery Services

First-class mail, second-class mail, third-class mail, fourth-class mail, priority mail, and express mail are examples of regular mail service. You need to be aware of which regular mail service you will need to use.

- **First-class:** Most of the mail sent out from the medical office will be sent first-class. First-class mail must weigh 13 ounces or less.

- **Second-class:** This class is used for mailing newspapers and periodicals only. It may be used in your practice if you send regular newsletters or magazines to patients.

- **Third-class:** This is bulk mail, used for mailing books, catalogs, and other printed material that weighs less than 16 ounces.

- **Fourth-class:** This is used for third-class mail items weighing over 1 pound.

- **Priority:** This is used for mail that needs to be delivered quicker than fourth class. Any mail that weighs between 13 ounces and 70 pounds may be sent via priority mail. Rates are based on weight and distance.

- **Express:** This is the quickest postal service available. Different types are available, including next-day and second-day delivery. Rates are based on weight and specific service.

Special postal services are also available.

- **Certified mail:** This service guarantees that the item has been received. It also requires the mail carrier to get a signature when it is delivered. The certified mail signature card becomes a legal document, which may be important in court.

- **Return receipt requested:** This is a request for a return receipt to get proof that a letter was delivered. This receipt shows who has received the item and when it was received.

- **Registered mail:** Valuable or irreplaceable items are sent by registered mail. This provides proof that the mail was sent and delivered.

- **Overnight delivery:** United Parcel Service (UPS), Federal Express, and DHL deliver overnight for quick delivery. The USPS also delivers overnight and is sometimes the least expensive option.

Opening and Sorting Mail in the Physician's Office

Another important job in the medical office is opening and sorting the mail. Your office may have unique rules as to how the mail should be handled, but the following are general guidelines that should be followed.

1. Check address to ensure that the letter has been delivered correctly

2. Sort the mail in piles by priority:
   - **Top priority:** sent by overnight mail, registered mail, certified mail, or special delivery; faxes and emails are also top priority
   - **Second priority:** personal or confidential mail
   - **Third priority:** all first-class mail, airmail, and priority mail
   - **Fourth priority:** packages
   - **Fifth priority:** magazines and newspapers
   - **Sixth priority:** advertisement and catalogs

Mail that is labeled "Personal" or "Confidential" is set aside to be given to the addressee and only the addressee should open it. Once the mail is sorted, deliver it to the correct recipients. Bills and statements that are received are stamped with the date. Only discard the envelope after carefully checking it for any additional information. It is a good idea to check the return address with the current address on file for that patient. The accounts receivable employee may do so when posting the payment.

All medical assistants should follow an established procedure that allows them to process and route the mail efficiently.

REVIEW QUESTIONS

1. Which type of appointment scheduling is most likely to be used for short patient visits in an office with multiple practitioners?

    (A) Double-booking

    (B) Wave

    (C) Modified-wave

    (D) Cluster

    (E) Time-specified

2. Which of the following completes the necessary paperwork for the insurance company on a referral?

    (A) Physician

    (B) Insurance company

    (C) Medical assistant

    (D) Patient

    (E) Specialist's office

3. A numeric filing system

    (A) is not used when patient confidentiality is especially important

    (B) organizes records according to the patient's last name

    (C) is the most commonly used filing system

    (D) may include portions of the patient's social security number

    (E) is the only practical system for a large practice

4. The policy and procedures manual is written jointly by

    (A) all the employees

    (B) the physician(s)

    (C) the physician and the staff

    (D) the medical assistants

    (E) using a manual from another office

5. Which of the following items is an output device?

    (A) Scanner

    (B) Monitor

    (C) Peripheral

    (D) Software

    (E) Keyboard

ANSWERS AND EXPLANATIONS

1. **A**

   With a double-booking system, two or more patients are scheduled for the same appointment slot. Wave scheduling (B) is based on the idea that some patients will be late and other patients require more time with the doctor. Modified-wave scheduling (C) can be used different ways. One way is to schedule in 15-minute slots, regardless of appointment type. Cluster scheduling (D) groups similar appointments together during the day or week. Time-specified scheduling (E) assumes a steady stream of patients all day at regular intervals.

2. **C**

   The medical assistant has the responsibility to complete the insurance portion of the referral. The physician (A) completes the procedure to be done. The insurance (B) receives the completed referral. The patient (D) does not have the responsibility to complete the referral. The specialist's office (E) would receive the completed referral.

3. **D**

   A numeric filing system may include the last four digits of a social security number. The numeric system is used when patient confidentiality is important (A). This system uses numbers, not names (B). This is not the most commonly used filing system (C). This system as well as the alphabetical system are good (E).

4. **C**

   A joint effort is used in creating a policy and procedures manual in a medical office between the physician and staff. The manual cannot be written by the employees only (A). The physician or physicians would need the assistance of the staff (B). The medical assistant alone (D) would not be the one to complete the policy and procedure manual. The help of the physician would be needed. Each medical office has its own circumstances and would require its own policy and procedures manual (E).

5. **B**

   A monitor is an output device. It displays information for the user. The scanner (A) is used to enter graphic information into the computer. Peripherals (C) are pieces of hardware that connect to the CPU. A peripheral may be an input or an output device. Software (D) refers to programs that tell the computer what to do. The keyboard (E) is used to enter text into a computer.

Chapter 11: **Financial Management**

An important aspect of a well-run medical office is sound financial management. Medical assistants need to be familiar with key financial and business activities including third-party reimbursement for health care, claims preparation and processing, and some basic accounting principles. In this section you will review these and other office activities related to financial management.

REIMBURSEMENT FOR MEDICAL CARE/THIRD-PARTY BILLING

Health care is costly, and most of the services provided to your patients will be reimbursed in full or in part by a third-party payer. The types of payers vary from government-funded programs to employer-sponsored insurance coverage and patients who do not have insurance coverage. You will need to understand the basic concepts associated with these forms of coverage for health care cost containment. It will also be important to know the type(s) of insurance coverage available to your patients, and for you to keep up-to-date records regarding their billing information.

Forms of Third-Party Coverage

Traditional Indemnity Health Insurance/Commercial Insurance Carriers

Medical assistants need to know about the different types of reimbursement systems available today to fund health care. Medical assistants will often be called upon to help patients and others understand how reimbursement systems function.

There are several different types of private health insurance. Traditional indemnity insurance policies include coverage on a fee-for-service basis. In this method of reimbursement, the insurer pays the provider a fee based on the cost of service. The insurance company creates a list of usual and customary charges for each type of service provided. The patient or the patient's employer, along with the patient, pays a monthly premium for health coverage. Employer-sponsored plans offer group coverage, while individuals who buy insurance on their own receive individual coverage (which may extend to family members as well). The patient is usually responsible for paying a deductible and a coinsurance amount. Bills are submitted to the insurance company and if the annual deductible has been met, the coinsurance is applied to the difference. Payment is made either to the physician (if the patient assigns benefits to the physician) or to both the insured and physician.

Most insurance policies cover payment only when there are diagnoses of illness, disease, or injury. Generally, they do not cover routine examinations. They may not cover tests or procedures for cosmetic or elective procedures such as fertility treatments. Only a small number of policies cover routine physicals or preventative health care.

Medical insurers often define two types of coverage: basic insurance and major medical insurance. Basic insurance covers a specific dollar amount for physicians' fees, hospital care, surgery, and anesthesia. Major medical coverage is designed to cover some of the costs of catastrophic expenses from illness or injury.

Blue Cross/Blue Shield indemnity policies are a well-known type of traditional insurance. Over the years, this company has grown into a nonprofit organization providing basic and major medical coverage. In most parts of the United States, Blue Cross and Blue Shield work in conjunction with each other. Blue Cross normally covers hospitalization, radiology, and other basic coverage under the health plan. Blue Shield covers the major medical portion and physician fees. In addition to traditional indemnity plans, Blue Cross and Blue Shield also offer several capitated prepaid health plans that feature managed benefits and managed care options. In a capitated plan, a managed care group makes a fixed per capita payment periodically to a medical service provider (such as a physician) in return for medical care provided to enrolled individuals. In the United States, the indemnity coverage business is shrinking as employers and insurers seek to control health care spending.

Prepaid Health Insurance Options

In an attempt to curb medical costs and create efficient use of medical resources, managed care is increasingly the method used to reimburse for health care services. In a managed care system, the insurers require that policyholders seek medical attention only from preferred providers. Preferred providers are physicians and other health care professionals who contract with the insurance carrier to provide patient care at a discounted rate. Patients pay lower premiums and copays when they use a preferred provider. These plans are becoming more common as employers look for ways to reduce their share of the insurance premium and the cost of medical care. Physicians look for a secure payment with a shorter turnaround time.

Managed care organizations (MCOs) such as health maintenance organizations (HMOs) are another form of prepaid insurance. HMO enrollment varies widely across the United States. The major principles of MCOs are to offer health insurance programs that ensure cost-effective services. To accomplish this, MCOs:

1. Use primary care providers or case mangers who are paid an incentive to save dollars for the insurer and who channel patients to the most affordable and effective care options.

2. Require preauthorization for medical services, prospective and retrospective view of treatment plans, and significant discharge planning.

3. Use specific treatment guidelines for high-cost chronic disorders.

4. Place emphasis on outpatient care versus hospitalization.

5. Use a drug formulary, or list of medications that may be prescribed without pre-approval.

6. Place emphasis on health education and preventive care.

7. Place emphasis on patient/family collaboration with health care providers to improve patient's compliance with treatment regimen.

8. Utilize selective contracting with all health care providers and institutions involved to achieve discounted rates.

Six primary MCO models operate across the country. They include:

1. Integrated delivery systems

2. Health maintenance organizations

3. Exclusive provider organizations

4. Preferred provider organizations

5. Physician-hospital organizations

6. Utilization review organizations

Integrated delivery systems are groups of affiliated provider sites that operate under single ownership to offer full and/or specialty services to their subscribers. The affiliated providers may include physician offices or clinics, hospitals, ambulatory surgery sites, and other ancillary allied health facilities.

Integrated delivery systems negotiate group rates for all providers with the insurance companies.

Health maintenance organizations (HMOs) are another form of managed health care. HMOs cover large groups of people for a monthly premium and a small copayment from the patient at each time of service. Sometimes, physicians are employed by the HMO and are paid according to the number of members enrolled (capitation) rather than the number of visits. When the HMO employs the physicians, it is called a closed-panel HMO. Open-panel HMOs establish a network of preferred providers who agree to a capitated contract fee schedule. Ideally, members can have all their medical needs met by the HMO. Members cannot see a physician outside the HMO setting unless they pay out-of-pocket or more expensive copays for services.

An EPO (exclusive provider organization) plan delivers in-network-only benefits through the national Blue Card PPO network. EPO members must seek care from participating Blue Card PPO providers, except in the case of a life- or limb-threatening emergency. If care is received from a nonparticipating provider, the claim will not be paid. It is the member's responsibility to confirm that the providers and specialists they are seeing participate in the network. Claims will not be paid if care is received from a provider who is not in the network.

A network of physicians and hospitals that have contracted together with insurance companies to provide health care at a discounted fee is known as a preferred provider organization (PPO). Usually, PPOs do not have contracts for laboratory or pharmacy services, but they do offer reduced rate contracts with specific hospitals. Patients have a greater out-of-pocket fee if they choose to receive health care from an out-of-network provider.

A hospital and selected physicians may form a business arrangement known as a physician-hospital organization (PHO). The primary function of the PHO is to contract with MCOs to provide health care to their subscribers at a reasonable rate of payment.

Utilization review organizations are also known as third-party administrators. They supervise funds set aside to cover medical expenses to employees under self-insured plans. The utilization review organization determines medically necessary treatments, approves or denies payment of claims for these services, and completes a retrospective utilization review.

Government Payers

The federal government funds the health insurance coverage for the aged and disabled in the United States under the Medicare program. Initiated by an act of Congress in 1965, Medicare was created to provide medical coverage to seniors and disabled adults. Many Medicare recipients also buy supplementary insurance policies through private carriers, which are known as Medigap policies.

Medicare is administered by the Centers for Medicare and Medicaid Services (CMS). Individuals who are 65 or older can file for Medicare coverage Part A, which covers hospital care, skilled nursing home care, and home health care. Those seniors who select to do so can also purchase low-cost Part B coverage for outpatient care and physician services. Medicare claims are processed by a fiscal intermediary, or insurance carrier that has signed a contract with Medicare to handle all claims for a particular region of the country. In some areas of the country, Medicare has contracted with managed care companies to administer benefits.

When a physician agrees to accept Medicare assignment, Medicare's allowable charge is accepted as payment in full for that particular service. Medicare pays 80 percent of that amount and the patient pays the remaining 20 percent for a Part B claim. The difference between the physician's charge and the Medicare allowable charge is submitted to the patient. The benefits to the physician are that Medicare makes a direct payment to the physician.

At this time, an annual deductible of $100 must be paid by the patient before Medicare will begin to pay the patient's bills. The rate at which Medicare then reimburses is 80 percent of the Medicare fee schedule for medical care and 100 percent for laboratory fees. Laboratory fees are paid based on a scale of payment known as resource-based relative value scale (RBRVS).

Medicare, as well as many other insurance companies, uses a fee schedule based upon usual, customary, and reasonable (UCR) fees. "Usual" refers to the fee that the specific physician charges most of his patients for the same treatment. "Reasonable" refers to the midrange of fees charged for this type of procedure or visit. "Customary" is based on the average charge for a specific procedure by all the physicians practicing the same specialty in a specific geographical location.

The Medicaid program is another form of government-funded health insurance for people who are unable to work due to illness or life circumstance. Medicaid is funded by both the federal and the state government. Each state has a unique list of covered benefits for Medicaid coverage. Eligibility for coverage is based on income, employment status, and state-specific requirements. Physicians and medical offices are not required to accept Medicaid patients in their practices.

People who are on aid for families with dependent children and supplemental security income (SSI), single women who are pregnant and whose income is at or below the national poverty level, and people who for many reasons due to physical, emotional, or mental difficulties are unable to work may qualify for this program. The patient is given an identification card that is presented to the medical provider at the time of the office visit. A claim form is then completed and a copy of the card is attached to the form and mailed to the state-specific address. Some states have a requirement for a copayment by the recipient at the time of service. When a patient has both Medicare and Medicaid, charges are submitted first to Medicare and then to Medicaid. Both federal programs require strict adherence to correct billing. Errors in billing could be construed as fraud, for which criminal penalties apply. It is very important that all billing practices conform to the legal requirements for accuracy.

Military personnel are covered by the medical personnel in the armed services. However, their dependents (spouse and children) often are not able to receive medical care on the base. When dependents need medical care and no military medical care is easily available to them or they need emergency medical care, they may seek medical care from nonmilitary medical providers without prior authorization. TRICARE covers dependents of active-duty personnel, retired personnel, dependents of retired personnel, and dependents of personnel who died on active duty.

The Civilian Health and Medical Program of the Department of Veterans Affairs (CHAMPVA) covers spouses and unmarried dependent children of veterans with permanent total disabilities from service-related injuries and the surviving spouses and children of veterans who died of service-related disabilities.

Each person covered by TRICARE or CHAMPVA will have an identification card showing his or her name, identification number, and the program covered. A person cannot be covered by both TRICARE and CHAMPVA. TRICARE and CHAMPVA are billed after all other insurance coverage except Medicaid.

Workers' Compensation

When an on-the-job accident or illness results in injury and/or disability, workers' compensation insurance pays the medical bills and a significant portion of the lost wages if the patient was covered by a workers' compensation policy. In most states, employers are required to pay premiums to an insurance carrier for a policy known as workers' compensation insurance. The premium is based upon the number of workers employed and the degree of occupational risk a job entails.

The medical office establishes and maintains separate medical records for workers' compensation claims and routine health care. Health issues not related to the workers' compensation claim will not be covered under workers' compensation. When a claim is made, a workers' compensation claim form is completed and sent to the insurance carrier or to the state fund for reimbursement. The injured worker receives no bills, pays no deductible or coinsurance, and is covered 100 percent for medical expenses related specifically to the injury.

Self-Insurance

Many larger companies, nonprofit organizations, and state and county governments choose to self-insure in an attempt to reduce the costs of medical insurance and to gain more control over the finances. In self-insured plans, special accounts are established and rather than paying premiums to an insurance carrier, the entity makes payments into the plan. Each self-insured plan will differ in its organization and claim filing requirements; if a patient is covered by a self-insured plan, call the plan administrator before scheduling a patient appointment.

Physician Fee Schedules

Your office will have a list of published fees charged for common services and products used in practice. This list should be reviewed at least once a year or if any federal or state payment systems are significantly altered. The fees should be based on the actual cost of the physician's time, and the cost of goods and services used in the office. Fees should be set so that office overhead costs such as rent, utilities, equipment, and supplies are reimbursed. Your practice will not continue to remain in business if fees are set or maintained at or below the actual cost of service. Before entering into a capitated payment contract, financial staff or advisors should determine if the payment rate is going to be above or at the level of cost. Fee schedules should be made available to patients, and need to be provided to any insurance companies with which your practice contracts.

The physician rates may be verified by reviewing them against national and state-specific usual and customary charge schedules. The federal government publishes relative value units (RVUs) that identify a range of charges for varying degrees of common office procedures and activities. These RVUs are set for all forms of general practitioners and medical specialty services.

Another system to use in establishing fee schedules is RBRVS (resource based relative value scale). These scales help rank a variety of laboratory tests and medical products relative to the intensity of labor and goods used to produce them.

Your office will likely have a coded encounter form that will be used each time a patient is seen. This form will be used to bill the patient or third-party payer for a variety of goods and services used during their visit. Most practices charge more for an initial history and physical exam as it takes more time to complete and document the findings. The encounter form will also include a spot to check for supplies and medications used in care and treatment of patients in the office.

As a medical assistant, you should also be familiar with the basis of inpatient hospital reimbursement. Since the late 1980s, hospitals have been reimbursed based on a system known as DRGs or diagnostic-related groups. In this system, the government, under the Medicare program, pays a flat fee to the hospital based on a patient's diagnosis, age, and presence of comorbidities. As patients leave the hospital, medical record specialists review the clinical record and classify the patient into a correct payment classification group based on these variables. Payment is then made to the hospital, regardless of the actual costs incurred in the episode of illness.

BOOKKEEPING AND PATIENT ACCOUNTING PRACTICES

Daily financial management in the ambulatory care setting is most important to the functioning of the office as it directly affects overall accounting and bookkeeping procedures. Bookkeeping, the actual daily recording of the accounts or transactions of the business, is the major part of this accounting process.

One aspect of this recordkeeping in a medical practice is maintaining patient accounts. Encounter forms mentioned earlier should identify any and all products and services for which the patient and/or third-party payer will be charged. The money owed to the office by third-party payers or patients is known as accounts receivable, and must be carefully monitored. Good record keeping is needed to ensure that the physician is paid for services and that patients are properly credited for payments made. Accounts receivable balances should be managed to ensure that cash is flowing into the office to cover expenses and generate a level of profit for the practice.

The other important aspect of bookkeeping is maintaining a record of accounts payable. Accounts payable are amounts of money due for goods and services provided to the practice office. Payroll costs are an example of an accounts payable item. Additionally, charges for rent, utilities, consumable supplies, and housekeeping are other examples of accounts payable. The office manager, accountant, or medical assistant may be asked to keep track of incoming bills and assist with sending in payments to keep the payable accounts up to date.

Patient Accounts

The two most common ways to track patient accounts are the pegboard system and computerized systems. Converting from manual to computerized recordkeeping is initially expensive, requires thorough retraining of staff, and takes a great deal of time at the beginning. However, it offers great versatility and reduces the need to record and re-record entries. A well-prepared medical assistant needs to be fully versed in both bookkeeping systems. When changing over from manual to computerized, both systems should be run simultaneously for at least 60 days.

The pegboard system consists of day sheets, ledger cards, charge slips, and receipt forms. All of the forms will have matching columns that align and are held in place on the pegboard when the system is in use. The forms are generally filled out in multiple copies (e.g., carbon copies), which permit entering (or posting) such information as charges, credits, or adjustments onto the day sheet, charge slip or receipt, and the patient's ledger card simultaneously. Two major advantages of the pegboard system are its efficiency and minimal use of time. By only having to enter information once, errors are reduced or minimized. This can also be a major disadvantage when an error is made and the entry appears on all forms. The day sheet provides complete and up-to-date information about accounts receivable status at a glance. A pegboard system is relatively inexpensive to establish and maintain.

The day sheet is used to list or post each day's charges, payments, credits, and adjustments. At the end of each business day, the day sheet will be balanced to provide a complete picture of all financial activity for that day. Those balances carried over from day to day will provide the accumulated data needed for month-end closing. The day sheet has five sections. The first three are used when posting transactions and the last two are for balancing, proof of posting, accounts receivable control, and accounts receivable proof.

Section 1 is where individual transactions are posted, using the ledger card and charge slips, or receipt forms. The information here includes the date, patient name, description of transaction or service, charges, credits, and previous and current balances. This is the write-it-once portion of the day sheet. Section 2 is the deposit portion. If a transaction includes payment, the payment amount will be listed under the appropriate right-hand column showing method of payment after the ledger portion is posted. Section 3 is for business analysis. These columns might be used for recording payments or charges to be credited to different physicians or they are often used as a breakdown for types of service. Section 4 is where transactions are totaled and balanced at the end of the day. Section 5 is used to verify the daily balances and to balance and track cumulative accounts receivable figures. The total accounts receivable figure shows how much is owed to the practice by all patients to date.

Ledger cards record services provided and charges and payments for each individual seen in the office or hospital. A separate card is created for each patient household. The columns on the front of the ledger card will show the date of activity, name of patient, a clear description of type of activity, charge or credit amount, adjustments (if any), and the family's total balance due. The back of the ledger card shows all pertinent patient demographic information and insurance information needed for bill collection. The ledger is placed under the charge slip or receipt, directly on the day sheet, and aligned prior to posting.

The encounter form (also called a charge slip or superbill) is a three-part form that provides patients with a record of account activity for the day, may eliminate the need for separate insurance forms, and provides the office with a copy of services, which will be filed in the individual's chart. Charge slips can be ordered to fit the specific needs of the practice. The information on the charge slip includes not only the amount of the day's transaction, but procedure codes and diagnosis codes that satisfy the requirements for most insurance companies to reimburse for the care provided. After seeing a patient, the physician places a check mark beside the services rendered. There is also an area for the diagnosis code to be filled in by the physician or assistant at the same time. The charge slip is printed with the name, address, and telephone number of the practice.

The receipt form is only used when someone makes a payment on the account and no services were rendered that day. There is only one copy of this form, which is given to the patient after the payment is recorded.

Adjustments are entries made to change the patient's balance but do not represent charges or payments. The adjustment column is a credit column, and therefore entries here normally reduce the balance due.

Day sheets are always balanced at the end of each workday. If more than one day sheet is required to record all of the transactions for a full day, balance each day sheet as if it were the end of the day and carry the standard information forward to the next day sheet as if it were a new day. On the last day of the month it will be necessary to verify that the month-end figures on the day sheet agree with patient's ledgers.

A software management program offers many advantages in managing patient accounts. The program automatically creates a charge slip at the time of each patient's visit. After the physician's examination, the program calculates the charges for the monthly billing statement. The management program also creates and updates the ledger card; adds new names to the list of patients and to the daily log; and transfers data to produce insurance forms, statements, lists of checks received each day, and deposit slips. The program also automatically ages the accounts at each billing cycle and creates billing statements. The computerized patient ledger contains personal information about each patient, including name, address, and telephone number; the person responsible for payment; and all insurance carriers.

BILLING AND CLAIMS PROCESSING

The best method of billing and collections is customized to the practice and regards the patient as a consumer who should be respected. Patients want to know in advance what charges and fees to expect whenever possible. Accurate billing techniques will make the cash flow and collection process smoother in the medical office. The best time for collection is at the time of service. This assures prompt collection, eliminates further bookkeeping work, and provides better cash flow for the practice.

In those cases where a payment schedule is arranged, it must be determined by the office whether or not interest will be charged. Ambulatory care settings may decide to charge interest for installment arrangements. The Truth-in-Lending Act (also called the Consumer Credit Protection Act of 1968) was established to protect consumers by requiring that providers of installment credit state the charges clearly in writing and express the interest as an annual rate. When there is a bilateral agreement between the physician and patient to pay more than four installments, the physician must disclose finance charges in writing. Even if no finance charges are made, the forms must still be completed.

The billing schedule is often determined by the size of the medical practice. In monthly billing, all accounts are billed at the same time each month. In a cycle billing system, all accounts are divided alphabetically into groups, with each group billed at a different time. In this way, personnel in a large practice with numerous bills to process each month will be able to handle them in a more efficient manner.

Preparing Medical Claims

Demographic Information

It is important for the medical office to provide accurate information on the bills. Demographic information regarding the patient will include the correct spelling of the name, the date of birth, the social security number, mailing address, and phone number. The office will also need to provide the third-party payer with the correct address, name and provider number of the physician, date of service, and the date of submission of the claim.

Coding

Coding is the basis for establishing the charges listed on the claim form. Medical coding is mandatory for the accurate transmission of procedures and diagnosis information between health care providers and the insurance companies or other payers. Codes are assigned both to identify the diagnoses of the patient and to specify the treatment or procedure that was provided as care and treatment.

The process of converting descriptions of diseases, injuries, and procedures into numerical designations is termed coding. Current Procedural Terminology (CPT) was developed by the American Medical Association (AMA) to convert commonly accepted, uniform descriptions of medical, surgical, and diagnostic services rendered by health care providers into five-digit numeric codes. These codes must be listed correctly on claim forms and bills to specify what services were rendered to patients.

The International Classification of Disease, 10th Revision, Clinical Modification (ICD-10-CM) was compiled by the World Health Organization (WHO). It is designed for the classification of patient diagnostic morbidity and mortality information. ICD codes are assigned for disease states, surgical procedures, and the full range of causative events such as injuries and poisonings. Level II HCPCS codes identify services and supplies that lack CPT-4 codes but are covered by many insurers.

Procedure codes and codes for patient encounters of all kinds—office, hospital, nursing facility, home services—are found in Current Procedural Terminology (CPT). This listing is updated annually. The CPT manual is divided into six sections, and each CPT code is five digits long:

- Evaluation and Management (codes start with **99**)
- Anesthesia (codes start with **0**)
- Surgery (codes start with **1–6**)
- Radiology (codes start with **7**)
- Pathology and Laboratory (codes start with **8**)
- Medicine (codes start with **9**)

For the insurance company to understand what is being billed, the claim form is completed by the medical assistant in the office setting. The physician completes a charge slip at the time of the visit. As discussed earlier in this chapter, the charge slip includes the date of service, the visit or consult code, diagnosis for this visit, procedures performed, and lab tests collected. This information is then translated onto the claim form.

The CMS1500 is the claim form accepted by most insurance carriers. This form is prepared using both name identifiers and CPT codes for procedures performed and ICD-10-CM codes for pertinent patient diagnoses. If the coding is omitted, incomplete, or noted to be in error, payment may be denied or delayed. Coding must correlate with the physician's note in the chart and the actual status of the patient. It is likely that individual insurance companies will require some unique information or procedures for correctly submitting medical claims information.

Figure 11.1—Universal Claim Form

The Move to ICD-10-CM and ICD-10- PCS Coding

In October 2015, the health care industry transitioned to an entirely new coding system that brought major changes to systems, processes, and staff involved in health information and health care delivery. As a medical assistant, you should remain current on changes to the new coding system to ensure appropriate billing that maximizes provider reimbursement.

Rationale for the Change

In 1979, the federal government—through the Health Care Financing Administration (HCFA)—adopted a procedure coding system to use in tandem with the *International Classification of Diseases, 9th Revision*, as established by the World Health Organization (WHO). Since that time, all health care providers in the United States have used the ICD-9-CM to code and track medical diagnoses for billing purposes and for epidemiologic tracking of diseases and conditions that befall the population. Since 1983, government and private payers have used the system of diagnostic and procedure coding for reimbursement of health care services. As the complexity of healthcare grows, the need for accuracy and specificity of coding systems has escalated. The code sets designed in the 1970s are no longer an adequate reflection of the care and treatment rendered in the United States in the 21st century. In addition, the structure of the coding system has run out of space and it has been difficult for experts to accommodate changes and additions that reflect new medical practice and newer disease states. It has also been determined that the ICD-9 system does not allow enough detail to describe complex patient statuses or account for the variety of health care encounters that occur in practice. The need to replace the ICD-9 system was recognized in the 1990s when the National Committee on Vital and Health Statistics studied the need for a more accurate and updated system and made recommendations for change.

Key Changes and Benefits of ICD-10 System Enhancements

The National Center for Health Statistics worked with a variety of professional organizations and experts to devise the U.S. Clinical Modifications in the ICD-10-CM system. A major effort was made to add detail and specificity to the system and to add language that fits the current clinical practice activities in health care. The new ICD-10-CM system uses 68,069 codes, up from the 14,025 in use with ICD-9-CM conventions. Extensive testing and public and professional input were sought in forming this new coding system. In addition to adding more levels of detail to the codes, professionals are better able to work with the system to add new codes and revise as medical advances occur. The new coding system is able to provide better and more detailed information to evaluate the quality of patient care. It provides more detail on patient complications, clinical outcomes, and comparison of treatments and conditions across the globe. In addition, the system enables public health officials to track disease outbreaks and bioterrorism events internationally and allows more sharing of practice patterns used to treat disease states.

The following items are proposed as the areas for data improvement based on the ICD-10 coding systems:

- Ability to measure patient care quality, safety, and outcomes of care
- Potential to design payment stems that improve claims processing

- Information availability for health research, epidemiology and clinical trials

- Establishing health policy based on detailed information

- Improvement in health care planning and tracking of health care resource use

- Tracking and reporting public health and medical risk factors

In addition to these improvements, it is anticipated that the new ICD-10 systems will contribute to lowering the cost of health care and improving operating efficiency of health systems through the following means:

- Increasing the use of automation in clinical coding

- Decreasing the claims associated requests for additional detailed medical information

- Decreasing rejected or improper claims for payment of health care

- Decreasing need for manual clinical record reviews

- Reducing coding and billing errors

- Potentially reducing labor costs and increasing staff productivity

Specific Changes Included in ICD-10-CM

The WHO ICD-10 system contains a completely new alphanumeric, structure for coding. The first character in all codes is a letter. All letters are used except U, which has been set aside for new diseases with uncertain causes or causes from bacterial agents that are resistant to antibiotics. The ICD-10-CM includes a tabular list organized alphabetically with indentations for qualifiers and descriptors. Unlike codes in the ICD-9 system, which contain up to five digits, the ICD-10 system uses seven digits. Below is a comparison of the coding structures across the two systems.

ICD-9 Coding Format

XXX.XX, where the first three digits signify the category of the disease and the last two digits (after the decimal) signify the etiology of the disease, the anatomic site and the manifestations presented.

ICD-10 Coding Format

XXX.XXXX, where the first three digits signify the category of the disease; the fourth, fifth and sixth digits signify the etiology, anatomic site, and severity; and the seventh digit signifies the extension.

In addition to the coding structure noted above, the following major changes have been made in the organization of the codes, the structure of the codes and the level of detail of coding.

- The order of the chapters of codes has been rearranged and the number of chapters has expanded to 21.

- All code titles are provided with no references to common fourth and fifth digits in earlier codes.

- All supplementary codes used in ICD-9 CM (E CODES and V CODES) are incorporated into the main classifications of the manual.

- Conditions with newly discovered etiology or treatments have been reclassified into their appropriate chapters.

- Postoperative complication codes have been expanded; those occurring during a procedure and those occurring postprocedure have been separated.

- Dummy placeholders using an X are used in some codes to allow for future expansion.

- Instructional notes to coders have been expanded.

- Extensions have been added in the seventh digit to describe the type of encounter for injuries and treatment of externally caused injuries and illnesses.

- Details for ambulatory and managed care encounters have been expanded.

In addition to the changes listed, many chapters have been updated and changed significantly from the ICD-9-CM system. These include injuries, diabetes, substance abuse, and postoperative complications. Along with changes in the coding of diseases and illnesses, significant changes also have been made to the ICD-10-PCS (procedural coding system). These changes, however, will only be used in inpatient facilities and are thus outside of the scope of this manual. Medical offices and clinics will continue to use the current CPT (Current Procedural Terminology) and HCPCS codes.

Medical assistants should keep their knowledge of ICD-10 implementation fresh by attending professional conferences, doing independent reading, or taking advantage of training and education provided by billing or software vendors.

Claims Processing

With the implementation of electronic health records, the use of manual claim submission has decreased dramatically. Regardless of the method of submission, it is important that to file claims in a timely fashion, as close to the date of service as possible. Claims should be numbered and tracked in a filing system for review. Once the claim is submitted, an accounting record should be made of the amount due in the accounts receivable system as money due to the practice. As a general rule, the older the account is from the date of payment, the less likely the practice is to collect the money. Some third-party payers may take time to submit claims payment. In order to keep a steady cash flow, an office should track payments through a claims register.

In filing claims, it may be that more than one payer is billed. Initially, the office practice should submit the bill to the patient's identified primary insurer or governmental payer. If the primary payer denies coverage, you may need to bill a secondary source. Many practices require the patient to sign a statement indicating that they will pay for any charges not covered by their insurance (or third-party payer). Most third parties require that claims be submitted in a sequential or chronological order based on the date of service. It is common for high-cost services to require supplemental documentation or clinical records to justify payment.

As claims are paid, the office staff will need to post the payments onto the patient's account records and determine if any unpaid balances are due. If all or part of the claim goes unpaid, the payer should be contacted for an explanation of benefits. The physician should then determine if the partial payment will be accepted or if another party should be billed for the balance.

In working with managed care organizations (MCO), you will still need to provide accurate and timely billing records. Each MCO will have unique forms and systems for payment that you must follow as part of your contractual obligation. Most MCOs require prior authorization for specialty referrals, elective surgery, or any needed patient equipment and supplies. You need to refer to the specific processes of each event or patient need as required for your patients and their insurance companies and third-party payers.

THE AFFORDABLE CARE ACT

This law, sometimes informally called "Obamacare," was signed in March 2010. It is composed of two parts: The Patient Protection and Affordable Care Act, and The Health Care and Reconciliation Act. It also includes additional amendments to other laws including the Food, Drug, and Cosmetic Act, and the Health and Public Services Act.

The Affordable Care Act is designed to reform the health care system by providing affordable insurance coverage and access to quality health care for all Americans while curbing or controlling the cost of health care spending. In addition, it is designed to eliminate discrimination in delivering services and charging for those services.

At press time, the administration of President Donald J. Trump had initiated action to repeal and replace Obamacare.

Impact of the Affordable Care Act on Medical Assisting

Health care reform in the United States has increased the emphasis on primary care. It has also dramatically expanded the number of people with health care coverage to more than 32 million. As a result, it is anticipated that the number of patients seeking outpatient care will also rise, expanding the need for qualified providers and allied health professionals to deliver these services. To contain costs, nurse practitioners, physician assistants, and medical assistants will play valuable and increasingly important roles in the U.S. health care system.

Medical assistants must be familiar with all insurance plans and understand provider and patient responsibilities, both to deliver the highest level of customer service and to assure that payment is received in a timely manner. Continuing education in the area of health care coverage is imperative in this ever-changing arena.

PAYROLL

The medical assistant may be involved in making certain the W-4 form (Employee's Withholding Allowance Certificate) is completed by all employees. If the medical assistant is also the office manger, then he or she has the responsibility to prepare payroll checks for each employee and record all deductions withheld. An up-to-date record on every employee is very important when complying with government regulations. Information should be gathered from new employees and updated every year and upon any change in employee status. Every employee file should contain a copy of an I-9 form, copy of social security card, number of exemptions claimed on the W-4 form, the employee's gross salary, and all deductions withheld for all taxes including social security, federal, state, local, plus unemployment tax (where applicable), and disability insurance (where applicable). When preparing payroll checks, it is important to keep a record of all tax and insurance amounts deducted from an employee's earnings.

Each paycheck stub should contain:

- Number of hours worked, including regular and overtime (if hourly)
- Date of pay periods
- Date of check
- Gross salary
- Itemized deductions for federal income tax, social security (FICA) tax, state taxes, city or local taxes
- Itemized deductions for health insurance
- Itemized deductions for disability insurance
- Other deductions such as uniforms, loan payments, and net salary (gross earnings minus taxes and deductions)

When figuring out federal income taxes and social security taxes, use the charts provided by the Internal Revenue Service. Federal tax amount is based on amount earned, marital status, number of exemptions claimed, and length of pay period. State and city or local taxes are typically a percentage of the gross earnings.

Benefits, or additional remuneration to the salary earned by full-time employees, must also be managed and records maintained for each employee. Examples of benefits may include paid vacation, paid holidays, health/dental insurance, disability, profit-sharing options, and complimentary health care.

REVIEW QUESTIONS

1. Which of the following was developed to cover the costs of catastrophic expenses from illness or injury?

    (A) Medicaid insurance

    (B) Medicare insurance

    (C) Primary care

    (D) Private insurance

    (E) Major medical insurance

2. Physicians and other health care professionals who contract with the insurance carrier to provide patient care are called

    (A) preferred providers

    (B) managed care organizations

    (C) assignment of benefits

    (D) primary care physician

    (E) exclusive provider organization

3. The process of using the number of members enrolled in a plan to determine salary of the physician is called

    (A) basic insurance

    (B) HMO

    (C) capitation

    (D) catchment

    (E) CHAMPVA

4. The dependents of active-duty personnel, retired personnel, dependents of retired personnel, and dependents of personnel who died while on active duty are covered by

    (A) CHAMPVA

    (B) TRICARE

    (C) SSI

    (D) EPO

    (E) HMO

5. In most states, the employer pays a premium to an insurance carrier for a policy known as

    (A) workers' compensation insurance

    (B) private insurance

    (C) TRICARE

    (D) Medicaid

    (E) Medicare

6. The EOB document may include all the of the following EXCEPT
   (A) allowed amounts
   (B) coding updates
   (C) deductible
   (D) patient name
   (E) payment responsibilities

7. Medicare is a federal health insurance program for the following categories of people EXCEPT
   (A) blind individuals
   (B) disabled widows
   (C) patients with end-stage renal disease
   (D) people 65 years or older
   (E) preschool children

8. ICD-9-CM codes that may be assigned during an encounter that are not necessarily a diagnosis but are factors that may influence a patient's health status are referred to as
   (A) E&M codes
   (B) E-codes
   (C) V-codes
   (D) Volume I codes
   (E) Volume II codes

9. An agreement in which the health care provider is paid a fixed amount for each person in a specific contract within the practice, regardless of service provided, is called
   (A) capitation
   (B) fixed coverage
   (C) total coverage
   (D) universal coverage
   (E) utilization review

10. Inquiry with an insurance company into the maximum dollar amount that will be paid for a procedure is called an insurance
    (A) coinsurance
    (B) preauthorization
    (C) precertification
    (D) predetermination
    (E) reimbursement

ANSWERS AND EXPLANATIONS

1. **E**

   Major medical insurance was developed to cover the costs of catastrophic expenses from illness or injury. Medicaid (A) was created to help those who are on aid for families with dependent children and supplemental security income. Medicare (B) was created to give all seniors access to health care. Primary care (C) is given by a general practitioner. In an HMO, all care is coordinated through the patient's primary care physician. Private insurance (D) is when a person pays for insurance on his own and not through an employer.

2. **A**

   Preferred providers are physicians and other health care professionals who contract with the insurance carrier to provide patient care. Managed care organizations (MCOs) (B) offer health insurance programs that ensure cost-effective services by employing case managers or primary care providers to keep costs down. Assigning of benefits (C) is signing over of benefits by the beneficiary to another party. Primary care physicians (D) serve as the key point of care for their patients. Primary care physicians may be responsible for any or all referrals to other specialty practices. Exclusive provider organizations (EPOs) (E) often require the provider to work exclusively for the EPO organization.

3. **C**

   Capitation is the use of the members enrolled in a plan to determine salary of the physician; the physician is paid a fixed fee for each member no matter how many times that member is seen by the physician. Basic insurance (A) is medical insurance that covers most physician fees, hospital expenses, and surgical fees according to the terms of the policy. The patient is usually responsible for a deductible. A health maintenance organization (HMO) (B) is the type of managed care operation that is typically set up as a for-profit corporation with salaried employees. A catchment (D) is a 40-mile radius of a military base where medical care is available to military dependents. Civilian Health and Medical Program of the Department of Veterans Affairs (CHAMPVA) (E) covers the spouse and unmarried dependent children of a veteran with permanent total disability from service-related injury and the surviving spouse and children of veterans who died of a service-related disability.

4. **B**

   TRICARE is the insurance that covers the dependents of active-duty personnel, retired personnel, dependents of retired personnel, and dependents of personnel who died while on duty. Civilian Health and Medical Program of the Department of Veterans Affairs or CHAMPVA (A), covers the spouse and unmarried dependent children of a veteran with permanent total disability from service-related injury and the surviving spouse and children of veterans who died of a service-related disability. Supplemental Security Income or SSI (C) is a federally funded program that assists single women who are pregnant and whose income is at or below the national poverty level, and people who for many reasons due to physical, emotional, or mental difficulties are unable to work. An exclusive provider organization or EPO (D) is a type of insurance. It usually requires that the physician work for the EPO organization. Health maintenance organization or HMO (E) is a type of managed care facility. It is very different from the traditional insurance.

5. **A**

   When an on-the-job accident or illness results in injury and/or disability, workers' compensation insurance (A) pays the medical bills. In most states, the employer pays a premium to an insurance carrier for a policy. Private insurance (B) is when a person pays for insurance on his own and not through an employer. TRICARE (C) is the insurance that covers the dependents of active-duty personnel, retired personnel, dependents of retired personnel, and dependents of personnel who died while on duty. Medicaid (D) was created to help those who are on aid for families with dependent children and supplemental security income. Medicare (E) was created to give all seniors access to health care.

6. **B**

   An EOB is an Explanation of Benefits. This patient-facing document does not include coding updates. The insurance company provides the EOB to the patient under the patient's name (D) following a claim by a provider. The EOB includes the amount of deductible (C) the patient has met and has yet to meet before additional coverage is included. It also demonstrates how much the insurance company allowed (A) and how much was paid, as well as any additional obligations the patient has for payment (E). If the provider has entered an agreement with the insurance company, the provider is obligated to accept the paid amount and not bill for the higher amount, excluding any deductible that may be required to be paid. The EOB would also note any exclusions and explain why a particular claim was not covered.

7. **E**

   Medicare is a federally funded health insurance program under the Social Security Act. Preschool children would not qualify for Medicare but may qualify for Medicaid, another federal program that works in conjunction with the individual states. Medicare covers all the other categories of people listed. In addition, patients with amyotrophic lateral sclerosis (ALS, also known as Lou Gehrig's disease) may qualify for Medicare after a waiting period.

8. **C**

    ICD coding is important for efficient and proper reimbursement for services rendered and is also used for statistical purposes. V-codes record a patient encounter for something other than disease or injury; they can be used as primary or secondary codes in billing and include health information such as exposure to a contagious disease like tuberculosis, even if the patient is not currently sick. E&M codes (A) are evaluation and management billing codes that are derived from reading the medical record and determining the services provided, the medical necessity and appropriateness of the services, and the location of services. E-codes (B) are supplemental codes that identify the external cause of an injury or poisoning. Volume I codes (D) are those found in the ICD book, which contains the tabular list of diseases and is numerically coded. Volume II codes (E) are an alphabetical listing of diseases and disorders.

9. **A**

    The root *capit* means "head," and *capitation* means that payment is per head or per patient. This type of a provider/insurance agreement pays the practitioner per patient, usually on a monthly basis, whether the patient is seen multiple times or not at all. Fixed coverage plans (B) are sold by insurance companies to patients; they are designed to provide the patient with a fixed amount of payment each time they see a provider. Fixed coverage plans are becoming less common because they tend not to meet minimal essential coverage needs. Total coverage (C) is a plan that covers all aspects of a patient's care. This type of coverage is unusual today given the rising cost of health care; often a copayment or coinsurance is required. Universal coverage (D) is usually offered to all citizens of the same country with the goal of assuring all citizens receive health care. Utilization review (E) is a periodic evaluation to determine if billing and other insurance components are being administered correctly.

10. **D**

    Patients have a right to know how much they will have to pay out of pocket for a particular procedure or service; predetermination is a means of providing that information to the patient. If an elective procedure is planned, the patient may then choose to establish a payment plan with the provider prior to services being performed. Coinsurance (A) is a percentage of the fee that the patient may be required to pay for the procedure. Preauthorization (B) is the process of getting permission from the patient's insurance company for procedures, tests, and other medical services. Precertification (C) is often used for hospitalization admissions to determine the maximum length of stay allowed for a particular procedure. Reimbursement (E) is repayment for the patient's out-of-pocket expenses after expenses have been incurred.

Chapter 12: **Patients in the Clinical Setting**

This chapter will review important information about clinical practice activities in the medical office. The topics include basic infection control procedures, treatments, and preparation of treatment areas. In addition, you will review patient history taking and strategies of assisting physicians with patient examination.

PRINCIPLES OF INFECTION CONTROL

An important aspect of health care is to avoid doing harm to the patient. Infection control is critical to successful patient outcomes, as well as to your own health and well-being as a provider of care.

Infectious disease is caused by pathogens or agents. These pathogens are microorganisms or organisms that are too small to be seen without a microscope. Methods must be used to halt the transmission of these organisms in the medical office.

The Chain of Infection

The spread of disease is dependent on a series of factors called the chain of infection. All of the links of this chain must be intact for infectious disease to spread. The goal of infection control is to stop the chain of infection from completing this series to prevent disease

The first link in the chain is the infective agent. The agent may be a virus, bacterium, protozoa, fungus, or rickettsia. The second link in the chain is the reservoir host. Potential hosts include contaminated people, insects, animals, food, water, or other objects including medical equipment. The reservoir host is where the pathogen resides prior to infecting a person. The third link is the portal of exit, which is how the agent leaves the host and spreads to another. The pathogen is then transmitted to the infected patient. Transmission (the fourth link) can occur with either direct or indirect contact. The pathogen might be expelled into the air from the host, transmitted by contaminated food or drink, or deposited on an inanimate object called a fomite. The pathogen is then picked up and deposited in the portal of entry. The pathogen may also be spread by a vector, which is an insect or animal that is capable of passing the pathogen on to a human host.

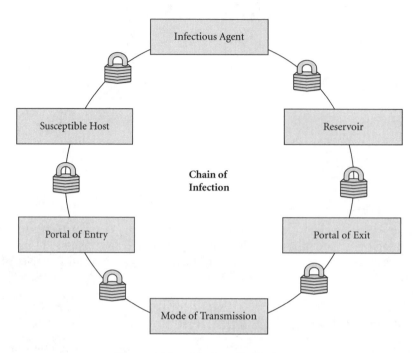

Figure 12.1—Chain of Infection

The portal of entry, the fifth link in the chain, could be the respiratory system, gastrointestinal system, reproductive system, or any open area in the skin of the susceptible host. The sixth link in the chain is a susceptible host. The pathogen must be able to survive in the environment of the host. Many different factors affect host susceptibility. If the host has immunity, the pathogen is not strong enough to fight the immune response of the host. If the host is not able to support the growth of the pathogen, the cycle will not complete. If there is no break in this chain, the cycle of infection will repeat itself over and over again. The actions that you take as a medical assistant are designed to prevent the spread of infection by breaking the links in this chain. Following is a list of examples of common pathogens and their methods of transmission to a susceptible host.

Organism	Disease	Method of Transmission
Virus	HIV	Blood, body fluids
Bacterium	Neisseria gonorrhoeae (gonorrhea)	Sexual transmission
Fungus	Tinia (athlete's foot, ringworm)	Direct contact, clothing, moist environment
Protozoa	Malaria	Vector (Anopheles mosquito)
Rickettsia	Lyme disease	Vector (tick)

Table 12.1—Spread of Infectious Disease

Types of Infections

There are several types of infections caused by the cycle of infection in humans. They include the following.

- **Acute infections** have a rapid onset of symptoms but the illness lasts only a short time; the common cold is an example of an acute infection
- **Chronic infections** last for an extended amount of time and may be lifelong infections; hepatitis B is an example of a chronic infection
- **Latent infections** persist with periods of activity and latency; herpes simplex is a latent infection
- **Slow infections** progress slowly over a long period; untreated Lyme disease and syphilis are examples of slow infections

Preventing Infection

Universal precautions are methods that are mandated by the Centers for Disease Control (CDC) to prevent the spread of infectious diseases in human populations. The CDC guidelines must be followed to protect the health and safety of the public and the health care worker. Universal precautions or standard precautions were first introduced in 1985 by the CDC in response to the concern about the spread of infectious disease and the safety of health care workers. Standard precautions are part the system of barrier precautions that are used with all patients regardless of their diagnosis by health care workers. These precautions include exposure to all blood, bodily fluids, skin that is not intact, and mucous membranes. Additionally, in July of 1992, the Occupational Safety and Health Administration (OSHA) began enforcing work practice controls in order to reduce or eliminate the risk of on-the-job exposure.

Potentially infectious body fluids include:

- Cerebrospinal fluid
- Synovial fluid
- Pleural fluid
- Pericardial fluid
- Peritoneal fluid
- Amniotic fluid
- Liquid or semi-liquid blood
- Mucous
- Vaginal or seminal secretions
- Saliva
- Any body fluid that is contaminated with blood, whether visible or not
- Human tissue
- Pus

Barrier protection or personal protective equipment (PPE) must be available and worn when there is any possibility of contact with any of the listed body fluids. The type of PPE worn is dependent upon the possibility of contamination. Gloves must be worn at all times. Gown, eye protection, and masks are used if possible exposure is anticipated. As a result of the increase in use of latex gloves, there has also been an increase in the incidence of latex allergies. Hypersensitivity reactions to the latex or the powder in the gloves can cause localized reactions with dermatitis, urticaria, and rhinitis or systemic reactions such as anaphylaxis.

OSHA standards require that all employees who are at risk for exposure to blood-borne pathogens must be offered vaccination for hepatitis B free of charge by the employer. The vaccine is given in a series of three injections. Employees may refuse the vaccination, but must sign a declination form that the employer will maintain in their employee file. Employees can always receive the vaccine at a later date if they change their mind.

OSHA also directs that certain procedures must be followed if there is a workplace exposure to body fluids. The procedures to manage the contamination include the following.

1. First aid is given including washing or flushing of the exposed area.

2. Report of the incident must be provided to the employee's supervisor immediately.

3. The employee must receive a medical evaluation.

4. An incident report is filed containing information about the exposure and the identity of the source patient if known.

5. The exposed worker and the source patient are screened for HIV and HBV if consent is given after counseling.

6. The health care worker must be offered HBV vaccination if not vaccinated or testing to assure immunity.

7. The worker must receive an opinion from the health care provider within 15 days of the medical evaluation.

8. Counseling is given to the exposed worker.

OSHA standards also apply to the disposal of biohazardous waste and specific housekeeping controls to make sure that your work areas are clean and maintained in a sanitary manner. Biohazardous waste includes any bodily fluid that comes from a patient, as well as any soiled or used equipment that came into contact with a patient. There must be a posted schedule of cleaning in work areas where there is possible exposure to biohazardous materials. Sharps containers must be used to contain waste such as glass, needles, scalpels, and syringes. These are rigid containers that must be sealed and disposed of properly by professional waste management companies. They may not be emptied by hand and should be monitored and changed before they become overly filled to prevent accidental injury. There must be a policy to clean biohazardous spills and materials to contain the spills for disposal. Garbage that is contaminated must be placed in a red bag marked with a biohazard sign and be disposed of by a specialized handler of biohazardous trash. It must be separated from noncontaminated trash to ensure it is taken care of in the correct manner and to keep costs down for the organization. It is much more expensive to dispose of contaminated waste than regular garbage. Soiled linens must be placed in an impervious bag without contaminating the surrounding area or your clothing. Gloves should always be worn when handling any item soiled with biohazardous waste.

Aseptic Techniques

Asepsis is the absence of infection or infectious material. *Medical asepsis* comprises the removal or destruction of pathogens after they leave the body. Examples of this are proper disposal of a soiled dressing into a red bag or a used sharp into a rigid biohazard container. *Surgical asepsis* is the removal or destruction of pathogens before they enter the body. Examples of this include the use of sterile instruments in a surgical procedure or a sterile syringe to give an injection.

Hand Washing

The cornerstone of infection control is hand washing. Routine hand washing in the medical office is necessary before and after treating a patient, even if gloves are used in a procedure. Hands should be washed with an antimicrobial soap. An extended hand wash should take place the first thing in the morning and the last thing before leaving work. This extended hand wash should last about twice as long as other times during the day. Soap, friction, and warm running water are the most important aspects of hand washing. Jewelry should be minimal, consisting of only a simple band and a watch. Hands should point downward to allow contaminates to run off the fingers. A nailbrush may be used or nails may be rubbed against the opposite hand to work the soap under the nails. Medical hand washing should last between 1 and 2 minutes and be done at any time contamination of the hands is apparent or suspected. If you are going to participate in a sterile procedure, there is another, more involved hand wash that must be done (see Chapter 15 for more information.). An alcohol-based hand rub can replace soap-and-water hand washing in some cases. It is not appropriate for use for the first hand washing of the morning, after using the restroom, or when there is visible material on your hands.

Sanitization

The process of preparing instruments to be disinfected or sterilized is called sanitization. All blood and debris from the instruments must be removed prior to any further processing. You should wear thick gloves to prevent puncture by sharp instruments along with eye protection and a protective gown or lab coat to prevent soiling of clothing. Ultrasonic sterilization uses a special cleanser in a bath, which cleans the instruments with bubbles caused by sound vibrations. This is especially useful for delicate instruments that cannot be scrubbed and eliminates the need for handling of soiled instruments.

Disinfection

Disinfection is the process of killing or inactivating pathogens on objects. Disinfectants can be purchased commercially or made fresh daily using a 1:10 solution of bleach and water. You must follow the manufacturer's directions very carefully when using chemical disinfectants to ensure the best results possible. Disinfection also can be achieved by boiling materials that are able to withstand the temperature of 212°F for 15 minutes. This process will not sterilize. Ultraviolet radiation using ultraviolet light and desiccation or drying are other methods of disinfection.

Antiseptics are used on the skin. The most common is 70 percent alcohol, which is commonly used to clean the skin and to decrease the number of organisms at the site of injections. Betadine is also safe to use for antisepsis on skin, as long as the patient does not have an allergy to iodine.

Sterilization

Sterilization completely removes all microorganisms from objects. It can be done chemically, by autoclave, or by gas sterilization. Gas sterilization rarely takes place in the medical office. The method most often used in a medical office is the autoclave. Chemical sterilization is done using manufacturer specifications and must be used immediately after taking the item from the sterilization solution. The autoclave uses a combination of steam, heat, and pressure for a prescribed amount of time to sterilize different items. This method kills all organisms and spores.

Items to be sterilized in the autoclave must be wrapped in special disposable autoclave paper or packaged in special materials. Hinged instruments must be opened to allow steam to penetrate all areas of the item. Sharp points must be wrapped in gauze to prevent tearing of the protective packaging. If instruments are packaged in bags, the handle should be inserted first to be properly displayed for use when the package is peeled open. All packaging must include indicator strips to monitor the sterilization process and ensure that it was successful. Labeling with the name of the instrument, the date of sterilization, and the name of the person performing the procedure is necessary.

Sterilization indicators may be incorporated with the bags in which the instruments are packaged. Indicator strips are also used. They have special inks that become visible when the conditions for sterilization have been achieved. They should be placed in wrapped packs in order to determine that the steam has reached all areas of the pack. Finally, packs should be secured with autoclave tape, which will also turns colors when the appropriate conditions have been reached. Autoclaving should be done according to manufacturers' directions. Control testing should be done in order to ensure that the autoclave is functioning properly.

Items that have been autoclaved are considered sterile for 28 days only. If the items have also been sealed in impervious plastic wrap, they will remain sterile for a longer period. The sterilized items must be stored properly and in a protected area. An item that has been autoclaved must be re-sterilized if the 28-day period has expired, the pack becomes wet, is dropped onto the floor, there is any tear in the packaging, or it is exposed to moisture. If there is any question about the integrity of the pack, it should be opened, the instruments re-cleaned, packed, and re-sterilized.

PATIENT PREPARATION

Measurement of Vital Signs

Accurate measurements of the vital signs are a very important part of patient assessment. Vital signs include temperature, pulse, respirations, and blood pressure. They are abbreviated TPR and BP and may also be called cardinal signs. Other measurements called anthropometric measurements may be taken when the patient comes to the physician's office. These are measurements of height, weight, BMI, body fat composition, and head and chest circumference. While measurements of vital signs are part of every office visit, they must not be considered routine or unimportant. Variation from normal can give important information about the patient's state of health.

Vital signs can be altered by a number of factors other than illness. Caffeine intake, smoking, medications, emotional stress, eating or drinking foods that are hot or cold, or exercise are just a few factors that can influence a patient's vital signs. The assessment of the patient's pain is sometimes called the fifth vital sign. Pain is assessed using a numeric scale from 0 to 10. Zero indicates that no pain is present, while 10 reflects the worst pain the patient has experienced. For those patients unable to understand the numeric scale or to participate in an interview, there are facial expression scales that allow the observer to rate the level of pain based on behavior or facial expression.

Vocabulary of Common Vital Signs

Apnea: absence of respirations

Arrythmia: irregular heart rate

Bradycardia: heart rate less than normal

Tachycardia: heart rate above normal

Bradypnea: respirations less than normal

Tachypnea: respiratory rate above normal

Dyspnea: difficult breathing

Febrile: pertaining to fever

Afebrile: without fever

Hypertension: blood pressure above the normal range

Hypotension: blood pressure below the normal range

Orthopnea: difficulty breathing in a reclining position

Orthostatic hypotension: temporary decrease in blood pressure readings when changing positions

Normal Vital Sign Ranges

Temperature:

Oral/Aural/Temporal: 98.6 +/– 1 degree

Axillary: 97.6 +/– 1 degree

Rectal: 99.6 +/– 1 degree

Age	Pulse	Respirations	Blood Pressure
Newborn	120–160	30–50	60–96/30–62
1–3 years	90–140	20–30	78–112/48–78
4–6 years	80–110	18–26	78–112/50–82
7–11 years	75–110	16–22	85–114/52–85
12–16 years	60–110	14–20	94–136/58–88
Adult	60–100	12–20	90–140/60–90

Table 12.2—Normal Vital Signs

Temperature

Temperature can be assessed with a variety of thermometers. Glass thermometers are no longer used according to OSHA guidelines due to the danger of breakage and need to disinfect between patients. Digital thermometers are used most frequently and temperature can be measured in the mouth, axilla, rectum, or ear canal. Disposable covers are used to prevent transmission of pathogens between patients. A separate probe is used for rectal temperature and color-coded in red to identify it. Rectal temperatures are the most accurate, but also the most invasive. Rectal temperatures should not be taken in patients with diarrhea, recent rectal surgery, or hemorrhoids, or if the patient is uncooperative. Tympanic or temporal readings are the least invasive but must be performed carefully in order to obtain accurate results.

Disposable thermometers can also be used to obtain body temperature using heat sensitive material that changes color. These are good screening devices and are accurate if used correctly. Care must be taken to check for expiration dates prior to use. Disposable thermometers and probe covers must be disposed of according to biohazard waste regulations.

Health care providers in the United States use both Fahrenheit and Celsius (metric) measurement systems. Medical assistants must be familiar with conversion formulas in order to interpret and assess the observed results.

°F to °C	Subtract 32, then multiply by 5, then divide by 9
°C to °F	Multiply by 9, then divide by 5, then add 32

Table 12.3—Formulas for Temperature Conversion

Normal body temperature	98.6°F = 37°C
Autoclave temperature	250°F = 121°C
Incubator temperature	95°F = 35°C
Refrigerator temperature	41°F = 5°C

Table 12.4—Common Temperature Conversions

Pulse

Pulse rates are the count of the palpable beats against the walls of the arteries. There are several areas in the body where the pulses can easily be palpated.

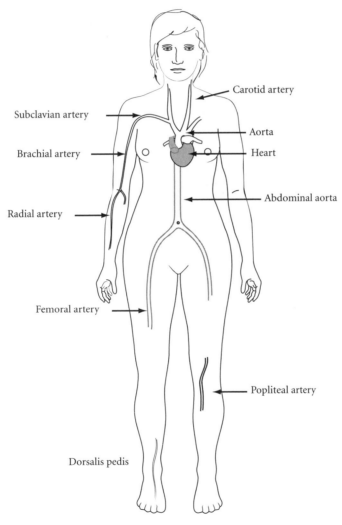

Figure 12.2—Adult Pulse Points

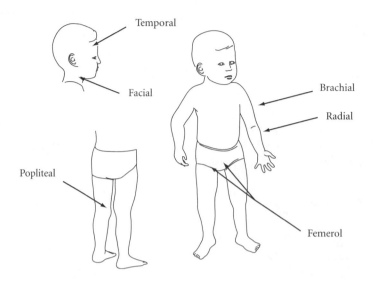

Figure 12.3—Child Pulse Points

Pulse Points

Temporal: the temporal area of the skull

Carotid: in the neck between the larynx and the sternocleomastoid muscle; most frequently used in emergencies and to evaluate the effectiveness of cardiopulmonary resuscitation

Apical: located at the apex of the heart; auscultated with a stethoscope and often used in infants and young children and for adults who have a rapid or irregular pulse. It is used to evaluate certain medications. The apical pulse can also be used to monitor for the pulse deficit by simultaneously measuring the apical and radial pulse and comparing the readings. The apical pulse should be counted for 1 minute.

Brachial: located in the inner aspect of the arm at the elbow level and frequently used in small children where the radial artery is difficult to palpate

Radial: located at the thumb side of the hand; most frequent point of use to palpate the pulse

Femoral: located in the groin below the inguinal ligament

Popliteal: located at the back of the knee; used to measure the blood pressure in the leg

Dorsalis pedis: located in the top of the foot

Evaluation of the Pulse

Rate: the measure of the number of beats felt per minute

Rhythm: the time between each pulse beat. Normally this is regular. If the rhythm is irregular, it is called an arrhythmia. Arrhythmia may be due to transient effects of caffeine, medication, stress, or exercise. It may also be due to disease.

Volume: the force of the beat against the artery wall. It is measured on a scale of +1, +2, or +3. A measurement of +1 is defined as weak and thready, +2 as normal, and +3 as bounding. This is usually only recorded in the chart if the pulse is not normal.

Respiration

Respirations are measured as the complete cycle of inspiration and expiration being counted as one. The respiratory rate is controlled by the brain, but the individual can control the respiratory rate to some degree. For this reason, you should not inform the patient that you are counting his respirations during the procedure as to not affect the rate. Respirations may be counted by observing the rise and fall of the chest or by feeling the rise and fall by placing your hand on the chest or back of the patient. Observation can be done at the time that the pulse count is being done by continuing to keep the fingers on the pulse, remembering the pulse count, and then counting the respirations. The respirations can also be counted during the patient interview as you observe the patient. In an infant or a small child, both the pulse rate and the respirations may be counted by auscultation of the chest while the parent holds the child on their lap.

Evaluation of Respiration

Rate: the measurement of the number of cycles of inspiration and expiration per minute

Rhythm: the breathing pattern. Irregular respirations are common in infants and young children. In adults you will expect the rhythm at rest to be regular.

Depth: measurement of the amount of air per respiratory cycle. You would expect this to be even in the healthy person. Respirations that are shallow, deep, or irregular may be a symptom of disease.

Blood Pressure

Careful evaluation of the blood pressure with comparison to previous readings is very important in evaluation of the patient. Comparison readings give information about changes in condition and effectiveness of medications. Changes in the blood pressure may indicate problems with the cardiovascular and other body systems. Hypertension is a serious health problem that does not have overt symptoms in the early stages except for elevated readings when the blood pressure is checked. Care must be taken to use correct technique and equipment when checking the blood pressure readings and recording in the chart.

The arm should be at or about heart level and resting comfortably when the reading is taken. The cuff must be the correct size. The cuff should be checked for any defects and for correct calibration prior to using. The arterial markings should be used to make sure that it is applied to the arm correctly. If the reading is not what you expect it to be, you should ask the patient about medications taken, caffeine intake, or stress situations that may be affecting the reading. Never hesitate to have another practitioner in the office check the reading if you have any doubt about your results.

Heart sounds: Sounds heard when the blood pressure is measured are called heart sounds or Korotkoff sounds. These sounds are classified into five phases:

> **Phase I:** the first sound heard, which should be a sharp tapping sound

> **Phase II:** a swishing sound that is made as the cuff continues to deflate and more blood enters the artery

> **Phase III:** distinct tapping sounds that are heard as the pressure is released in the blood pressure cuff

> **Phase IV:** the point at which the distinct tapping sounds disappear and usually where the diastolic number is read

> **Phase V:** the point where the sound disappears completely

Blood pressure readings that are very weak or faint can be measured by palpation or by use of a Doppler device. In this case, there is only an initial systolic reading available and the blood pressure should be recorded as the systolic number over P for palpation or D for Doppler.

Anthropometric Measurements

Height and weight are normally measured at every physician visit. These are very important measurements and must be carefully calculated and recorded in the patient chart. Results are measured in feet, inches, pounds, and ounces or in the metric system using kilograms and centimeters. You should be able to convert between the two systems to interpret results. Remember that 1 kg equals 2.2 lbs.

Weight should be measured in an area that ensures some privacy. Many people are sensitive about their weight and do not want to be weighed publicly or have the results of the measurement announced where others could overhear. Shoes may be taken off or not as the patient prefers, but if weight is done without shoes, measures should be taken to prevent transmission of pathogens to the surface of the scale, which could be passed on to the next patient.

Height is another important measurement that is taken at each office visit. In children, this measurement gives information about normal growth and development. In older adults, it can indicate bone loss with aging. Measurements are taken by using a ruler-type device attached to the scale or attached to the wall of the office.

Once height and weight are obtained, you can also calculate and record the BMI or body mass index of the patient. With obesity becoming a problem in all age groups, this measurement is used more often for evaluation. You can calculate the BMI by using a formula, online calculator, or app.

PATIENT HISTORY INTERVIEW

After the patient's vital signs have been taken and accurately recorded, you may be expected to obtain a patient health history. This will be done in detail at the first visit and then reviewed and updated with every subsequent visit. The process may start prior to the first visit with a brief telephone history when the initial appointment is scheduled. The gathering of information should be done in a comfortable and private setting. Recording of the information should be complete and not reflect any opinion or interpretation by the medical assistant.

Components of the Medical History

Personal data: You must make sure that you have the correct name, address, telephone number, date of birth, and insurance information. This should be reviewed at every visit. Other parts of the personal database may include the initial physical, lab work, and medication list for the patient. The medication list should also be checked and updated with every visit and in the event that the patient calls into the office with a question or a request for the physician.

Chief complaint: This is the patient's reason for seeking medical care in her own words. This should contain onset of symptoms, a description of any pain or discomfort, what type of treatment the patient has tried at home, what the patient's opinion of the problem is, and any other medical treatment that has been sought for this problem.

Past medical history: This would include immunization, childhood illnesses, allergies, accidents, surgeries, past hospitalizations, and any major illnesses.

Family history: Here information about the immediate family members and their state of health or cause of death would be recorded. Information about genetic or familial diseases would be placed in this section.

Social history: This section would include information about employment; education; lifestyle choices; diet and exercise; use of alcohol, tobacco, or drugs; and sleep habits. This information can help the care provider to assist the patient in making changes in this area to increase wellness and prevent disease.

Systems review: This is the area where the present illness is discussed and charted. It is a head-to-toe systemic assessment that looks at all aspects of the patient. By reviewing all body systems, the provider may discover valuable clues that the patient did not think were relevant to the current situation. This may also uncover early signs of problems that can be addressed before they become problematic for the patient.

All areas of the medical history should be documented carefully in the patient chart. Care should be taken to use correct accepted medical terminology and only approved abbreviations when documenting in the chart. Unclear or unapproved abbreviations can lead to problems with communication between health care workers. All entries must be signed and legible.

Patient education and teaching also must be documented in the chart. There should be notations about the patient response to education and teaching so follow-up can be continued on subsequent visits. Referrals to other agencies or support services for follow-up should be documented.

THE PHYSICAL EXAM

The purpose of the physical examination is to determine the state of health of the individual and to evaluate health problems. A diagnosis is then made by the physician and a plan of care is developed. Testing and medication may be ordered. Follow-up is scheduled to evaluate the results of treatment.

Your role as the medical assistant in the physical examination includes the following steps:

1. Prepare the exam room and the equipment used to do the physical exam. The medical assistant must make sure that the room is clean and all equipment is available.

2. Prepare the patient for the exam. The patient must be greeted and chart information confirmed. The patient then will be interviewed and vital signs checked. It may be necessary to help the patient into a gown and give instruction pertinent to the type of exam being done.

3. Assist the physician with the exam. The role of the assistant is to help the physician with equipment, patient movement, specimen procurement, and draping and controlling the exam environment. In addition, you are there to provide a sense of security and support to the patient.

Methods of Examination

Inspection: using visualization to detect physical data. This includes the general physical examination, posture, mannerisms, grooming, gait, visible injuries, rashes, color changes, and deformities or asymmetries.

Palpation: examination using touch. Palpation may allow the examiner to feel the surface of the body or to press deeper and palpate internal organs. Pulses would be evaluated using this method of examination.

Percussion: using the method of tapping or striking to hear sounds or feel vibrations. It can be used to evaluate the abdominal organs or the lungs.

Auscultation: listening to sounds of the body. An example of this would be using the stethoscope to listen to the apical pulse.

Mensuration: the process of measuring. This would include characteristics such as recording height, weight, or the size of a wound.

Common Tests: Vision, Hearing, and EKG

Several screening exams can be done in the physician's office. While not complete exams, they may point out areas that need further investigation.

Vision Tests

Visual acuity is performed with a Snellen chart to measure distance vision. The Snellen chart uses predetermined numbers that indicate the distance from which an individual with normal vision can see a particular line of letters. For testing, the patient stands 20 feet from the chart. The patient covers one eye and reads the lowest line possible. Normal vision is expressed as 20/20 and is considered normal for an individual viewing a particular line of the chart from 20 feet away. The results are recorded as a fraction. For example, in the fraction 20/60, the first number denotes that the patient was standing at 20 feet and the second number is the distance an individual with normal vision could view those same images. Pictorial eye charts are used to test vision of children and nonreading adults. Both eyes are tested independently and then together. The patient should be given an eye shield to prevent squinting while reading the chart. If the patient wears corrective lenses, the testing can be done with the corrective lenses. Modified charts are available for patients who cannot read and for children. If the patient's vision at maximum correction is 20/200 or greater, the patient is considered legally blind. The results should be recorded in the chart and carefully labeled.

Near vision testing can also be done using a chart that approximates the size of print in several different types of reading material. The chart is held about 14 to 16 inches away.

Colorblindness is mainly an inherited condition, and it occurs 20 times more often in males than females. Inheritance is sex-linked, meaning that the defective gene resides on the X chromosome, so females can carry the gene for colorblindness without ever developing the condition. The most common deficiency is red/green colorblindness, but there are other forms in which yellows and blues are distorted or the patient perceives only black and white. To evaluate color vision, illustrations such as the Ishihara color system are used. This system contains numbers or symbols made up of colored dots that appear among other colored dots. The patient is asked to identify what item is seen. A patient who is colorblind is unable to see the number or symbol within the colored dots. To test, you will need to have the patient trace the pattern that they see using their finger. In the chart, you will document how many patterns the patient is able to distinguish.

Hearing Tests

Evaluation of hearing can be done using audiometer or tuning-fork testing in the office. The Weber test is done to test if hearing is better in one ear than the other. The audiometer measures the sound intensity in decibels (dB) and the tone in cycles per second (cpc) or hertz (Hz). The patient is asked to indicate when they hear a tone, usually by raising a hand. A tuning fork is struck on the palm of the hand to facilitate vibration. The tuning fork is then placed on the center of the head and the patient is asked if there is a difference in the sound in one ear or the other. The tuning fork can also be used to compare bone conduction with air conduction. This test is called the Rinne test. The tuning fork is made to vibrate and then placed on the mastoid process. When the sound disappears, the tuning fork is turned to the front of the ear canal and the sound will normally still be able to be heard.

Tympanometry is a noninvasive procedure designed to evaluate the mobility of the eardrum and ascertain middle ear function through inducing air pressure variations into the ear canal. It is not a test of hearing and should not be confused with audiometry. This test is often used to screen tympanic membrane function in infants and small children who would be unable to complete audiometry and assist in diagnosing otitis media. Tympanometry also aids in diagnosing sensory or conductive hearing loss.

EKG Testing

An electrocardiogram (EKG) is a visual picture of the electrical activity of the heart created by placing electrodes on the body. Ten electrodes are placed, six on the chest and one on each limb, as shown in Figure 12.5. Each electrode, or lead, presents a picture of the electrical activity at its particular position on the body. Positions are identified as bipolar, augmented, unipolar, or precordial, as shown in Table 12.5. Care must be taken to place the electrodes precisely and make sure they are attached securely. It may be necessary to remove hair or otherwise prepare the skin to make sure that there is good connection to the skin. Other things that can interfere with recording are patient movement, tremor, talking, and electrical interference.

The EKG machine uses specialized paper that is heat and pressure sensitive. It is marked in 1-mm squares, which are also marked in groups of five by five squares. In normal mode, the paper will move through the EKG machine at 25 mm per second.

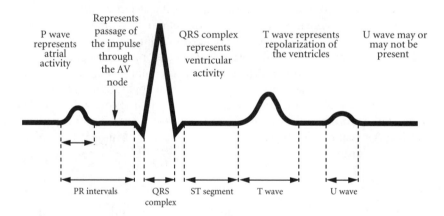

Figure 12.4—EKG Tracing

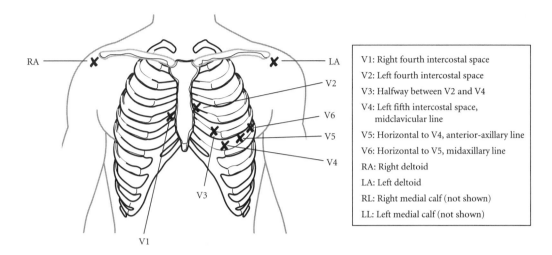

| | V1: Right fourth intercostal space |
| V2: Left fourth intercostal space |
| V3: Halfway between V2 and V4 |
| V4: Left fifth intercostal space, midclavicular line |
| V5: Horizontal to V4, anterior-axillary line |
| V6: Horizontal to V5, midaxillary line |
| RA: Right deltoid |
| LA: Left deltoid |
| RL: Right medial calf (not shown) |
| LL: Left medial calf (not shown) |

Figure 12.5—EKG Placement

Lead	Polarity	Electrical Conduction Location
I	Bipolar	Left arm/right arm
II	Bipolar	Right arm/left leg
III	Bipolar	Left leg/left arm
AVR	Augmented	Midpoint between the left arm and left leg to right arm
AVL	Augmented	Midpoint between the left leg and right arm to left arm
AVF	Augmented	Midpoint between the left arm and left leg to the left foot
V1–V6	Unipolar	See Figure 12.5 above

Table 12.5—Electrode Involvement in the EKG Recording

Terminology. It is important for the medical assistant to know common terminology related to EKGs in order to support patient education and document information accurately.

1. **Depolarization** occurs when the heart muscle contracts. On an EKG tracing, the P wave represents atrial depolarization, and the QRS wave represents ventricular depolarization.

2. **Repolarization** occurs when the heart muscle relaxes. On an EKG tracing, the atria are relaxing when the ventricles are contracting, so repolarization occurs during the QRS wave. The T wave represents ventricular relaxation.

3. The **stylus** is the heated instrument on the EKG machine that burns the recording into the heat-sensitive paper. If the recording is too thick or dark, the stylus heat can be reduced; if too light, stylus heat can be increased.

4. **Electrodes** are devices attached to the arms, legs, and chest that sense electrical impulses. They either include an electrolyte conduction material impregnated within the pads or have a connection, such as a metal plate or a suction bulb, to which electrolyte gel is added as a conductor.

5. **Leads** are the wires that transmit the signals for the EKG recording from the various electrode locations on the arms, legs, and chest.

6. A **standard** is the mark that appears at the beginning or end of an EKG tracing that is a universal signal of the speed and sensitivity of the tracing. The typical standard mark is 10 mm high by 5 mm wide, representing an EKG with a sensitivity of 1 and a speed of 25 mm per second.

7. Electrical conduction that comes from one specific location (such as a chest lead) is **unipolar**. It travels in only one direction.

8. Electrical conduction that occurs between two poles is **bipolar**; it travels in both directions between the poles. The first three leads (I, II, III) are bipolar.

9. The electrical conduction of unipolar leads needs to be **augmented**, or enhanced, to produce a clear tracing. Augmentation is used in the arm and leg leads with aVR (augmented vector right), aVL (augmented vector left), and aVF (augmented vector foot).

Artifacts. Artifacts are unwanted disturbances that can interfere with accurate interpretation of an EKG tracing. Machine malfunction, body movements, electrical interference, or poor contact of the electrodes can lead to artifacts. The medical assistant needs to know what these artifacts are and how to troubleshoot them in order to produce a clear EKG recording for interpretation by the health care provider.

Body movements cause an EKG tracing artifact known as **somatic tremor**. Sources of somatic tremor include shivering, coughing, sneezing, talking, and moving, as well as disorders that cause uncontrollable movement, such as Parkinson's disease. It is important that you properly instruct the patient to limit movement during the procedure, ensure the patient stays covered and warm, and (if needed) have the patient slip their hands, palms down, under the buttocks. These measures tend to promote relaxation and reduce somatic tremors.

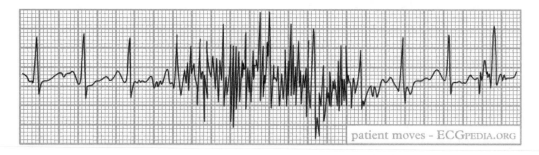

Figure 12.6—Somatic Tremor (*Source:* Cafer Zorkun, wikidoc.org)

Alternating current (AC) interference is caused by improper grounding or by a machine that is not equipped to filter out extraneous electrical currents. A tracing with AC interference will have a thickened appearance, with relatively even, sharp spikes. To reduce electrical interference, confirm that the ground wire on the right leg is attached appropriately and that the EKG machine has a three-pronged outlet connector, and move the patient away from the source of electricity (for instance, walls with electrical wiring or other electrical equipment in the room). Note that if a total break in the tracing, the likely problem is a broken lead wire or loss of connection of one of the electrodes.

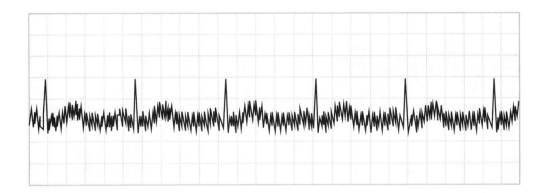

Figure 12.7—AC Interference

Poor lead contact with the skin produces a **wandering baseline** in the EKG tracing. In this artifact, the baseline "wanders" up and down on the EKG paper, interfering with accurate recording. Possible sources of wandering baseline (sometimes called "baseline drift") include lotions, powder, oils, or ointments on the client's skin; nylon stockings that the client is wearing (stockings should be removed along with the client's other clothing prior to EKG testing); and expired or poor-quality electrolyte gel, dry electrolyte pads, or dirty/loose wires or electrodes. Wiping the attachment areas with alcohol to ensure that the skin is clean and dry will often reduce this unwanted tracing artifact. A related artifact that may be seen is an **interrupted baseline**, in which there is a sharp break in the tracing. This artifact is typically seen when a wire is broken or a lead becomes disconnected.

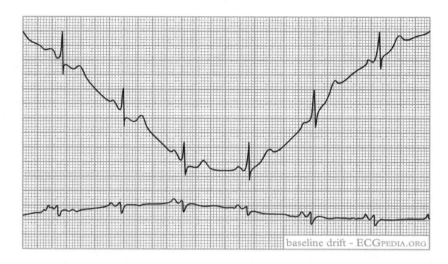

Figure 12.8—Wandering Baseline (*Source:* Cafer Zorkun, wikidoc.org)

Patient Positioning

There are a variety of positions that facilitate patient examination. You must be able to instruct the patient on how to assume the correct position and assist him with the positioning. You will then drape the patient in a manner to maintain dignity and privacy while allowing the physician to do the examination. If it is necessary for the patient to wear a gown for the examination, you must be sure that it fits correctly and is in good repair. If the gown is disposable, it is used for one patient only and then discarded in the appropriate waste container. The exam table should be cleaned with disinfectant and covered with clean paper prior to the patient entering the exam room. The exam table should be checked periodically to make sure that all features are in good working order and the covering is intact.

The primary purpose of draping is to provide the patient privacy and dignity. Only the parts being examined should be exposed. A blanket should be available for the patient to keep him warm and comfortable. The medical assistant should be available to assist the patient in assuming positions on the exam table and to prevent falls.

In an erect position, the patient is standing. This position is used for evaluation of gait and neurological testing. No draping is needed. If the patient is wearing a gown for this position, make sure that is it secured for dignity and privacy.

In a sitting position, the patient sits on a chair or on the edge of the exam table. This position can be used for a number of examinations including the nervous system, head and neck, lower extremities, chest, upper extremities, and the back. Draping may be necessary to cover the lower extremities for patient comfort.

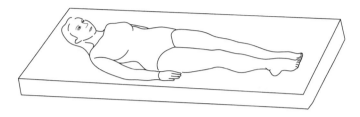

Figure 12.9—Supine Position

The supine position, also called horizontal recumbent, is when the patient is lying flat on the back with arms at the sides. This position can be used to assess the chest, breasts, abdomen, heart, and extremities. Draping is done from under the arms downward.

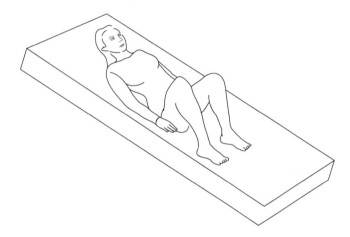

Figure 12.10—Dorsal-Recumbent Position

In the dorsal-recumbent position, the patient is supine with the legs bent at the knees and feet flat on the exam table and spread about shoulder width. This position can be used to examine the abdomen, genital, and rectal areas. It may be more comfortable than the supine positions for patients with back or abdominal pain. Draping is done in a diamond fashion with a point facing toward the head and the feet. The points that extend to the sides can be positioned to wrap around the legs when the patient is being examined.

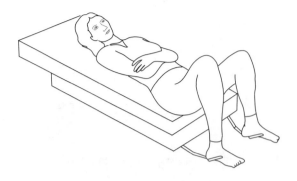

Figure 12.11—Lithotomy Position

The lithotomy position is similar to the dorsal-recumbent, except that the feet are placed in stirrups. This is done for vaginal exams, pap smears, and pelvic exams and procedures. Draping is done in the same manner as the dorsal-recumbent position.

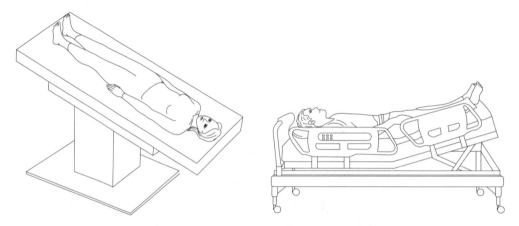

Figure 12.12—Trendelenburg Position and Modified Trendelenburg Position

The patient is positioned with the head lower than the feet in the Trendelenburg position. It is used for shock, fainting, or to delay a precipitous delivery. Draping is done from the shoulders downward. Alternatively, the modified Trendelenburg position may be used, in which the feet are elevated 45 degrees and the head remains level with the rest of the body.

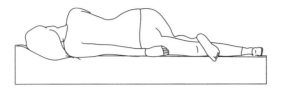

Figure 12.13—Sims's Position

Sims's position is also called the left lateral position and calls for the patient to be on his left side with the left arm behind the body and the right arm in front of the face. The legs are flexed; the right more than the left so that access to the rectal area is exposed. This position is used for enemas, suppositories, rectal temperature, and rectal exams. It may be used for proctologic exams in those patients who cannot tolerate the knee-chest position.

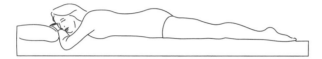

Figure 12.14—Prone Position

In the prone position, the patient lies flat on the abdomen with neck turned to one side. Arms are down by the side. This position is used to examine the spine, back, and lower extremities. The patient is draped from the mid-back downward.

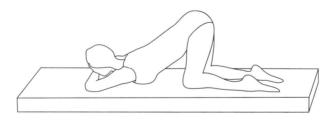

Figure 12.15—Knee-Chest Position

In knee-chest position, the patient is positioned on the knees with the head and chest on the table and the buttocks elevated. This position may be assumed with or without the use of a special table. It is used for rectal exams and proctologic exams and procedures. This position is difficult to assume for a large patient or an elderly patient. You should stay by the patient's side and assist the patient when moving out of this position to prevent falls. Orthostatic hypotension may be a problem after assuming this position for a period of time. Draping is done to cover the buttocks.

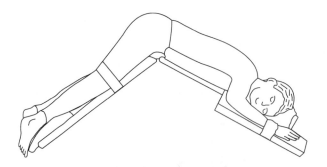

Figure 12.16—"Jack-Knife" Position

The "jack-knife" position is used for surgical procedures involving the rectal area.

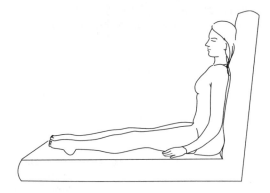

Figure 12.17—Fowler's Position

When in Fowler's position, the patient is sitting at a 90-degree angle with lower extremities elevated. The table supports the back. It is used for examination of the chest, head, and neck. It may also be used for someone who has problems breathing in a flat position. Draping is done from the mid-chest downward.

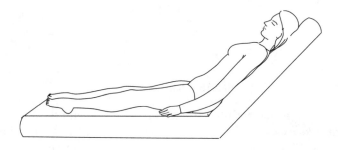

Figure 12.18—Semi-Fowler's Position

Semi-Fowler's position is similar to Fowler's position, but the head is elevated at a 45-degree angle. It is used for the same procedures in which Fowler's position is used and draping is the same.

Instruments and Equipment

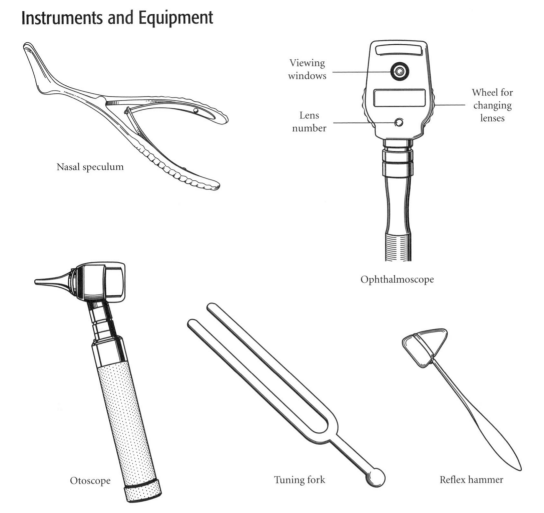

Figure 12.19—Instruments Commonly Used in the Physical Exam

Otoscope and ophthalmoscope: used to examine the ears and eyes. Disposable covers should be used prior to examining the ears with the otoscope. These instruments may be handheld or wall-mounted. If they are portable, you must make sure that they are fully charged and ready to use.

Nasal speculum: dilates the nares for examination of the internal structures

Tongue depressor: a flat wooden stick used to depress the tongue for examination of the throat

Reflex hammer: a small hammer with a rubber head used to test reflexes in a neurological examination

Tuning fork: used to test for bone vibration and auditory acuity

Stethoscope: used to take blood pressure and listen to the heart, lung, and abdominal sounds

Gloves: disposable exam gloves of various sizes

Lubricant: a water-soluble lubricant available to be used for rectal or vaginal exams

Hemocult cards and developer: to check stools for blood after a rectal exam

Tape measure: disposable paper measures can be used to measure body parts, wounds, areas of skin rash or excoriation, ulcers, and other areas of the body

Other objects that should be available are gauze sponges, waste containers, specimen containers with labels, plastic bags with biohazard labeling for specimen transport, culture tubes, cotton applicators, and any other supplies that are relevant to the physician practice or exam being done.

Body Mechanics

You must protect yourself while caring for and moving patients and equipment. Learning and practicing proper lifting and moving techniques may help prevent injury. You must also make sure that equipment in the office is in proper working order. That will include the exam table, scales, wheelchairs, and other equipment used for patient care.

Lifting Techniques

- Do not attempt to lift objects by yourself that are too heavy to manage easily. Ask for help.
- Do not lift items above your head. Get as close as you can to the object that will be lifted.
- Bend at the knees and keep your back straight when you lift objects. Use your leg muscles to assist in the lift.
- Carry heavy objects as close to your body as possible
- Move your feet in the direction of the lift. Do not twist at the waist.
- Bend your knees when lowering the load that you are putting down.
- When assisting a patient, do not allow the patient to put his arms around your neck. When transferring a patient to a wheelchair, make sure that the wheelchair is locked. Encourage the patient to do all that she can for herself. When assisting the patient, always stand at the stronger side if one is stronger than the other.
- If you must move an object that is too heavy for you to lift, push it rather than pull it.

REVIEW QUESTIONS

1. The normal speed for an EKG machine is
   (A) 5 mm/second
   (B) 25 mm/second
   (C) 25 mm/minute
   (D) 50 mm/second
   (E) 50 mm/minute

2. To take vital signs on an infant, the medical assistant should
   (A) have the parent place the child on the exam table
   (B) ask the parent to leave the room
   (C) take the pulse using the radial artery and place your hand on the child's chest to feel the respiration
   (D) use the stethoscope to listen to the heart and lungs while the parent holds the child
   (E) ask the parent to take the vital signs and record them in the chart

3. If a patient has orthopnea, the medical assistant should position them on the exam table in the
   (A) lithotomy position
   (B) Sims's position
   (C) Trendelenburg position
   (D) Fowler's position
   (E) supine position

4. The Snellen test measures
   (A) visual acuity
   (B) bone conduction
   (C) color vision
   (D) near vision
   (E) nerve conduction

5. In which section of the chart would information about the patient's smoking habits and employment be documented?
   (A) Review of systems
   (B) Family history
   (C) Social history
   (D) Miscellaneous
   (E) Plan of care

6. It is appropriate to check the carotid pulse if

   (A) the patient is uncooperative
   (B) the patient has a cast on the left arm
   (C) the patient has fainted
   (D) the patient refuses to have a rectal temperature taken
   (E) the patient has just drunk a cold beverage

7. Screening for osteoporosis would include

   (A) plotting the weight and height graph of all children until age 18
   (B) calculating the BMI for all patients
   (C) carefully measuring the height of older adult patients
   (D) using a tape measure to measure the uterine fundus in a pregnant patient
   (E) asking all patients about their sleep habits

8. Which of the following would the medical assistant hand to the physician if she wanted to check the pupils of the eye?

   (A) Otoscope
   (B) Tuning fork
   (C) Speculum
   (D) Ophthalmoscope
   (E) Snellen test

9. The agency that sets standards for the disposal of infectious waste is

   (A) CDC
   (B) DEA
   (C) OSHA
   (D) CBC
   (E) FBI

10. All of the following are artifacts in an EKG tracing EXCEPT:

    (A) AC interference
    (B) DC interference
    (C) interrupted baseline
    (D) somatic tremor
    (E) wandering baseline

11. An instrument that would be used to examine the eyes is a(n)

    (A) audiometer

    (B) ophthalmoscope

    (C) otoscope

    (D) Ishihara chart

    (E) Snellen chart

12. Which of the following is NOT an example of proper body mechanics?

    (A) Avoid lifting items over your head.

    (B) Bend at the knees and keep your back straight when lifting objects.

    (C) Instruct the patient to put both arms around your neck for stability as you help the patient to stand.

    (D) Instruct the patient to assist as much as possible and use a gait belt as you help the patient to stand.

    (E) Stand on the patient's stronger side when assisting in ambulation.

13. Which of the following sequences represents the waveforms of the EKG in correct order?

    (A) A, B, C, D, E

    (B) P, Q, R, S, T

    (C) P, T, Q, R, S

    (D) Q, R, S, T, P

    (E) R, S, T, P, Q

14. The aseptic process that is aimed at removing all microorganisms, including spores, is called

    (A) sanitization

    (B) sterilization

    (C) disinfection

    (D) hand washing

    (E) gloving

15. A patient has developed antibodies to varicella (chickenpox). What part of the chain of infection has been broken in this case that would provide protection from disease?

    (A) Infectious agent

    (B) Portal of entry

    (C) Portal of exit

    (D) Susceptible host

    (E) Reservoir

ANSWERS AND EXPLANATIONS

1. **B**

    At normal speed on the standard setting, the EKG paper moves through the machine at 25 mm/second.

2. **D**

    The parent should be with and hold the child in order to decrease the child's anxiety and increase cooperativeness. The brachial artery is usually used in the young child due to the body makeup making it difficult to palpate the radial artery. Using the stethoscope while the parent distracts the child will be the least invasive method. The parents can assist with obtaining the child's cooperation, but obtaining accurate vital signs is the responsibility of the medical assistant.

3. **D**

    Fowler's position is a seated position with legs elevated and the head up at a 90-degree angle. If the patient has orthopnea, they will have difficulty breathing, so the upright position would be the position of choice.

4. **A**

    The Snellen test is a measure of vision. It measures the visual acuity by using the eye chart to compare the patient's vision to what can normally be read at 20 feet away.

5. **C**

    This information would be found in the social history along with other personal information about the patient. Family history (B) would provide information about the immediate family. The review of systems (A) is done by the physician when he examines that patient about the current issue.

6. **C**

    The carotid pulse is used more frequently in an emergency, such as when a patient has fainted, or evaluating the effectiveness of CPR.

7. **C**

    Measuring the height of older adult patients is a general screening for osteoporosis, which can cause bone degeneration that results in a decline in stature. This condition does not commonly occur in children, so (A) is incorrect. Item (B) is a metabolic index used to calculate body fat in patients. Uterine fundus measurement (D) is a gross measure of fetal growth during pregnancy. Item (E) is not related to osteoporosis.

8. **D**

   The ophthalmoscope would be used to examine the eye. The Snellen test (E) measures visual acuity. The tuning fork (B) and the otoscope (A) would be used to evaluate the ears.

9. **C**

   OSHA or the Occupational Safety and Health Administration is responsible for the OSHA standard precaution guidelines that were established in 1992.

10. **B**

    Artifacts are unwanted distortions in an EKG tracing that interfere with diagnostic interpretation of the tracing. AC interference (A) is caused by improper grounding or electrical currents in a room that may cause sharp spikes in the tracing. To avoid this artifact, ensure that the bed is not close to the wall, that a three-prong outlet is used, and that the patient's right leg lead is properly attached. An interrupted baseline (C) is a sharp break in the tracing that appears when a wire is broken or a lead detached from the skin. Somatic tremor (D) is caused by muscle movement and is associated with motions like shivering or symptoms of Parkinson's disease. A wandering baseline (E) is often caused by poor electrode connections; possible causes of this problem are lotions, powders, or stockings worn on the skin and poor-quality electrolytes on the electrodes.

11. **B**

    The word *ophthalmoscope* breaks down into the root *ophthalm*, meaning "eyes," and *scope*, meaning "an instrument that views." An audiometer (A) tests hearing, while an otoscope (C) is used to examine the ears. An Ishihara chart (D) is used to test for colorblindness, and a Snellen chart (E) is used to screen vision, but neither is used to examine the eyes.

12. **C**

    Patients should not be encouraged or allowed to put their arms around your neck as you assist them with standing; this could lead to injury of your neck and back. While a patient may need to put their arms on your shoulders (depending on the situation), you should have patients do as much as they can for themselves. If in doubt, get assistance from someone else in order to avoid injuring yourself. Avoiding lifting objects over your head (A), bending at the knees to lift objects (B), and using a gait belt when helping patients to stand (D) are all examples of proper body mechanics. The patient will be much more stable and able to contribute to ambulation if you provide stability to their stronger side when assisting (E).

13. **B**

    From the beginning of the P wave to the end of the T wave is one cardiac cycle (or one heartbeat). The P wave represents atrial depolarization, the QRS wave represents ventricular depolarization and atrial repolarization, and the T wave represents ventricular repolarization.

14. **B**

Sterilization aims to remove all microorganisms, including spores. Sanitization (A) should be viewed as the preparatory phase for sterilization as items are physically cleaned. Disinfection (C) is more aggressive than sanitization and removes a great deal of microorganisms, but not all of them. Hand washing (D) is the most effective means for preventing the spread of germs, but it does not remove all microorganisms. Gloving (E) is a means to prevent the spread of infections and protect both yourself and the patient but will not remove any microorganisms.

15. **D**

A patient who has developed antibodies to a disease, either by being infected with the disease and recovering or by receiving a vaccine, is no longer a susceptible host. Therefore the chain is broken at this stage, and the patient would not get the infection. The infectious agent (A) is still present, and the portals of entry (B) and exit (C) are still in place; without susceptibility, however, the individual will not get the disease. The infectious agent will continue to grow within the reservoir (E), or body of the infected individual, which can be spread to others via the portal of entry and exit.

Chapter 13: **Laboratory Work**

Clinical laboratory testing is an important part of a medical office. Laboratory tests are often used to provide vital information regarding the body's functions and its ability to maintain homeostasis. When the human body is unable to maintain homeostasis, certain biological changes can alter the chemical content of blood and urine. These changes can trigger the production of antibodies or influence the size, shape, and counts of specific cells in the body. These changes are measured and compared to normal ranges or reference numbers for that particular patient. The physician utilizes specific laboratory tests, a health history, and a thorough physical examination to help make an accurate diagnosis or manage a patient's existing condition.

CLINICAL LABORATORY IMPROVEMENT AMENDMENTS

The Clinical Laboratory Improvement Amendments (CLIA) were passed by Congress in 1988 and were developed to improve the quality of laboratory testing. Laboratories that are not CLIA-compliant cannot receive Medicare and Medicaid reimbursement. The amendments established quality assurance standards for all laboratories providing patient testing regardless of their location within the United States. Quality assurance requirements include written policies, employee training, documented maintenance of instruments, documented procedures, and quality control. Laboratories also must participate in proficiency testing. The Food and Drug Administration (FDA) is responsible for regulating each laboratory under CLIA guidelines the guidelines are centered on three specific categories of tests, which are based on the potential risk to the public's health: waived, moderate complexity and provider performed microscopy tests, and high-complexity tests.

Personnel and quality assurance requirements do not apply to waived tests. Waived tests include tests approved by the FDA that a patient can perform at home, procedures with a low or insignificant risk of errors if performed incorrectly, or tests that pose little risk of harm to the patient if performed incorrectly. The following are waived tests: dipstick or tablet reagent urinalysis, fecal occult blood, ovulation testing, urine pregnancy test, blood glucose, erythrocyte sedimentation rate (ESR), hemoglobin (HGB), hematocrit (Hct), and CLIA-approved strep A tests.

Moderate-complexity tests account for approximately 75 percent of all lab tests performed today. Most of the testing takes place in physician's office laboratories (POL). These tests include hematology and blood chemistry performed with an automated analyzer, pinworm preparation, Gram's staining, and microscopic analysis of urine sediment. High-complexity tests are usually not performed in a POL. These tests include pap smears, blood typing, blood cross matching, and cytology testing.

Quality control measures ensure accuracy in test results through careful monitoring of testing procedures. To comply with quality control standards, the POL must follow certain procedures including calibration, control samples, reagent control, maintenance, and documentation.

Calibration of the testing equipment must be performed according to manufacturers' guidelines. Each calibration should be recorded in a quality control log. Calibration procedures require that the equipment generate the correct results for the standards (a specimen with a known value) supplied.

Control samples are specimens with known values used prior to processing a patient sample that checks for the accuracy of the test. If the control is not within the prescribed range, the patient sample is not analyzed. Control samples can show normal and abnormal results and can generate qualitative test response (substances being tested are present or absent) or quantitative response (the concentration of a test substance is given).

Reagents are chemicals used in test procedures that will react in specific ways when exposed to certain substances. To ensure the quality of reagents, the medical assistant should keep a reagent control log.

Maintenance of the testing equipment and instruments is an important part of the laboratory and must be documented. It is best to use manufacturers' guidelines and keep a complete record of all work performed.

Documentation of quality control depends on adherence to the procedures designed to identify problems with equipment calibration, errors in designed procedures, and defective testing supplies. Documentation of all procedures includes a log of all mentioned quality control measures and a daily workload log and reference laboratory log (specimen sent to an outside lab for testing).

SPECIMEN COLLECTION

The medical assistant's primary responsibility in the laboratory is the skillful collection of a specimen. The clinical lab results are only as reliable as the received specimen. The most common specimens collected in offices today are blood, urine, and swab samples from mucous membranes or wounds. The medical assistant should be familiar with commonly performed laboratory tests, the purpose and performance of each test, the normal range, the patient preparation, and any special instructions for collecting, handling, and storage of the specimen. Practicing quality control and laboratory safety is of the utmost importance to the medical assistant.

There are vital steps the medical assistant should follow to avoid errors. The medical assistant must correctly identify each patient prior to the collection and labeling of the obtained specimen. Each label should include the patient's name, date, time of collection, type of specimen, and tentative diagnosis. The label should be placed directly on the container and not on the lid or cover to avoid separation of the specimen and the identification. The medical assistant should follow guidelines to avoid contaminating the specimen or themselves. Expiration dates of collection items (swabs, tubes, and transport media) should be checked. Standard or universal precautions should be followed at all times. All blood specimens and other body fluids from patients should be considered infective. The Occupational Safety and Health Administration (OSHA) Bloodborne Pathogens Standard of 1991 was designed to reduce the risk to employees from exposure to infectious disease.

The OSHA standards include the following.

- **Hand washing:** used when performing clinical procedures, before and after patient contact, before and after applying gloves, and after contact with blood or other potentially infectious materials
- **Biohazard containers:** place infectious waste in these containers that are closable, leak proof, and properly constructed to contain the contents during handling, storage, transport, or shipping
- **Clean disposable gloves:** gloves should be worn when in contact with blood and other potentially infectious material, mucous membranes, non-intact skin, and contaminated articles or surfaces
- **Appropriate protective clothing:** gowns, aprons, and laboratory coats
- **Face shields or masks in combination with eye protection devices:** in case of splashes, spray, spatter, or droplets of blood or other potentially infectious materials

MICROBIOLOGY

The compound microscope is the most common type of magnification instrument used in the medical office. Microscopes permit visualization of structures that cannot be seen with the unaided eye. Microscopes consist of three main components: the magnification system, the illumination system, and the framework.

The magnification system of the microscope includes the ocular and objective lenses. The eyepiece, or ocular, is located at the top of the instrument and contains a lens to magnify approximately 10 times (10×). The objectives are on the revolving nosepiece. Most microscopes contain three objectives. Each objective provides a different magnifying power. The shortest objective has the lowest power at 10× magnification. This objective is used to bring objects into initial focus. The next objective is the high power, which brings objects into view at 40× magnification. The longest objective is the oil immersion (100×) allowing for the fine focusing of the object and requires the use of special oil that is placed directly on the slide. To determine total magnification, multiply the power of the ocular lens and the objective lens.

Example: 10× (ocular) 10× (lowest objective) = 100× total magnification of the viewed object

The illumination system includes the light source, the condenser, and the iris diaphragm. The light source is on the base of the microscope. Light is directed to the condenser then through the objective lens. The condenser collects and concentrates light rays then directs them up onto the objective lens. The diaphragm regulates the amount of light passing through the specimen. The diaphragm can be located within or beneath the condenser. A lever increases or decreases the light by changing the size of the aperture.

The framework includes stage, arm, and the adjustment knobs. The arm of the microscope connects the objectives and oculars to the base. The stage is a flat, horizontal platform that holds the slide. The stage has a mechanical adjustment knob that allows vertical or horizontal movement of the slide. Just above the base of the microscope are the two adjustment knobs. Coarse adjustment is used to approximate focus quickly and find the object under the low power objective. The fine adjustment allows for precise focus to produce sharp, clear images with high power and oil-immersion lenses.

Focusing the microscope is done through movement of the objective or stage. Stage focus is more common and involves movement of the stage while the body tube is stationary. Movement is controlled by the adjustment knobs located on both sides of the microscope. Proper focusing begins with the lowest power objective, which is used for initial focus and observation. The course adjustment moves the object into approximate focus quickly. Once the specimen is in view, the objective nosepiece is rotated to the high power objective and the fine adjustment knob is used for precise focus.

Classifications of Microorganisms

The following groups of microorganisms are known to contain species capable of causing human disease and include bacteria, viruses, fungi (yeast and molds), protozoa, and parasites.

Bacteria are single-celled microorganisms found throughout the environment. Once a bacterial specimen reaches the laboratory, it will be analyzed for certain criteria used for identification. This criterion includes morphology and staining reaction.

Bacteria can be classified into three basic groups according to morphological shape. Spherical bacteria are called cocci, rod-shaped bacteria are called bacilli, and spiral-shaped bacteria are called spirilla.

Bacilli are rod-shaped bacteria that are frequently found in the soil and air. Some are able to form spores, a characteristic that enables them to resist adverse conditions such as heat and disinfectants. *Escherichia coli* is a species of bacillus that is found in vast numbers among the normal flora of the intestinal tract.

Spirilla are spiral or curved bacteria. *Treponema pallidum* is a spirochete (tightly coiled spirilla) and the causative agent of syphilis. *Vibrio cholerae* causes cholera.

Staphylo- is a Greek term that denotes "bunch of grapes." *Staphylococci* are round bacteria that grow in grapelike clusters. The Greek term streptos means twisted. *Streptococci* are round bacteria that grow in chains. *Diplococci* are round bacteria that grow in pairs (*diplo-* means double) and are associated with disease such as pneumonia, gonorrhea, and meningitis.

Chemical composition of the cell wall determines if the bacteria will stain. Three types of cell wall structures exist among pathogenic bacteria: gram positive, gram negative, and acid fast. The most common type of staining is gram staining. The stain is a solution of a dye or group of dyes that imparts a color to the microorganisms. A gram positive stain results in a bluish-purple color based on cell-wall structure. A gram negative stain results in a pink-red color because the cell wall is a thinner structure with distinct layers. Acid-fast staining is a procedure used for identifying bacteria with a waxy cell wall. These organisms retain stains despite being rinsed with acid. The bacteria that cause TB can be stained with this procedure.

Viruses are the smallest living organisms and cannot be seen with a regular microscope. Viruses are considered non-cellular and consist of nucleic acid surrounded by a protein coat. Viruses cannot grow independently (without a host). Viruses cause many conditions in people and are classified by diseases they produce. The following list outlines the categories of viral conditions and examples of each.

- **Dermotrophic:** smallpox, rubeola, rubella, chicken pox, shingles
- **Pneumotrophic:** influenza, common cold, infectious mono
- **Neurotrophic:** rabies, encephalitis, polio
- **Enterotrophic:** hepatitis
- **Immunotrophic:** AIDS

Mycology is the study of fungus and the associated diseases. Fungi are a diverse group of microorganisms that produce spores and sometimes filaments. Fungi are present in the soil, air, and water but only some are pathogenic. The two primary forms of fungi are yeasts and molds. Yeasts are single-celled fungi that reproduce by budding. Molds are multicellular forms that depend on plants or animals for food.

Parasitology is the study of parasitic organisms that live on or in the human body. Parasites are transmitted by ingestion during the infective stage, direct penetration of the skin, and inoculation by an arthropod vector. Helminths are parasitic worms and are large enough to see with the naked eye. Roundworms can occur in the intestines (pinworms) or muscle tissue (*Trichinella spiralis*, a form of roundworm, enters the body in infected meat eaten raw or insufficiently cooked). Tapeworms and flatworms are obtained from ingestion of undercooked meat.

Protozoa are single-celled microorganisms lacking a cell wall and most have some form of locomotion (cilia or flagella). These microorganisms are found in soil and water and most do not cause disease in humans. Pathogenic forms include malaria, amebic dysentery, and Trichomoniasis vaginitis (venereal disease).

Collection of Microbiological Specimens

The medical assistant should follow standard guidelines for proper specimen collection. The specimen should be collected with great care to avoid causing the patient harm, discomfort, or embarrassment. The specimen should be collected from a site where the organism is most likely to be found and where contamination is least likely to occur. There are site-specific devices to help ensure optimal collection, transportation, and processing of microorganisms. The most common types of cultured specimens include the throat, urine, sputum, wound, and stool.

Throat culture specimens are frequently performed in medical offices. Identification of the microorganism responsible for the infection allows for proper treatment of the patient for upper respiratory, throat, or sinus infections. When obtaining a throat specimen, the medical assistant must avoid touching any other structures inside the oropharynx to avoid contamination.

Sputum specimen collection involves the patient coughing mucus from the lungs into a container. The specimen must not come into contact with saliva and should be refrigerated or cultured immediately. Care must be taken when collecting these items, especially if the patient is coughing. Always use universal precautions.

Wound specimens are collected from infected wounds and lesions by using a sterile swab. The sterile swab is placed deep into the infected area and surface areas of the wound without contaminating the swab by touching any areas outside the suspected area. The medical assistant's job is to collect the specimen and place it in transport medium.

Medical assistants may assist in the collection of vaginal specimens. Women should not douche within 24 hours of collection of a cervical or vaginal culture. The physician inserts a sterile, cotton-tipped swab into the vagina and samples of fluid are placed on a slide for testing.

Culturing blood requires two or three samples collected 30 to 60 minutes apart. Blood samples can be drawn into sterile, yellow stopper evacuated tubes and transferred to culture media. An anticoagulant must be present in the tube or blood culture bottle to prevent microorganism from being trapped within a clot. The venipuncture technique for collecting blood cultures follows the routine procedure, except for an increase in the antiseptic preparation at the puncture site. There should be at least a 1:10 ratio of blood to culture media as the number of organisms present is usually small.

When the patient is suspected of having certain types of digestive disorders, cancer, bacterial or parasitic infections, a stool specimen may be obtained. The patient must take care not to contaminate with urine or water from the toilet. If a physician requests an Ova and Parasites (O&P), a protozoal or parasitic infection is suspected. Culture collection swabs may be used to collect a rectal specimen or a swab of fecal material, then the swab should be placed in a C&S vial (fecal transport system).

Culture and sensitivity (C&S) testing is a procedure performed on a patient suspected of having a bacterial infection. To identify the microorganism, the medical assistant may perform a culture in which a sample of a specimen is placed in or on a substance (medium) that allows it to grow. For optimal growth, the specimen is placed in an incubator set to a specific temperature and humidity.

Sensitivity testing is utilized to isolate the bacterium's sensitivity to antibiotics. This will assist the doctor in determining which antibiotics might be most effective in treating the infection.

URINALYSIS

Collection of Urine Specimens

Urine can reveal a considerable amount of information regarding the function of the body and its ability to regulate fluid, balance electrolytes, and remove waste products. Urine is composed of 95 percent water and 5 percent organic and inorganic waste products.

The medical assistant must obtain an adequate volume (30–50 mL) of urine to be able to perform the physical, chemical, and microscopic evaluation of the collected specimen. The specimen cup should be properly labeled with the patient's name, date, and time of collection. If possible, urinalysis should be avoided during menstruation.

There are several ways to collect urine for laboratory testing. The random specimen is collected in a clean, dry container and is tested immediately. The first-voided morning specimen contains the greatest concentration of dissolved substances and is utilized for accuracy in pregnancy testing. A clean catch midstream specimen should be obtained if a bacterial urinary tract infection is suspected or if the specimen is to be cultured. This type of specimen should be collected in a sterile container. Two-hour postprandial urine specimens are collected two hours after a meal and are used for diabetic screening. The 24-hour specimen measures specific urinary components such as calcium, creatine, lead, potassium, urea, and nitrogen. The 24-hour specimen utilizes a 3,000-mL container that is kept refrigerated.

Physical Analysis of Urine

Assessment of urine includes physical, chemical, and microscopic analysis. The first component of a complete urinalysis is the physical assessment of color, turbidity, volume, odor, and specific gravity. The color of urine can range from pale straw to amber, but typically is a shade of yellow. If the sample is diluted, the color will be much paler. If the sample is concentrated, the color will be darker. The color of urine can be influenced by fluid intake, diet (beets can tint urine red), medication, and disease.

Turbidity is the cloudiness of the urine sample. Cloudiness can result from the accumulation of cells, yeast, bacteria, crystals, or possibly contamination. If a clear urine sample is not tested within one hour after voiding, it will become cloudy as crystals form and precipitate. Foam may also be seen in urine samples as bubbles that persist for some time after the specimen has been shaken. White foam can indicate the presence of a large amount of protein. Green/yellow foam can indicate bilirubinuria, possibly associated with viral hepatitis.

Volume is measured when assessing a timed specimen collection. Once the volume is assessed and recorded, a small amount, called an aliquot, is removed and tested. The normal volume varies according to the age of the individual. The normal adult urine volume is between 750 to 2,000 mL in a 24-hour period.

Urine usually has a slight odor. Standing for a long time breaks down the urea, which gives urine an ammonia odor. Diabetic patients may have urine that tends to smell fruity due to the amount of ketones that are present. Patients with urinary tract infections have foul-smelling urine that becomes worse after standing. Certain foods can cause changes in urine smell, such as asparagus, which leads to a musty urine smell.

Specific gravity compares the weight of urine with an equal amount of distilled water. This measurement indicates the amount of dissolved substances in the urine and illustrates the ability of the kidneys to dilute or concentrate urine. The specific gravity of distilled water is 1.000 and is used to calibrate the refractometer. The normal range for specific gravity is 1.005–1.030. A decrease in a patient's specific gravity may indicate chronic renal insufficiency, or hypertension. An increase may imply chronic heart failure, diabetes, or dehydration. To measure specific gravity, laboratories use a reagent strip, refractometer, or urinometer.

Chemical Analysis of Urine

The chemical analysis of urine can detect abnormal amounts of substances in the blood that should be removed by the kidneys. Tests are available for pH, glucose, protein, ketones, blood, leukocytes, nitrites, bilirubin, urobilinogen, and other chemicals. The presence of these chemicals in the urine provides information on the status of several body functions. Testing strips are dipped into the urine and assessed for an abnormal color change as the reagent reacts with chemicals in the specimen after a specific time. The reagent strips are sensitive to light, heat, and moisture. Once dipped into urine, the medical assistant should compare the strip to the color chart in good lighting. Quality control strips should be used prior to testing patient urine each time a new container is opened. The reagent strip should never be touch by the medical assistant's hands.

Potential hydrogen, or pH, is a measurement of the amount of acidity or alkalinity of urine. A pH of 7.0 is considered neutral. A number less than 7.0 is acidic and greater than 7.0 is alkaline. The normal range for freshly voided urine is 4.5–8.0. Measuring the pH can indicate the possibility of crystals in the urine sediment.

Glucose should never be detected in urine. Glucose is filtered by the glomerulus and under normal conditions, most of it is reabsorbed by the renal tubules. If glucose is detected in the urine (glycosuria), then there is excess glucose in the blood and the kidneys cannot reabsorb it into the bloodstream. Positive glucose is a common finding in urine from diabetic patients and may be the first indication of the disease.

Protein does not normally occur in urine. Proteinuria is one of the first signs of renal disease. Protein excretion in high amount can be caused by unusually high stress or strenuous exercise. Proteinuria is a common finding during pregnancy, especially in cases of toxemia.

Ketones are by-products of fat metabolism in the body and include three types; beta hydroxy-butyric, acetoacetic acid, and acetone. Ketosis occurs when the body burns fat for energy. The ketones will accumulate in the body tissues and fluids. Ketonuria is observed with diabetes mellitus, low-carbohydrate diets, excessive vomiting, and starvation. Because ketone bodies evaporate at room temperature, urine should be tested immediately after collection.

Blood is an abnormal finding in urine and may indicate trauma or infection of the urinary tract or bleeding in the kidneys. Hematuria may be associated with injury, cystitis, tumors, or kidney stones. The reagent strip pad can react with intact red blood cells, hemoglobin from red blood cells, and myoglobin to give positive results.

Leukocytes are also abnormal when found in urine. This finding may indicate inflammation in the lower urinary tract, kidneys, or infection of the urinary tract. White blood cells may also be present as a result of contamination, often from the vagina.

Nitrates are normally found in urine. Nitrites occur in urine when bacteria convert or reduce nitrates to nitrites. A positive reagent strip test may indicate the presence of nitrites, which may indicate a bacterial urinary tract infection. Escherichia coli bacterium is the most common cause of urinary tract infections and can reduce nitrate to nitrite.

The average life of a red blood cell (RBC) is between 100 and 120 days. When the RBC dies, it releases a yellow substance called bilirubin, which is transported to the liver and excreted into the bile leaving the body via the intestines. Bilirubin is a bile pigment not normally found in urine. Bilirubinuria may be an indication of liver disease and can result from gallstones, hepatitis, or cirrhosis. The urine appears yellow-brown or greenish in color. The urine sample must be tested immediately or must be protected from light as direct light leads to decomposition of bilirubin.

Urobilinogen is a normal component of urine in small amounts. An increase in the production of bilirubin (increased red blood cell destruction) increases the amount of urobilinogen in the urine.

Other diagnostic tests that can be performed on urine include Phenistix for phenylketonuria, Clinitest for glucose, and urine pregnancy tests for human chorionic gonadotropin (hCG).

Pregnancy tests detect the presence of human chorionic gonadotropin (hCG). This hormone is released by the placenta and will be present in the urine during pregnancy. An enzyme immunoassay (EIA) test is the most common type of pregnancy test. EIA tests are sensitive enough to detect the presence of hCG as early as one week after implantation or four to five days before a missed menstrual period. The test should be performed on the first-morning voided specimen.

Urine cultures are used to assist in the diagnosis of bacterial urinary tract infection and assess the effectiveness of the antibiotic therapy. A clean catch midstream specimen should be obtained in a sterile container. The container incubates at 37°C (body temperature) for 18 to 24 hours, after which the density of the bacterial colony growth is compared to a density chart.

Microscopic Analysis of Urine

The microscopic examination of urine consists of counting cells, recognizing casts, crystals, and other components of the sediment obtained after a portion of the urine is centrifuged. The clear upper portion of the centrifuged sample, called supernatant, is decanted, leaving concentrated sediment for staining and examination under a microscope. Many formed elements will be found in urine and should correlate to the physical and chemical analysis.

Cellular elements that are found in urine may include red blood cells (RBCs), white blood cells (WBCs), and epithelial cells. Red blood cells can enter the urinary tract at the site of trauma or inflammation. These cells are round, colorless, nongranular, and are biconcave discs. The presence of zero to five is considered normal for this type of cell. White blood cells are larger than red blood cells and will appear as round, granular cells with a nucleus. More than 5/HPF (high power field) is associated with inflammation or contamination of the urine specimen. Squamous epithelial cells line the lower portion of the urinary tract. These cells are normally present in small numbers. A large number present in a female patient usually indicates vaginal contamination. Squamous epithelial cells are large, clear and flat with an irregular shape and a single, small, round, centrally located nucleus. Renal tubular or round epithelial cells are large and round with a large nucleus. They are found in the deeper layers of the urinary tract. Presence of a large number indicates tubular damage. Transitional epithelial cells are found from the renal pelvis to the upper portion of the urethra. Transitional cells are large, round to oval, and may contain a tail and two nuclei. Presence of these cells in large amounts indicates pathology.

Casts are formed when protein accumulates and hardens in the lumen of the tubules that make up the nephron. The precipitated protein hardens, takes on the size and shape of the tubules, and is washed out into the urine. Casts are cylindrical with flat or rounded edges and are classified by their contents. Casts are observed and counted under low-power magnification. Casts may dissolve in alkaline urine; therefore, examination of a freshly voided specimen is important. Hyaline casts are pale, colorless cylinders with rounded edges. Hyaline casts can be found in patients with kidney disease or those who engage in strenuous exercise. Granular casts are hyaline casts that contain granules. Presence of these casts is also associated with heavy exercise or possible renal disease. Cellular casts are hyaline that contain a certain clump of cells (WBC, RBC, epithelial cells, bacteria). Red blood cell casts appear brown due to the color of the cellular inclusions. RBC casts indicate pathology and occur with glomerulonephritis. White blood cell casts contain leukocytes and are seen with pyelonephritis. Renal tubular epithelial cell casts may be confused with white blood cell casts. These casts are found with shock, heavy-metal poisoning, and allergic reactions. Fatty casts are hyaline casts that contain fatty deposits. Fatty casts are characteristic of nephritic syndrome. Waxy casts appear glassy, light yellow, and brittle with serrated edges. Waxy casts are found with severe renal disease.

Crystals are a common component of urinary sediment. Most crystals are not considered significant unless they are found in large numbers. Identification of crystals begins with pH determination. Most abnormal crystals are found in acidic urine. Crystals are recognized by color, shape, and refractivity. Amorphous urate crystals are salts of uric acid and are shapeless granular substances found in acidic urine. Amorphous phosphates are fluffy white precipitate and are found in alkaline urine.

HEMATOLOGY

Hematology is the study of blood and includes the morphologic appearance of cells, function of blood, and diseases of blood and blood-forming tissues. Blood is composed of plasma, red blood cells, white blood cells, and platelets.

Plasma is a straw-colored liquid that makes up 55 percent of the total volume of blood. Plasma functions include transporting nutrients to the tissues of the body and picking up wastes from the tissues. Plasma is composed of 91 percent water and 9 percent plasma proteins.

Erythrocytes (*red blood cells*) transport oxygen from the lungs to body tissues. The normal adult range is between 4.2 to 6.3 million per mm^3. Red blood cells are biconcave in shape and do not contain a nucleus. The biconcave shape provides a greater surface area for the exchange of substances. Hemoglobin is the important component of red blood cells, which binds with and transports oxygen.

Leukocytes (*white blood cells*) are clear, colorless cells that contain a nucleus. These cells help protect the body from infections. White blood cells attempt to destroy invading pathogens and remove them from the body. The average white blood cell count is between 4,500 and 11,000 per mm^3. A level above 11,000 may be indicative of an infection or disease.

Platelets (*clotting cells*) or thrombocytes are small, clear cells that lack a nucleus. Platelets are formed in the red bone marrow from giant cells known as megakaryocytes. These cells also produce thrombokinase, an enzyme utilized in the clotting process. The average platelet count is between 150,000 and 350,000 per mm^3.

Collection of Blood Specimens

The two most common ways to collect blood are phlebotomy and capillary puncture. Phlebotomy or venipuncture requires insertion of a needle into a superficial vein to withdraw blood. Phlebotomy is performed primarily for diagnosis and monitoring a patient's condition. Capillary puncture involves a puncture (prick) of the skin with a lancet, which causes the body to release a small amount of blood.

If a large blood specimen is needed, venipuncture is the preferred method. A vein is punctured with a needle and blood is collected utilizing the evacuated tube method, the syringe method, and/or the butterfly method. The evacuated tube method allows for the collection of several samples from one venipuncture site using interchangeable vacuum collection tubes. Collection tubes are calibrated by evacuation to collect the exact amount of blood required for a specific test. Tube volumes range from 2 to 15 mL. Some tubes are prepared with additives to correctly process blood samples for testing. There is no need to transfer materials from a collection syringe or a sample tube.

The evacuated tube system includes an evacuated closed glass or plastic tube containing a vacuum, a special double-pointed needle, and a plastic needle holder/adapter. The vacuum tubes contain several different additives such as clot activators, anticoagulants, and thixotropic gels.

The size and content of the tubes depends upon the test to be performed. With the exception of the red-stoppered tubes, all tubes contain an additive. Clot activators promote clotting of blood by providing a surface for platelet activation. Thrombin encourages clotting and is used in tubes drawn for stat chemistry testing. Anticoagulants prevent blood from clotting and can be used to collect whole blood and plasma.

Order of Draw

Despite the method of blood collection, the samples must be mixed with the appropriate additive in the correct collection tubes before they are transported to the lab for testing. Each tube stopper has a different color, each color identifying the type of additives they contain. Tubes should be filled in a specific order to preserve the integrity of the blood sample. The following table outlines the National Committee for Clinical Laboratory Standards recommended order of draw.

Order	Tube stopper color	Additive	Tests
1	Yellow	Sodium polyanetholesulfonate	Blood cultures
2	Light blue*	Sodium citrate additive	Coagulation studies
3	Red	No additive	Chemistry, AIDS antibody, viral studies, serology, blood typing
4	Red/gray ("tiger")	Silicone serum separator	Serum testing
5	Green	Sodium heparin (anticoagulant)	Electrolytes, arterial blood gases
6	Lavender/purple/ pink	EDTA**	Hematology, blood bank crossmatching
7	Gray	Potassium oxalate or sodium fluoride	Blood glucose

* If a light blue–stoppered tube is the first or only tube to be drawn, a 5-mL, red-stoppered tube should be drawn first and discarded to eliminate contamination. This is because the needle may pick up thromboplastin (clotting factor) from the patient's body when it penetrates the skin. Thromboplastin can then enter the blood specimen, affecting test results.

**EDTA = ethylenediaminetetraacetic acid

Table 13.1—Order of Draw

Capillary blood specimen is used when a small amount of blood is required. Small blood samples can be collected for testing hemoglobin, hematocrit, and glucose. The skin puncture technique can also be used for adults if there are no accessible veins suitable for venipuncture. Infants and children typically have low blood volume and removing large quantities may result in anemia.

Puncture sites will vary depending on the age of the patient. For adults and children, the typical site is the distal phalynx of the middle (3) or ring finger (4) on the nondominant hand. Capillary puncture on infants (birth to one year) is performed on the outer edge of the plantar surface of the heel or the big toe. Capillary puncture is not performed on the finger because the amount of tissue between skin surface and bone is too small and may injure the bone. Once a child begins to walk, the fingertip is the preferred site.

The skin puncture technique is performed using a disposable semiautomatic lancet. The disposable semiautomatic lancet is a spring-loaded plastic holder with a metal blade. This device is available in various sized blades, which are used to control the pierce depth. Blades are approximately 1.0 mm wide and produce a small cut that results in an ample blood flow. The blade itself is concealed within a plastic case. The typical puncture depth should not penetrate deeper than 3.1 mm on an adult and 2.4 mm on infants and children.

Blood specimens can be collected directly onto a reagent strip (glucose testing), into capillary tubes, and/or microcollection tubes. Capillary tubes are disposable glass or plastic tubes that can hold 5 to 75 microliters of blood. These tubes are most often used for hematocrit determination, but have many other uses, such as cholesterol testing. Microcollection tubes are small plastic tubes having a removable collector tip. The tip is designed to collect capillary blood from a skin puncture.

The patient should be seated comfortably. The patient's arm is extended with the palm surface of the hand facing upward, exposing the lateral part of the tip of the third or fourth finger on the nondominant hand. Gently massage the finger or place in warm water to increase blood flow. The first drop of blood is wiped away with gauze, as the sample is diluted with alcohol and is unsuitable for testing. The medical assistant should allow a large drop of blood to form. The blood droplet should then be collected and placed in the appropriate device.

Diagnostic Testing

Several blood tests are routinely ordered as part of a complete examination to determine a patient's health. Medical assistants must understand the chemical properties, the purpose, and the normal ranges for each of those tests. Hematologic tests include blood cell counts, morphologic studies, coagulation tests, and erythrocyte sedimentation rates. These tests can be performed on venous or capillary whole blood samples. A complete blood cell count (CBC) includes the following items: white blood cell count (WBC), red blood cell count (RBC), platelet count, hemoglobin (Hgb), hematocrit (Hct), differential white blood cells count (Diff), and red blood cell indices.

Morphological studies assess the shape or form of cells. A blood smear is examined and the cells are studied for appearance and shape. Abnormal size, shape, content, and color are noted. A morphologic study is often performed on the same blood smear slide after the differential count and platelet estimate.

Erythrocyte sedimentation rate (ESR) measures the rate (time) it takes red blood cells to settle to the bottom of a blood sample. A freshly collected sample of anticoagulated blood is transferred to a calibrated tube and placed in a sedimentation rack on a counter free of vibrations and away from sunlight. The tube is examined exactly one hour later to determine the distance the red blood cells have fallen. Tests results are recorded as millimeters per hour (mm/hr). This test can indicate inflammation within the body.

Hemoglobin (Hgb or Hb) measures the oxygen-carrying capacity of the blood. The normal range for an adult woman is 12–16 g/dL and for an adult man is 14–18 g/dL. A decreased level occurs with anemia (especially iron deficiency), hyperthyroidism, and certain systemic diseases such as leukemia. Increased levels of hemoglobin are present with polycythemia, chronic obstructive pulmonary disease (COPD), and congestive heart failure.

Hematocrit (Hct) means to separate blood. The solid or cellular elements are separated from the plasma by centrifuging an anticoagulated blood specimen. Red blood cells settle at the bottom of the tube. The top layer contains plasma. Hematocrit measures the volume of packed red blood cells in whole blood. The normal range for an adult woman is 37–47 percent and for an adult male is 40–54 percent. A low level may indicate anemia and an elevated level may indicate polycythemia. Calculating the hematocrit requires dividing the amount of packed red blood cells by the amount of the whole blood volume and multiplying by 100.

White blood cell differential count is used to identity the five types of white blood cells within a sample. A blood cell counter is used to determine the number of neutrophils, lymphocytes monocytes, eosinophils, and basophils. *Neutrophils* are granulocytes that have a purple, multi-lobed nucleus. Neutrophils are seen with acute infection. *Lymphocytes* are agranulocytes with a round or slightly indented nucleus that almost completely fills the cell and stains a deep purplish blue. Lymphocytes are seen with viral disease, infectious mono, mumps, chicken pox, rubella, and viral hepatitis. *Monocytes* are agranulocytes that contain a large nucleus that is kidney or horseshoe-shaped. Monocytes are the largest phagocytic white blood cell. *Eosinophils* are granulocytes with a segmented nucleus. These cells are seen with allergic conditions and parasitic infestation. Basophils are also granulocytes that contain an s-shaped nucleus.

Chemical Testing of Blood

Blood chemistry testing involves the quantitative measurement of chemical substances present in the blood. These chemicals are dissolved in the liquid portion of the blood; therefore, most blood chemistry tests require a serum specimen for analysis. Automated blood chemistry analyzers consist of a reflectance photometer that quantitatively measures the amount of chemical substances or analytes in the blood.

Several blood chemistry tests are routinely performed in the physician's office laboratory. Glucose monitoring is usually performed on a capillary blood specimen and the level is determined by comparing the color on a reagent strip to a standard or by using an automated device. Hemoglobin A1c is another test used to monitor diabetic patients. The test measures the amount of glycosylated hemoglobin in the blood. As blood glucose levels rise, the glucose molecules bind with hemoglobin to form hemoglobin A1c (HgBA1c). This test can be performed without fasting. HgBA1c gives information over a period of two to three months. The ideal range for HgBA1c is less than 7 percent.

Fasting blood sugar (FBS) involves collecting a fasting blood sample and measuring the amount of glucose present. The patient should not have anything to eat or drink, except water, for 12 hours preceding the test. Certain medications (do not take for three days prior) interfere with FBS. These medications include salicylates (aspirin), diuretics, and steroids. A normal range is 70–100 mg/dL. FBS above 120 mg/dL is considered the dividing point between normal and hyperglycemic. Hyperglycemia is often indicative of diabetes mellitus.

The two-hour postprandial blood sugar test is used to screen for the presence of diabetes mellitus and to monitor the effects of insulin dosage in diagnosed diabetics. The patient is required to fast. A blood specimen is collected two hours after consumption of a 100-gram test-load glucose solution. In a nondiabetic patient, the glucose level returns to the fasting level within one and a half to two hours from the time of glucose consumption. The glucose level in the diabetic patient does not return to the fasting level. A postprandial glucose level of 140 mg/dL or higher is suggestive of diabetes mellitus.

Glucose tolerance test (GTT) provides more detailed information about the ability of the body to metabolize glucose by assessing the insulin response to a glucose load. The patient is required to consume a high carbohydrate diet for three days, consisting of 150 grams of carbohydrates per day. The patient must be in the fasting state when the test begins. After the FBS has been performed, the patient is instructed to drink a measured amount of a glucose solution (1.75 grams of glucose per kilogram of body weight, or the standard adult dose of 100 grams). Thereafter, at regular intervals (30, 60, 120, and 180 minutes), blood and urine samples are taken. The patient should not consume food or fluid (except water) during the test to assist in producing urine samples. Smoking is not permitted because it acts as a stimulant that increases the blood glucose level. The patient should remain at the site because activity affects the test results by utilizing glucose. In a nondiabetic patient, the blood glucose level rises to a range between 160 and 180 mg/dL approximately 30 to 60 minutes after the glucose solution is consumed, but should return to normal levels within two hours.

Cholesterol is a white, waxy, fat-like substance (lipid) that is essential for normal functioning of the body. Cholesterol levels are a combined measurement of the amount of low-density lipid cholesterol ("bad cholesterol") and high-density lipid cholesterol ("good cholesterol") in the blood. Cholesterol test results are interpreted as follows: under 200 mg/dL is desirable, levels 200–239 mg/dL are considered borderline high, and 240 mg/dL and above are considered high. Patients are not required to fast for total cholesterol and HDL testing; however, for a complete lipid profile, the patient must fast. Total cholesterol and high-density lipid cholesterol determinations are not affected significantly by food consumption. If the patient is getting a lipid profile done, they must be in a fasting state. The lipid profile includes total cholesterol, triglycerides, high density lipoprotein (HDL), and low density lipoprotein (LDL). Triglycerides are affected by food intake; a level higher than 250 mg/dL is considered dangerous.

The two most common blood tests for kidney function are the blood urea nitrogen test (BUN) and the creatinine test. These two substances are produced by cellular metabolism and the kidney should clear them out of the blood via urine. High levels of these substances in the blood therefore suggest that kidney dysfunction.

Another group of tests indirectly assesses the health of liver cells by measuring enzymes levels and substances produced by the liver. Liver function tests include alanine aminotransferase (ALT), aspartate aminotransferase (AST), gamma-glutamyltranspeptidase (GGT), bilirubin levels, albumin levels, and prothrombin time (PT).

ALT is an enzyme produced in hepatocytes, the major cell type in the liver. AST is an enzyme found in muscle. In many cases of liver inflammation, the ALT and AST activities are elevated roughly in a 1:1 ratio. GGT is an enzyme produced in the bile ducts that may be elevated in the serum of patients with bile duct diseases. Bilirubin is removed from the blood by the liver. Bilirubin concentrations are elevated in the blood either by increased production, decreased uptake by the liver, decreased secretion from the liver, or blockage of the bile ducts. Albumin is synthesized by the liver and secreted into the blood. Low serum albumin concentrations indicate poor liver function. Prothrombin time (PT) is necessary for blood clotting and is made in the liver. In chronic liver diseases, the prothrombin time is usually not elevated until cirrhosis is present.

Serology

Serology is defined as the scientific study of serum of the blood. Mononucleosis is caused by the Epstein-Barr virus. Individuals with mononucleosis produce an antibody called heterophile antibody, usually by the 6th to 10th day of the illness. Rapid mono tests are able to detect the presence of this antibody within five minutes.

ABO and Rh blood typing is performed to determine an individual's ABO and Rh blood type. Blood typing helps to prevent transfusion and transplant reactions, helps identify problems such as hemolytic disease of newborns, and can assist in determining parentage. The Rh Antibody Titer detects the amount of circulating Rh antibodies against red blood cells. These antibodies can occur in a pregnant woman who is Rh– and is carrying an Rh+ fetus.

RADIOGRAPHIC TESTING

X-rays are used to visualize internal organs and structures and to serve as a diagnostic aid. Radiation is also used therapeutically in the treatment of malignancy. A radiograph is a permanent record of the picture produced on a radiographic film. Items in the body that obstruct the passage of x-ray, such as bone, are termed radiopaque. A structure, such as lung tissue, that permits the passage of x-rays is considered radiolucent. Contrast medium is used to make a particular structure visible on the radiograph.

The patient's position is determined by the purpose of the examination and the area examined. The various types of radiographic views include anteroposterior, posteroanterior, lateral, oblique, supine, and prone. X-rays that are directed from the front to the back of the body are called anteroposterior views. The patient is facing the x-ray tube and the posterior aspect is against the radiographic film. The patient's back would face the x-ray tube for a posteroanterior view. When performing the lateral view, the x-ray beam passes from one side of the patient's body to the other. For an oblique view, the body is positioned at an angle or in a semilateral position. Supine positioning has the patient lying on his back for the x-ray. The patient is positioned face down for a prone radiograph.

The medical assistant should understand the purpose and proper instructions for commonly performed radiographic examinations. Other types of radiological testing that may be performed in a medical office include the following.

- **Angiography:** insertion of a catheter into a patient's vein or artery. Dye is then injected and a series of x-rays helps assess the vessel's blood flow and condition.

- **Barium studies:** a lower GI series or barium enema requires barium sulfate to be instilled through the anus into the rectum and the colon to help diagnose and evaluate obstruction. The upper GI series or barium swallow involves oral administration of barium sulfate to visualize the esophagus, stomach, duodenum, and small intestines.

- **Computed tomography (CT):** allows cross-sectional views of the area in question. The x-ray camera rotates around the patient and produces a series of views of a body part.

- **Magnetic resonance imaging (MRI):** a combination of nonionizing radiation and a strong magnetic field allow for examination of internal structures and soft tissues of the body based on water content of tissue.

- **Intravenous pyelogram (IVP):** also called excretory urography; involves injection of contrast medium into a vein. A series of x-rays are taken as the medium travels through the kidneys, ureters, and bladder.

- **Kidney, ureter, and bladder (KUB) radiography:** also called flat plate of the abdomen; x-ray of the abdomen to assess the size, shape, and position of the urinary organs. No contrast medium is used.

- **Ultrasound:** uses high-frequency inaudible sound waves through the skin over the area being examined and produces an image based on echoes.

OTHER COMMONLY PERFORMED TESTS

Respiratory Testing

Pulmonary function tests (PFT) measure the volume and flow of air by utilizing a spirometer and compares against normal values. A spirometer is a device attached to a computer that measures the capacity of the lungs while the patient blows exhaled air from the lungs into the disposable mouthpiece.

Tuberculosis Testing

The Mantoux tuberculin test, or purified protein derivative (PPD), is a type of intradermal skin test. A small extract from the tubercle bacillus is injected into the skin and results are read in 48–72 hours. Raising and hardening of the skin (called an induration) of 10 mm or more around the area indicates a possible positive reaction. Less than 5 mm induration is not considered a positive test; induration of 5–10 mm is equivocal (likely needs repeat or further testing). However, individuals vaccinated with bacille Calmette-Guerin (BCG) will also test positive even if they are not infected with TB; many foreign-born individuals have received BCG vaccination. When the tuberculin test is positive, other testing is then required, including a chest x-ray and sputum culture.

Guaiac Testing

Guaiac reagent strips are used to detect the presence of occult blood in the stool. The test may detect bleeding in the GI tract that is undetectable with a visual inspection. This test is designed to detect hidden blood in the stool early enough for corrective measures to be taken. The patient collects stool samples on the reagent paper and sends the test in a leak-proof envelope to the laboratory.

Hemoglobin and Hematocrit Determination

The hemoglobin and hematocrit tests are used to detect iron-deficiency anemia and are often conducted in an office setting. They can be obtained simply and rapidly using the finger-stick method of blood collection. Hemoglobin (Hb) is the protein in red blood cells that carries oxygen to the tissues. It is measured using a device called a HemoCue and expressed in grams per deciliter (g/dl). Normal hemoglobin values vary based on gender and age, but adult hemoglobin is typically in the range of 12–18 g/dl. Hematocrit is the ratio of red blood cell volume to total blood volume and is expressed as a percentage of red blood cells. The specimen is collected into a micro-capillary tube and then centrifuged, which concentrates the red blood cells at the bottom of the tube so that the total can be read on a scale. Normal adult hematocrit values are 36–55 percent.

Streptococcus Testing

Beta-hemolytic streptococcus group A is a major cause of serious bacterial throat infections. Left untreated, streptococcus can lead to rheumatic fever with associated heart and kidney complications, among other health problems. There are two tests for streptococcus: a throat swab placed in culture media and incubated for 24–48 hours, and a CLIA-waived kit that provides immediate results. Whenever using a prepared kit for testing, use extreme care to avoid inaccurate results. This includes confirming that the kits are within their use dates (not expired), following the testing guidelines, and running positive and negative controls with the patient test.

Pregnancy Testing

Pregnancy testing can be rapidly and easily accomplished with a first morning urine specimen from the patient. A first morning urine specimen provides the greatest concentration of human chorionic gonadotropin (hCG), which is produced by the placenta shortly after embryonic attachment to the uterus. This test can detect pregnancy as early as two weeks after conception and is 97 percent accurate if performed correctly.

Epstein-Barr Virus Testing

The Epstein-Barr virus (EBV) is a one of the most common infectious viruses, perhaps best known as the cause of infectious mononucleosis (IM). A common contagious disease, IM is sometimes called "the kissing disease" because transmission occurs via saliva. IM is difficult to detect because of the vague symptoms it presents. After the primary infection, the virus establishes latency in the victim that lasts for a lifetime. Rapid detection kits using a small amount of blood obtained via a finger-stick are available, but serologic tests in conjunction with clinical observations of the patient may be required to confirm diagnosis.

REVIEW QUESTIONS

1. Which of the following states the purpose of laboratory testing?

   (A) Assists in the diagnosis of patient's condition

   (B) Takes the place of a hands-on examination

   (C) To practice the skills learned in school

   (D) To increase revenue for the laboratory

   (E) To overcome lack of confidence

2. Which of the following is within the normal range for pH of urine?

   (A) 0–1

   (B) 1–3

   (C) 4.5–8

   (D) 9–11

   (E) 12–14

3. A fruity smell to the urine may indicate the pathological condition of

   (A) diabetes mellitus

   (B) diabetes insipidus

   (C) a urinary tract infection

   (D) starvation

   (E) liver failure

4. Which of the following substances is a normal metabolic by-product of ketones?

   (A) Protein

   (B) Sugar

   (C) Fat

   (D) Carbohydrates

   (E) Cellular

5. Which of the following is the correct reason the foot is used as a puncture site for infants?

   (A) Gravity helps with blood flow.

   (B) They won't see it coming.

   (C) Blood flow is slower at this location.

   (D) Higher concentration of hemoglobin can be obtained.

   (E) The heel is soft, and puncture will avoid injury to bones.

6. Which of the following is considered an OSHA standard?

    (A) Placing needles in a biohazard sharps container
    (B) Throwing blood vials in the trash
    (C) Placing used syringes in the trash
    (D) Blood-stained gloves in the trash
    (E) Wearing a lab coat and mask when taking vital signs

7. Which cells settle to the bottom of the test tube after blood is centrifuged?

    (A) RBCs
    (B) Platelets
    (C) Bacteria
    (D) Plasma
    (E) Serum

8. Which of the following is the correct gauge range for venipuncture needles?

    (A) 13–15
    (B) 15–19
    (C) 19–21
    (D) 20–22
    (E) 23–25

9. The total magnification while looking through the high power objective (40×) is

    (A) 10
    (B) 40
    (C) 100
    (D) 400
    (E) 1,000

10. Which of the following is the proper order of draw when collecting multiple tubes of blood?

    (A) Lavender, yellow, blue, tiger
    (B) Red, blue, lavender, yellow
    (C) Red, lavender, green, yellow
    (D) Yellow, blue, red, tiger
    (E) Yellow, red, tiger, lavender

Read the following scenario to answer questions 11–14:

A 20-year-old female was experiencing urinary frequency, increased thirst, and nausea. She was instructed to bring in a first morning, clean-catch midstream urine specimen, and then she would be examined by the doctor.

11. What reason would the doctor have for requesting a first morning specimen?

    (A) The patient could be pregnant, and a first morning specimen has the highest concentration of dissolved substances.

    (B) The patient may not be able to urinate when in the office, and the provider requires a specimen to test.

    (C) A first morning specimen is the only accurate specimen when screening for infection.

    (D) A first morning specimen is the only specimen that can be collected via a clean-catch midstream technique.

    (E) The first morning specimen will be the baseline for comparison when another specimen is obtained in the office.

12. The patient does not have a commercial sterile container. What instructions should the medical assistant give the patient about how to collect the clean-catch midstream specimen at home?

    (A) Wash a glass jar, cleanse the perineum from front to back, and urinate in the jar. Do not collect the end of the stream in the jar.

    (B) Wash a glass jar and avoid putting hands in the cleaned jar. Cleanse the perineum, urinate, and catch the middle part of the stream in the jar.

    (C) Boil a glass jar, cleanse the perineum from front to back, begin to urinate, and then positon the jar to catch the middle part of the stream. Do not collect the end of the stream in the jar.

    (D) Boil a glass jar, cleanse the perineum from back to front, begin to urinate, and then position the jar to catch the middle part of the stream. Do not collect the end of the stream in the jar.

    (E) Do not collect the specimen at home, because it would not be valid for a screening test.

13. The urine specimen reveals a 2+ glucose level and ketones. What could these results indicate?

    (A) Nothing, because glucose and ketones in the urine are normal.

    (B) Diabetes, because glucose and ketones are symptomatic of this condition.

    (C) Infection, because the patient has urinary frequency, an indicator of infection. The glucose is a result of that infection.

    (D) Kidney damage, because ketones indicate protein breakdown.

    (E) Vomiting or anorexia nervosa, because ketones indicate fat breakdown.

14. Based on the results of the urine testing, the provider ordered a fasting blood sugar (FBS) test. Which of the following statements regarding this test is TRUE?

(A) FBS is a blood chemistry test, and the patient should fast except for water for 8–12 hours before testing.

(B) FBS is a hematology blood test, and the patient should have nothing to eat or drink for 8–12 hours before testing.

(C) FBS tests a blood sample that is collected 2 hours after a meal.

(D) FBS tests a blood sample that is collected via capillary puncture.

(E) If FBS test results are 120 mg/dL or less, the patient is not diabetic.

ANSWERS AND EXPLANATIONS

1. **A**

   Following a thorough health history and physical examination, the doctor orders lab tests to help confirm or rule out disease conditions. Laboratory tests are used in conjunction with hands-on examinations (B). Class time and internship time is the opportunity to practice skills learned in school (C). Laboratory testing usually requires a substantial budgetary allotment (D) from the office including testing supplies, equipment, and trained personnel. Lack of confidence (E) is a common problem with new graduates, especially in the arena of laboratory testing.

2. **C**

   The correct pH of urine is between 4.5 and 8. A pH of 0–1 (A) and 1–3 (B) are too acidic for a normal pH of urine. A pH of 9–11 (D) and 12–14 (E) are too basic or alkaline for a normal pH of urine.

3. **A**

   Uncontrolled diabetes mellitus will result in a fruity smell to urine due to excretion of acetone (a type of ketone) from the lungs. Diabetes insipidus (B) does not cause any change to body or urine odor. Urinary tract infection (C) can cause the urine to have a foul smelling odor. Starvation (D) does not cause any change to body or urine odor, but can lead to fat metabolism and the accumulation of ketone bodies in the body tissue. Liver failure (E) can produce a musty smelling urine sample.

4. **C**

   Ketones are by-products of fat metabolism. Urea and creatinine are by-products of protein metabolism (A). Monosaccharides are by-products of sugar (B) and carbohydrate (D) metabolism. Many items can result from cellular metabolism (E).

5. **E**

   The area between the skin and bone in the finger or the hand is too small in infants and puncturing with a lancet can cause injury to bone. Gravity (A) can help with blood flow despite the area of puncture. Infants are unaware regardless of the procedure (B) and the lancet is usually a concealed semiautomatic blade. Blood flow in the heel of the foot is usually ample if the puncture is substantial (C). Higher concentration of hemoglobin (D) was found in the earlobe; therefore, this site is not utilized any longer.

6. **A**

    OSHA standards state that needles and other sharps should be placed in a biohazard sharps container. Vials of blood (B) should be placed in a biohazard container. Used syringes (C) should be placed in the biohazard sharps container if there is a used needle or in a biohazard container if no needle is present but has been exposed to medication or bodily fluid. Blood-stained gloves (D) should be placed is a biohazard container. Wearing a lab coat and mask when taking vital signs (E) is unnecessary.

7. **A**

    Red blood cells (A) are heavy elements that will move to the bottom of the centrifuged sample of blood. Bacteria (C) should not be found in a blood sample. When blood is centrifuged, it forms into striated layers, from top to bottom: plasma, buffy coat, and red blood cells. Plasma (D) is the top layer. Platelets (B) and white blood cells are included in the buffy coat. Serum (E) is plasma from which the clotting factor fibrinogen has been removed.

8. **D**

    The typical range for needles used in venipuncture is 20–22 gauge. Gauge 13–15 (A) needles are too large for most superficial veins. Gauge 15–19 (B) needles are also too big for venipuncture, but may be used for intramuscular injections. Gauge 19–21 (C) includes needles that are still too large for comfortable phlebotomy procedures. Gauge 23–25 (E) needles are smaller. Butterfly winged infusion sets may have 23-gauge needles.

9. **D**

    Total magnification is calculated using the following formula: 10× (ocular) 40× (lowest objective) = 400× (total magnification of the viewed object). Magnification of 10× (A) is the strength of the eyepieces and the low power objective. Magnification of 40× (B) is the strength of the high power objective. Magnification of 100× (C) is the strength of the oil immersion objective. Magnification of 1000× (E) is the total magnification when using the oil immersion and the eyepieces.

10. **E**

    Yellow is always first if a sterile specimen must be obtained; the yellow tube is used for blood cultures and avoids the chance of contamination from other tubes and additives. Since the red tube has no additives, it comes second. The red/gray (tiger) tube contains a serum separator and is silicone, so would not contaminate other tubes; it should be drawn third. The lavender tube contains EDTA, and thus should be drawn last. It can be helpful to use a mnemonic to remember the order of draw. Try using "You bring really good lollipops, girl!" to remember: yellow, blue, red, green, lavender, gray.

11. **A**

Since people typically drink little at night and urinate less frequently at night, the first morning specimen contains a higher concentration of dissolved substances; thus it should be used when testing for pregnancy. A false negative pregnancy test, especially early in pregnancy, may occur if the patient has drunk a lot of fluids, which dilutes the urine. If a patient is unable to void immediately when in the office (B), the staff typically will offer water and have the patient wait until able to provide a specimen for testing. Although a first morning specimen may be used to screen for an infection (C), a sterile, clean-catch, midstream specimen freshly obtained in the office is desired for accuracy. The clean-catch midstream technique can be used at any time of day (D). Although the specimen could be used as a baseline for a later comparison, this is not the principal reason for collecting it.

12. **C**

If the patient has a boiled jar it can be used to collect a midstream specimen. Washing (A and B) does not remove all the germs in a jar. Before voiding, the patient should cleanse three separate times from front to back (*not* back to front, D) on each side of the urethral opening and then down the middle. The urine should be collected in the middle of the stream. This is because the first part of the stream will cleanse the urethra, and the end of the stream could contain residual sediment from the bladder. Although commercial sterile container is preferable, and it is likely that the provider will want a fresh specimen taken in the office, a sample taken at home is valid if properly collected (E) and may help determine what additional testing is necessary.

13. **B**

Although not a definitive diagnosis, glucose in the urine calls for further laboratory testing for diabetes. (Other clues are increased thirst and increased frequency of urination.) Ketones are a result of fat breakdown; in uncontrolled diabetes, a person's metabolism often breaks down fat for energy at a faster rate than average, spilling ketones into the urine. Glucose and ketones in urine are not normal (A). Infection (C) would likely be indicated by positive nitrites in the urine screening, not glucose. Patients with kidney damage (D) will likely have protein in their urine (i.e., albuminuria or proteinuria) as a result of the excessive stress on the kidneys, but not ketones. A patient who is experiencing excessive vomiting or anorexia nervosa (E) may spill ketones into the urine as a result of fat breakdown, but not glucose.

14. **A**

The FBS is a chemistry test, and the patient can drink water but should avoid some medications such as aspirin, diuretics, and steroids for several days prior to the blood draw. Although FBS is a good indicator of diabetes, it is not a definitive test; additional testing would still be warranted. Hematology tests (B) involve testing the cellular part of the blood; FBS is a chemistry test. A 2-hour postprandial test (C) may be ordered to aid diabetes diagnosis, but the specimen collected for this test is urine, not blood. The blood sample tested in FBS cannot be collected via capillary puncture (D) because this method would not provide enough blood for testing, and also because venous blood provides a more representative specimen of the amount of glucose circulating in the bloodstream. Normal blood sugar levels are in the range of 70–100 mg/dL; 120 mg/dL (E) is too high to rule out diabetes.

Chapter 14: **Medications**

As a member of the medical office team, you will work with the physicians and other staff to assist patients with medications. It is likely that you will assist the physicians with prescription orders, medication refills, and patient instruction regarding their medication schedules. In this chapter, you will review the basic principles of pharmacology and drug therapy. The major classifications of drugs will be covered, along with information about ensuring safe and effective use of prescribed medications.

PHARMACOLOGY

Pharmacology is the study of prescription drugs. As a medical assistant, you must have a basic understanding of commonly prescribed medication. You must be able to effectively use reference books to locate information about medications. Because of the vast array of available drugs, you will use reference material regularly. When administering medication to a patient, you will need to know why it is being used and how it should be administered. In addition, you will need to know the common side effects of the drug.

Several federal agencies control medication development and use. The Food and Drug Administration (FDA) controls the sale of over-the-counter medications (OTCs) as well as prescription drugs. The FDA also controls the development of new drugs and the process of these drugs being approved for distribution. Each drug has a name that corresponds to the chemical makeup of the drug. In addition, each drug is also given a unique generic name. This is the drug's official name and is not copyrighted by the drug manufacturer. The generic name is not capitalized in printed material. Once a medication is approved, the manufacturer is awarded a copyright for that drug for 17 years. During this time, the original manufacturer is the only company that can sell the medication. The manufacturer assigns each new drug a trade name that is used to market the drug under their company name. Trade names of medications are capitalized. Once the copyright expires, other manufacturers may market the drug. Thus, the drug may have many different trade names but the generic name will not change.

Medication History

When interviewing your patients, you will initiate and maintain an up-to-date list of the medications that are both prescribed and self-administered. Be sure to ask patients specifically about any pills, herbal remedies, or OTCs that they take regularly. It is common for patients to forget to tell their health care provider about self-administered medications, vitamins, and other remedies; however, these may cause complications or incompatibilities with prescription drugs. The doctor will want to review a comprehensive list of each patient's current medications.

Controlled Substances

Production and distribution of controlled substances or narcotics are monitored by the federal government through the Drug Enforcement Administration (DEA). The agency is responsible for regulating the use, storage, and recordkeeping involved with narcotics. The DEA also is involved with enforcement of drug abuse laws and drug abuse prevention. The DEA identifies which drugs are classified as controlled substance. The Controlled Substances Act designates a schedule in which all pertinent drugs are separated into five categories. Based on the schedule to which the drug is assigned there are specifications about how and when the drug can be prescribed. Schedule I drugs have no acceptable medical use and cannot be prescribed. Schedules II through V have limitations on prescriptions that must be followed. Meticulous records must be kept in the office when administering, destroying, and accounting for narcotics. Every physician who prescribes controlled substances must have a federal DEA registration number. Prescriptions are completed in triplicate with copies available to the pharmacist and to government regulators. Controlled substances must be stored in a locked area that is secure and procedures must be in place to track their use. Prescription forms should also be kept in a secured area to prevent access by unauthorized persons. If you work in an office where controlled substances are kept and administered, it is essential that you understand the state and federal laws that govern the storage and use of these drugs.

Drug abuse is also something that you should be aware of, and you should know your role in its prevention. All drugs, not only controlled substances, have the potential for misuse. Drug misuse is the improper administration of drugs that can cause physical dependence. Such dependence can occur with routine OTC medications such as laxatives or antihistamines. Drug abuse is the use of a drug in a manner that leads to physical or psychological dependence. When a person develops a physiological dependence to a substance and stops regular intake of the substance, withdrawal may occur. Symptoms of withdrawal can cause minor discomfort or may be life threatening. Patients with problems with drug abuse or family members who have concerns may seek information about treatment alternatives. You should be aware of treatment centers that patients can be referred to if they are having problems with drug abuse. To avoid drug abuse in the office setting, the medical assistant should monitor phone calls for narcotic refills and document requests in the clinical record.

Drug Reference Material

References for looking up medication information must be available in all medical offices. It is important to know the drug action, use, contraindications, precautions, adverse reactions, usual dosage, and available drug forms. Information is available in package inserts, the *Physicians' Desk Reference*, the U.S. Pharmacopeia, and other drug references. Your practice may use an online drug reference system. If you work in a specialty practice, you may want to have patient education material for commonly used drugs. It is likely that drug companies and sales staff can provide you with this material.

Basic Medication Information

There are four main sources of drugs:

1. **Plant:** obtained from plant parts or products (examples: digoxin, atropine)

2. **Animal:** glandular products (examples: insulin, vaccines)

3. **Mineral:** mineral sources (examples: sodium chloride, coal tar)

4. **Synthetic:** produced in a laboratory (examples: Demerol, oral contraceptives)

Medication uses vary widely. Some common examples are listed in the following table.

Type of Medication	Clinical Use
Diagnostic	Used to diagnose a health problem Example: allergy testing
Palliative	Provides relief from symptoms Example: pain medication
Prophylaxis	Provides prevention of illness or disease Example: immunizations
Replacement	Replaces substances needed to maintain health Example: insulin or thyroid replacement
Therapeutic	Used to treat and cure Example: antibiotics

Table 14.1—Clinical Uses of Medication

As the name implies, all prescription medications require an order from a physician or other licensed practitioner. Prescriptions can be handwritten, computer generated, or phoned in to a pharmacy. Controlled substances or narcotics require that the prescription must be handwritten, signed by the physician, and filled at the pharmacy within a certain period of time. Each prescription will include the following items:

1. Superscription: patient's name, address, date, and the symbol ℞

2. Inscription: name of drug, dose form, and strength

3. Subscription: directions for the pharmacist

4. Signature: directions for the patient

5. Refill information

6. Physician's signature

When your office staff provides a patient with a prescription, the information and date should be noted in the medical record and the medication list should be updated. When the drug is refilled, the date and name of the person confirming the refill should be noted in the record. At each appointment, it is important to review and update the medication list with relevant information.

Drug Administration and Absorption

The oral route is the most convenient and cost-effective method to administer most medications. However, some medications cannot be absorbed by the digestive system or are destroyed by the digestive enzymes. Sometimes patient problems such as nausea or vomiting prevent oral administration of medications. Food may slow or prevent absorption of some medications, so they may need to be given before or between meals. Some medications may be damaging to the digestive system and may need to be enteric coated so that they will not dissolve until they reach the small intestine.

The parenteral route refers to the delivery of medication by injection. Medications can be injected in a variety of ways. The most common ways include intramuscular injections into large muscles of the body and subcutaneous injections into the subcutaneous tissues of the body. Insulin is an example of a subcutaneous injection using a small-gauge needle. Other thicker medications such as penicillin require that a large, deep intramuscular injection be administered. Other forms of injection include intradermal or allergy testing, intraspinal, or intra-articular.

Some drugs are administered by mucous membrane absorption. The routes include the mouth, throat, nose, eyes, rectum, vagina, respiratory tract, and urinary tract. Sublingual administration refers to the absorption of medication from the blood vessels below the tongue. Respiratory inhalation and rectal suppository forms of administration are also included in the mucous membrane category.

Topical absorption includes all methods that use the skin to absorb medication. This includes ointments, creams, lotion, and dermal patches.

Other Drug-Related Definitions

Drug distribution refers to the transportation of the medication throughout the body once it is absorbed.

Drug action refers to how the medication works in the body. There are many different methods of drug action, dependant on the type of medication.

Drug metabolism is how the medication is converted for excretion from the body.

Drug excretion is the removal of medication from the body. The most common method of excretion is through the kidneys. The combination of metabolism and excretion of half of the medication dose is called the *half-life* of the medication. Physicians use the half-life of the drug to calculate the dosage schedule.

Factors That Affect Drug Action

Weight: In prescribing medication, the usual adult dose is based on a body weight of 150 pounds. Dosage for children may be based on body weight or on body surface area. Dosage for adults who vary a great deal in weight from the 150-pound average may also need to be adjusted.

Age: Dosage may need to be adjusted for children and the elderly due to differences in metabolism or immaturity of the body systems.

Physiological state: States such as pregnancy will change the safety of administration of medications. It is important to determine any potential harmful effects on the fetus of medication treatment in pregnant women. All medications are rated for their safety in pregnancy. The body distribution of fat to muscle differs between men and women, and this may also change the action of medications in the body.

Time of day: Some medications must be administered at the correct time to get the desired effect.

Pathological issues in the body: Disease processes change the dosage needs of the body. Disease of the kidney and liver will change metabolism and excretion and necessitate a decrease in either dosage strength or frequency.

Immune response: Development of antibodies to the medication may cause an allergic reaction to the medication if given again. The most severe reaction is anaphylactic shock, which is a medical emergency.

Psychological factors: Mental attitude may make a difference in how the medication works for the patient. For years, health care providers have given placebos, which contain no active ingredients. The placebo effect refers to the fact that if the patient believes a medication will be helpful, it may be effective even if what is administered is a placebo.

Tolerance: Over a period of time, patients may develop a lack of responsiveness to medications taken regularly.

Accumulation: This occurs if the medication is not adequately excreted from the body prior to another dosage being given. It can happen due to too-frequent dosing or to problems with metabolism and excretion.

Idiosyncrasy: Sometimes a medication will have an effect that is not expected or contradictory to what is expected.

Drug interactions: These may occur when patients take two or more medications. Such interactions may be beneficial or detrimental. If the effect is antagonistic, one of the medications shortens or decreases the intensity of the other. Synergism is when one drug increases or lengthens the action of the other. This can be a negative or positive effect. Potentiation is when one drug increases the action of the other.

Classification of Drugs

Drugs can be classified by several different methods and some medications will be part of more than one category. Drugs may be classified by their action in the body or by the body system that they affect. The following table comprises examples of classification by drug action.

Classification	Action	Example
Adrenergic	Constricts lumen of a vessel	Epinephrine
Anesthetic	Brings about inability to feel pain	Lidocaine
Antianxiety	Reduces anxiety	Ativan
Antibiotic	Kills pathogens	Amoxicillin
Anticoagulant	Decreases the clotting time	Coumadin
Antidepressant	Decreases depression	Zoloft
Antihistamine	Counteracts histamines	Zyrtec
Antihypertensive	Decreases blood pressure	Lopressor
Anti-inflammatory	Decreases inflammation	Advil
Anti-tussive	Decreases cough	Robitussin
Bronchodilator	Relaxes smooth muscle of respiratory system	Proventil
Cathartic	Irritates lining of the bowel	Dulcolax
Decongestant	Relieves congestion	Sudafed
Diuretic	Inhibits reabsorption of sodium, chloride, and water	Lasix
Hypnotic	Induces sleep	Dalmane
Hormone replacement	Replaces deficient hormones	Synthroid
Narcotic	Decreases central nervous system activity	Demerol

Table 14.2—Drug Classifications

Patients also must be given information about any medications that are prescribed for treatment of a medical condition. Patients should be given both verbal and written instructions about the name of their medications, the actions of the medication, the correct route of drug administration, as well as the time schedule and correct dosing. It is very important that patients be aware of side effects so they can be alert for signs and symptoms that they need to report back to your office. A list of commonly prescribed medications and information on each is available at rxlist.com.

MEDICATION ADMINISTRATION

To safely administer medication in the office, the medical assistant must follow a series of routine procedures. Medications should be prepared in a quiet and well-lit environment. Always make sure that you go through all the steps of drug preparation no matter how busy the day is. Shortcuts will not save time and may lead to a medication error. Make sure that the medication order you are filling is complete and legible. If you are in any doubt, double-check with the prescribing provider. Be sure to check the patient's allergies for any interaction with the ordered medication. Make sure that you check expiration dates on the medication labels prior to administration. Never substitute any medication without instruction from the physician. Always prepare the medication immediately prior to administering it and never ask anyone else to administer medication that you have prepared or administer medication that you have not prepared yourself. Patients should be observed for at least 20 minutes after a new medication is administered, unless ordered differently by the physician. In order to safely administer medications, the medical assistant should be familiar with and practice the Six Rights of Medication Administration:

1. **The right patient:** identify the patient using two identifiers such as name and date of birth

2. **The right drug:** check medication with the order three times when preparing the medication for administration. First check the medication when you have obtained it, then as you are preparing the dose for administration, and finally right before you administer to the patient.

3. **The right dosage:** check for an appropriate dosage for the patient and if you have to perform calculations in order to prepare the medication, make sure you check your calculations with another person.

4. **The right route:** how the medication is to be delivered

5. **The right time:** usually given immediately in the office setting, but must be checked prior to administration

6. **The right documentation:** immediate and complete documentation of all the details about the administration and patient tolerance of the medication

When administering medications to children, you should involve the caregiver if necessary. Explain the medication to the child and attempt to gain cooperation. Offer the child choices if possible. Do not make promises that you cannot keep such as, "This won't hurt." If you have to restrain the child to administer the medication, make sure that the child is safe and that adequate assistance is available. Do not scold the child for failure to cooperate; acknowledge that the child is scared. When the medication has been given, offer a reward and encouragement even if the child was not cooperative with the procedure.

Geriatric patients are also likely to have some special needs when it comes to medication administration. They are most likely to have multiple physicians and to take over-the-counter medications and home remedies in addition to prescription medication. You must have a complete list of all medications that they are taking from all physicians and include questions about other nonprescription items they use when taking the patient history. Update the medication list every time the patient comes into the office to ensure the list is correct. If a family member accompanies the patient, he should be educated also about medication schedules, and instructions should be written down and sent home with patients.

The patient should be encouraged to drink adequate fluids. If there is a problem in swallowing medications, check to see if the medication could be crushed and placed in food for administration. Patients should be encouraged to discard medications that they are not currently taking to prevent confusion or taking the wrong medications. If elderly patients are taking a lot of medications, they may benefit from a medication-dispensing system that can be filled by family or a visiting nurse on a weekly basis.

Drug Forms

Oral administration of solid forms includes pills, caplets, gelcaps, spansules, powders, tablets, capsules, and lozenges. Some medications are enteric coated so that they are not dissolved in the stomach, but in the small intestine. This is to prevent stomach upset or irritation. Tablets and pills should not be split in pieces unless they are scored and this should be done with a device in order to cut them equally. Some tablets can be crushed in order to administer to patients that cannot swallow, as long as the tablets are not coated or sustained release. Capsules are coated with gelatin and dissolve within the digestive system. Some capsules have smaller capsules within them that are coated to be dissolved at different times so there is a sustained release of medication. Lozenges are made to dissolve in the mouth to coat the mouth, throat, or upper part of the digestive tract. Oral medications can also be given in the liquid form. There are several different types of liquid medications available. The most common include:

1. **Syrups:** solutions of medication with sugar and water with a flavoring

2. **Elixirs:** solutions of medication with alcohol, sugar, water and a flavoring

3. **Suspensions:** a mixture of an insoluble drug in a liquid. Because the drug does not dissolve in the fluid, the mixture must be shaken well prior to administration. This category includes emulsions and gels.

4. **Solutions:** liquid preparations of one or more medications that are dissolved in a liquid.

Oral medications should be given with a sufficient supply of water unless ordered otherwise. When administering oral medications, you must stay with the patient as they take the medication and verify that the medication has been swallowed. Liquid medications can be measured out into a medicine cup or in a syringe.

Parenteral medication forms are injectable medications. They must be sterile and are often provided in sterile water or normal saline. Some medications that are released slowly are supplied in an oil base. Prior to administration of parenteral medications, you must check the expiration date of the medication. The medication must be examined closely to check for any discoloration or sediment in the medication. You must also follow all OSHA standard precautions guidelines when administering parenteral medications. Parenteral medications are supplied in many different forms. An ampule is a small glass vial that contains a single dose of medication. Ampules are scored at the neck and broken prior to use. Single-dose vials are small vials with rubber stoppers that deliver one dose of medication. Before removing medication from the vial, you must first clean the stopper carefully with alcohol. Multi-dose vials are vials with rubber stoppers that contain more than one dose of medication. You must be very careful not to contaminate the remaining medication in the vial when withdrawing a single dose. If you have any doubt as to the integrity of the remaining medication in a vial, discard it and use another.

When you remove medication from a multi-dose vial, you should inject air in the same amount that you are going to withdraw as fluid. A prefilled syringe will contain one dose in a disposable syringe. Often the syringe will be attached to a plunger mechanism that is reusable, and a disposable needle may be attached if the syringe does not come with a needle attached.

It is important to know what type of medication and the preferred area of injection to use when determining which syringe and needle type you need. Syringes vary from 0.5 mL to 60 mL. You should use the smallest appropriate syringe for the injection you are going to administer. Syringes are available marked in units in order to administer insulin. To administer small amounts of intradermal medications, 1-mL syringes are marked in 0.1 increments. The needle gauge must be appropriate for the medication that you are administering. The larger the gauge of the needle, the smaller the diameter of the needle is. Needle gauges range from 28 to 14. The smallest gauges are used for intradermal injections. The 25 and 26 gauges are commonly used for subcutaneous injection. The 20–23 gauge needles are the usual size for intramuscular injections, with the larger gauges used for thick or oil-based medications.

Needle length is based on the area where the medication is to be delivered and the size of the patient. The range is from $\frac{3}{8}$ inch to about 3 inches. Intradermal injections use the shortest needles. For subcutaneous injections, the needle length should be about $\frac{1}{2}$ to $\frac{5}{8}$ of an inch. Intramuscular injections should use the longest needles, and needle length should correspond to the site being used and the size of the patient.

KAPLAN

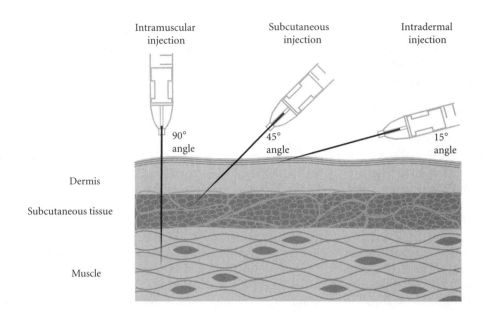

Intramuscular injection

Subcutaneous injection

Intradermal injection

90° angle

45° angle

15° angle

Dermis

Subcutaneous tissue

Muscle

Figure 14.1—Injection Administration

Some medications have their own delivery method. Insulin injectors have been developed to reduce the need to use a syringe and needle each time to draw up a dose of insulin. These injectors can be set to administer the correct amount of insulin with the turn of a dial. They resemble a pen and can be easily carried in a shirt pocket. They are ideal for diabetic patients who must inject themselves with insulin frequently. The Epi-pen is also available to self-administer epinephrine for patients who have had anaphylactic reactions to allergens in the past. The dosage is ordered by the doctor and carried by the patient in the case of an emergency.

There are similarities to administering any type of injection. Once again, you must be sure to use the Rights of Medication Administration when preparing the medication and administering it. Additionally, you must pick the injection site and prepare the skin. Using standard precautions and wearing gloves along with aseptic preparation of the medication and safe disposal of the syringe after administration are very important. Alcohol is the most common antiseptic used and the site of the injection should be swabbed from inside to outside and allowed to dry without blowing or fanning prior to giving the injection. After the injection is given, unless contraindicated, the site should be massaged to facilitate absorption and the patient should be checked for bleeding and a bandage applied. When giving an injection to a small child, you should have assistance to make sure that the child does not move during the injection. Never promise that the injection will not hurt the child. There usually will be some discomfort and you will lose the trust of your patient.

Giving an intradermal injection is accomplished by depositing the medication just under the epidermis. It is usually given in the forearm, upper back, or upper chest. When correctly administered, a raised white wheal will appear at the site of the injection. The needle should be inserted at a 15-degree angle and so the bevel is visible below the layer of skin. The medication is then injected. This method is used to perform the Mantoux test for tuberculosis and for allergy testing.

Subcutaneous injections are given in the subcutaneous layers underneath the skin, but above the muscle. The needle is inserted at a 45-degree angle. The most common drugs given in this manner are insulin and heparin. Insulin injections should be rotated between sites so that tissue damage is minimized to prevent problems with drug absorption. An injection site log can be kept to make sure that the sites are rotated. Heparin is commonly administered in the abdomen. When administering heparin and insulin, you should not aspirate prior to injection and you should not massage the area after administering heparin to prevent bruising in the tissues.

Intramuscular injections are given in large muscles in the body. In the adult, the preferred sites are the dorsogluteal, the vastus lateralis, the ventrogluteal, and the deltoid muscles. In children, the vastus lateralis is the preferred site. You must make sure that the needle that you have selected to give the injection is long enough to deliver the medication to the muscle.

Medications that are meant to be given in the muscle tissue may not adequately be absorbed if injected subcutaneously. IM injections should be given at a 90-degree angle, except in the vastus lateralis in small children. These should be given at 45 degrees.

Some medications that are given intramuscularly can be damaging to the subcutaneous tissues. They are given in the Z-track method to prevent leakage of the medication out of the muscle. This is accomplished by pushing the tissue to one side prior to inserting the needle, administering the injection, and then allowing the tissue to slide back into its original position once the needle has been removed. The Z-track method should only be used in large muscles.

Dosage Calculations

When preparing medications, it may be necessary to calculate dosage. The medical assistant should have a basic knowledge of the commonly used measurements in drug preparation. You should be able to convert between the systems of measurement, such as between ounces and pounds. Any calculations that you have to do to administer the medication should be double-checked with a coworker prior to administration. The most common method to use to calculate the dosage uses a formula into which information about the medication is applied:

$$\frac{\text{dosage that is ordered}}{\text{dosage that is available}} \times \text{quantity of vehicle}$$

This formula sets up a proportion in which you can insert the information you have available to you to calculate correct dose.

To administer medication to children when the adult dose of the medication is known, you can use Clark's Law. Clark's Law assumes the weight of the adult as 150 pounds.

$$\text{Pediatric dose} = \frac{\text{child's weight in pounds}}{\substack{\text{average adult weight} \\ \text{(150 lbs)}}} \times \text{adult dose of medication}$$

REVIEW QUESTIONS

1. Which of the following blood tests is used to monitor dosage of anticoagulant therapy?

   (A) CBC

   (B) PT/INR

   (C) Bleeding time

   (D) UA

   (E) Lipid profile

2. Medications in which of the following categories provide pain relief without sedation?

   (A) Hypnotics

   (B) Anesthetics

   (C) Analgesics

   (D) Antiemetics

   (E) Antibiotics

3. If the medical assistant has questions about the dosage of a medication order, he should

   (A) consult the reference book for the usual dosage for the patient

   (B) ask a coworker to read the order for him and verify the dosage

   (C) check the medication supply to see what dosage is available to administer

   (D) verify the dosage with the physician who wrote the order

   (E) call the pharmacy to verify the usual dosage for the medication

4. A parenteral medication is one that is administered

   (A) via injection

   (B) in pill form

   (C) topically

   (D) enteric coated

   (E) sublingually

5. The generic name of a medication is

   (A) always capitalized

   (B) trademarked by the manufacturer

   (C) related to the chemical makeup of the drug

   (D) protected by copyright

   (E) its assigned or official name

6. Transdermal medications are NOT available for

    (A) relief of pain
    (B) administration of nitroglycerin
    (C) delivery of birth control medications
    (D) administration of anticoagulants
    (E) use in smoking cessation programs

7. Sublingual medications are administered by

    (A) placing under the tongue
    (B) placing rectally
    (C) placing into the inner canthus of the eye
    (D) placing between the cheek and the gumline
    (E) placing in the intradermal area

8. The Rights of Medication Administration include all of the following EXCEPT

    (A) right medication
    (B) right route
    (C) right label
    (D) right time
    (E) right documentation

9. References for information about medications to be administered in the office should NOT be obtained from

    (A) *Physician's Desk Reference*
    (B) drug reference books
    (C) magazine articles
    (D) U.S. Pharmacopeia
    (E) package inserts

10. Factors that may affect the absorption, distribution, and metabolism of drugs include all of the following EXCEPT

    (A) age of the patient
    (B) other disease processes the patient is experiencing
    (C) sensitivity to the drug
    (D) time of day of administration
    (E) tolerance of the drug

11. Which of the following statements about controlled substances is TRUE?

    (A) All drugs classified as controlled substances are narcotics.

    (B) All drugs classified as controlled substances have the potential for physical and/or psychological dependency.

    (C) The Controlled Substance Act groups these substances into six categories.

    (D) The FDA controls the regulation and distribution of controlled substances.

    (E) Schedule V drugs have no acceptable medical use.

12. Which of the following drug forms would be INAPPROPRIATE for an alcoholic client?

    (A) Elixir

    (B) Lozenge

    (C) Solution

    (D) Suspension

    (E) Syrup

13. Which of the following length and gauge needles would the medical assistant choose to administer an intramuscular injection in the dorsogluteal muscle of an adult?

    (A) ½ inch, 22 gauge

    (B) ⅝ inch, 22 gauge

    (C) 1 inch, 18 gauge

    (D) 1 inch, 25 gauge

    (E) 1½ inch, 22 gauge

14. Which of the following terms denotes a medication that is used to relieve symptoms but not aimed at curing?

    (A) Diagnostic

    (B) Palliative

    (C) Prophylactic

    (D) Replacement

    (E) Therapeutic

15. What classification of medication would be used to promote rapid bowel evacuation?

    (A) Antidiarrheal

    (B) Antitussive

    (C) Cathartic

    (D) Diuretic

    (E) Laxative

ANSWERS AND EXPLANATIONS

1. **B**

    PT/INR is used for monitoring the anticoagulant therapy and should be preformed regularly in order to adjust the medication. The CBC (A) is a complete blood count and would be used for monitoring the blood cell counts. Bleeding time (C) measures the efficiency of clotting factors in the blood. A UA (D) is the urinalysis and would screen for a urinary tract infection or abnormal constituents in the urine. The lipid profile (E) measures the blood lipids such as cholesterol, HDL, LDL, and others.

2. **C**

    Analgesics are pain-relief medications that do not sedate the patient. Anesthetics (B) and hypnotics (A) do sedate the patient. Antibiotics (E) are used in the treatment of infections, and antiemetics (D) are used to control nausea.

3. **D**

    If there is any question about a medication order, you should consult the physician who wrote the order. While it is appropriate to use a reference book (A) to look up information about the medication prior to administration, it must not be used to determine dosage for a specific patient. The coworker (B) cannot advise you regarding the correct dosage. Having the pharmacy verify the usual dosage (E) does not confirm the dosage for this particular patient.

4. **A**

    A parenteral medication is one that is administered via injection, such as an intramuscular injection. Choices (B) and (D) use the digestive system to absorb the medication, Choice (C) refers to absorption through the skin, and (E) refers to medication that dissolves under the tongue.

5. **E**

    The generic name of a drug is the assigned or official name of the drug. This name is not capitalized (A) and not related to the drug manufacturer. The trade name is assigned by the manufacturer (B) and copyrighted (D). Once the drug is available to market as a generic drug, it may have many different trade names but the generic name will not change. The chemical name is related to the chemical makeup of the drug (C).

6. **D**

    Anticoagulants must be frequently monitored and dosages changed, and are not available in a transdermal form at this time. Transdermal medications are delivered in patches that are applied to the skin and are used for pain relief (A), birth control medications (C) and hormones, administration of some cardiac medications including nitroglycerin (B), and for nicotine replacement in smoking cessation programs (E).

7. **A**

Sublingual refers to under the tongue. The buccal area is located in the mouth between the gumline and the cheek (D). The canthus is the corner of the eye adjacent to the nose (C). Intradermal refers to an injection given into the layers of the skin (E). Placing rectally (B) refers to administering the medication through the anus.

8. **C**

The Six Rights of Medication Administration are right patient, right drug, right route, right time, right technique, and right documentation. You would check the medication's label to help determine if all the "rights" were followed correctly.

9. **C**

Magazine articles are not appropriate sources for information about administration of the medications, although if the magazine is a professional journal, you may learn about drug use and research. If you need information about administration, the best reference would be a drug reference book (B). There are many different types available. Package inserts (E) and the PDR (A) are also useful and are readily available. The U.S. Pharmacopeia (D) is not usually available in the office but is a reference if it is available.

10. **C**

A patient who is "sensitive" to a given drug is likely allergic and would not receive it. Sensitivity would not be involved in drug absorption, distribution, or metabolism. Age of the patient (A) affects metabolism; the elderly and young do not metabolize drugs the same way as a normal adult. Experiencing another disease process (B) can affect metabolism; for example, hepatitis would affect metabolism, because most meds are metabolized in the liver. Time of day (D) may be important to a drug's efficacy; for instance, the thyroid supplement levothyroxine must be taken in the morning to achieve its therapeutic effect. Prolonged use often builds up tolerance (E), which diminishes the patient's responsiveness to the medication. A patient with drug tolerance requires increasing doses in order to achieve the desired effect.

11. **B**

The Drug Enforcement Agency (DEA) is responsible for the regulation of controlled substances, and all those on the list have been identified as possibly leading to physical and/or psychological dependency. Although many of the controlled substances are narcotics (A), some are not; for example, valium has the potential to cause psychological dependency but is not a narcotic. There are five categories of controlled substances, not six (C). Ultimate responsibility for controlled substances lies with the DEA, not the U.S. Food and Drug Administration, or FDA (D), which focuses on the human safety aspects of drugs (e.g., monitoring drug research, manufacturing, and distribution). Schedule I drugs have the highest degree of addiction and have no use in medicine, not Schedule V drugs (E); drugs in this category include LSD and marijuana. Schedule V drugs have the least potential for dependency.

12.   **A**

An elixir is a solution of medication mixed with alcohol, sugar, water, and flavoring. An alcoholic should not receive any medication containing alcohol. A lozenge (B) is a solid drug form placed in the mouth and used for its local effects in the mouth or pharynx; it does not contain alcohol. A solution (C) is a medication dissolved in a liquid, usually water. A suspension (D) is a mixture of a medication that does not dissolve well in liquid; a suspension must be shaken prior to administration to distribute all the components. Syrups (E) are medications mixed with sugar and water; they may not be advisable for diabetics.

13.   **B**

An intramuscular (IM) injection requires relatively deep penetration into the body, and a 1½-inch needle is the most appropriate length for administering IM into the dorsogluteal muscle. A ½-inch (A) or a ⅝-inch needle length (B) would be too short for IM; either is appropriate for a subcutaneous or intradermal injection. A 1-inch needle (D) is too short for dorsogluteal administration but could be used for IM into the deltoid muscle. An 18-gauge needle (C) would be used only for an extremely thick (viscous) medication: The smaller the gauge size of the needle, the wider the lumen; a typical needle is 22–25 gauge. In general, the medication used for IM is only a little thicker than water, so a moderate 22-gauge size would be appropriate.

14.   **B**

A palliative drug simply relieves symptoms. For instance, a patient may take an antacid to relieve heartburn symptoms, but the drug does not cure the underlying cause of the heartburn. Diagnostic medications (A) are used in to help make a diagnosis. For instance, allergens are administered diagnostically to determine the cause of allergies. Prophylactic medications (C) are administered to prevent disease, often in the form of vaccines. Replacement medications (D) put something back into the body that is missing, such as insulin in a diabetic patient. Therapeutic medications (E) are aimed at treating and/or curing a condition. For instance, antibiotics are therapeutic drugs aimed at killing bacteria.

15.   **C**

A cathartic causes rapid evacuation of bowel contents and is often used in preparation for bowel testing and certain surgeries. Examples of cathartics include magnesium citrate (Citroma), polyethylene glycol (MoviPrep), and bisacodyl (Dulcolax). An antidiarrheal drug (A) such as loperamide (Imodium) inhibits bowel evacuation in order to relieve diarrhea. An antitussive (C) is aimed at decreasing coughing. A diuretic (D) causes an increased loss of fluid from the body through the kidneys. Although a laxative (E) does promote bowel evacuation by softening the stool, it tends to work gradually (over several hours or overnight) rather than "rapidly" (within a few hours).

Chapter 15: **Minor Surgery**

Minor surgery can be performed in an outpatient setting with local anesthesia. This chapter will provide you with a review of the types of minor surgery commonly seen in practice, the instruments used in surgical procedures, and the specifics of how you will assist in such procedures. The most common surgical procedures performed in office settings are suturing, incision and drainage of abscesses, biopsies, and cyst removal.

INFORMED CONSENT

Prior to any surgical procedure, patients must sign a consent form indicating that they have been informed of the benefits and risks of the procedure. This information about the procedure should come from the physician, and any questions should be answered by the physician. The medical assistant may then obtain a patient's signed consent. As a medical assistant, you can give general information to the patient and answer general questions that the patient may have, but any concerns about the procedure itself or concerns about the outcome of the procedure should be referred to the physician and resolved prior to obtaining the signed consent. Patients coming into the office for minor surgery may be scared or apprehensive. You should make sure that the patient is prepared for the procedure and that it will be performed in a timely fashion. The patient cannot sign an informed consent while under the influence of any sedating medication. The medical assistant can offer support and comfort to the patient prior to the procedure but should not guarantee a specific outcome. Avoid phrases such as "Everything will be okay" or "This won't hurt."

The medical assistant will ensure the patient is appropriately gowned and draped for the procedure. Positioning of the patient must be convenient for the physician and comfortable for the patient. Ensure that the patient can maintain any required position throughout the procedure. The patient should mark the anatomical site where the procedure is to be performed and the medical assistant should confirm that the site corresponds with the surgical permit.

SURGICAL ASEPSIS

Surgical asepsis refers to the use of sterile instrumentation and technique before entering the body. This technique prevents introduction of microorganisms into the body. (Medical asepsis refers to the proper disposal of biohazardous waste after it leaves the body.) You must be familiar with the general principles of sterile technique and comfortable with the setup of a sterile field. A sterile field is a work area specially prepared with sterile draping that will hold instruments used in a procedure.

Principles to remember in any minor surgery include the following:

1. Know which items are sterile and which are nonsterile, and keep them separated.

2. Take precautions to prevent accidental contamination of the sterile field once it is prepared. It is best not to leave the sterile field unattended but if you must, cover it with a sterile towel.

3. Any contamination of your sterile clothing, gloves, or the sterile field must quickly be addressed by replacing the contaminated items.

4. Carefully examine sterile objects prior to use. Check the expiration date of each object and ensure that the wrapping is intact and dry. If there is any doubt about the sterility of the object, re-sterilize.

5. The outside of sterile gloves must not be touched with bare hands. Once you have put on sterile gloves, you must not touch any nonsterile items. Nonsterile persons must not touch any sterile items unless they are using sterile transfer forceps. Once these forceps are used, they are considered contaminated and must be re-sterilized prior to being used again.

6. The sterile field, all sterile items, and your sterile gloved hands must be kept at or above waist level.

7. Keep movements around the sterile field to a minimum. Make sure that air currents are kept to a minimum. Avoid drafts and fans. Do not reach across a sterile field. Avoid coughing, sneezing, or talking directly over a sterile field. It is advisable to stand with your hands clasped in front of you above waist level when idle.

8. Avoid spilling anything wet on the sterile field. Areas that become wet allow microorganisms to migrate into the sterile area. Wet areas are considered contaminated and must be covered with sterile towels or the sterile field must be dismantled and set up again.

9. Outer wrapping of sterile packs are not sterile and must be opened by someone not wearing sterile gloves. The flaps of the sterile pack must be opened away from the body, being careful not to touch the inner wrappings with your clothing, your hand, or any other object. Once the outer wrapping is opened, the inner pack may be added to the sterile field by placing it in the center of the field without letting the outer wrapping touch the field.

10. Instruments in peel packs may be opened by peeling downward and allowing the article to be picked out by someone wearing sterile gloves or allowing the articles to slide from the pack onto the sterile field.

Setting Up a Sterile Field

A sterile field is set up on a flat, secure surface. The sterile field is often set up on a metal stand on wheels called a Mayo stand. The stand must be cleaned with disinfectant prior to use. Its outer one inch and any material that falls below the level of the sterile field are considered nonsterile. Liquids must be added to the sterile field in a specific manner. First the medical assistant must check the label of the bottle to make sure that it is the right solution. The lid is removed and held in the hand or placed on a hard surface with the lid downward without contaminating the sterile field. The label is rechecked and then placed in the hand to protect it. The liquid is poured from about six inches above the sterile field very carefully to prevent spilling onto the sterile field. The label is rechecked again and the lid replaced carefully without contaminating the bottle.

Surgical Hand Wash

A surgical hand wash should be done prior to gloving. All jewelry should be removed and hands and nails inspected. Ideally the water and soap will be controlled by foot pedals. A sponge and brush combination that is impregnated with antiseptic soap may be used. A file should be used to clean under fingernails. Hands should be pointed upward so that water runs off toward the elbows. The hands and arms (up to the elbows) should be washed for a total of 6 to 10 minutes. Avoid touching the inside of the sink. After washing for the proper amount of time, rinse well from fingertips to elbows. Turn off the water using the foot control. Dry your hands on a sterile towel using a patting motion. Use a separate end of the towel for each hand. Make sure hands are completely dry so that sterile gloves can easily be applied.

Applying Sterile Gloves

Applying sterile gloves must be practiced until the skill is mastered. It is important to make sure that you have the correct size of gloves. After opening the peel pack, carefully open the inner sterile pack using the tabs and avoid touching the inner surface of the paper. Pick up the cuff of the glove for the dominate hand. Lay the thumb flat against the palm of the hand and slip the hand into the glove. With the gloved hand, slide the fingers under the cuff of the other glove, taking care not to touch the inside surface of the glove. Again tuck the thumb into the palm and slide the hand into the glove. After both gloves are on, you may adjust the fit and link the fingers together to remove air and wrinkles in the gloves.

It is very important to properly remove soiled gloves after performing a procedure. Grasp the palm of the glove of the nondominant hand with the dominant hand and pull it into the gloved hand carefully in order to prevent splattering of any infectious material. Once the first glove is removed, insert the finger of the bare hand under the other glove and peel the glove in and down to prevent contact with the outside of the contaminated glove. Dispose of the gloves in a biohazard waste container. Wash your hands thoroughly.

Applying a Sterile Gown

After doing the hand scrub, you may need to apply a sterile gown. You should be gowned prior to putting on sterile gloves. The sterile gown should be carefully opened and picked up by the collar. It is then held away from the body to prevent contamination and allowed to unfold. Then slip your hands into the sleeve and touching only the insides of gown pull it onto the shoulder area. The hands should remain inside the sleeves to prevent contamination. An assistant should then come behind you and fasten the neckline and secure the ties around the waist. Sterile gloves are applied as described here and the cuffs pulled up over the cuffs of the gown.

Preparation of the Skin

The medical assistant is responsible for preparing the skin prior to the surgical procedure. Supplies to assemble in advance include draping materials, antiseptic soap, sterile sponges, sterile forceps, razor, and antiseptic solution. You must carefully check allergies prior to cleaning the skin. Betadine is frequently used as an antiseptic solution. Alternatives are available if the patient has an allergy to iodine. Cleaning should start from the inside of the affected area and move outward in a circular motion. If the area must be shaved, it should be done after cleaning. Shave in the direction of the hair growth to help prevent cuts in the skin. The area should then be rinsed and painted with the antiseptic solution using a sterile cotton swab. The surgical area should be draped in preparation for the procedure.

ANESTHESIA

Local anesthesia can be administered by infiltration, nerve block, or topical application. Before any anesthesia is administered, you should ask the patient about allergies and previous reactions to anesthesia. Emergency supplies should be available because of the chance of anaphylactic reaction when an anesthetic is administered.

Types of Local Anesthesia

1. **Infiltration:** injection of anesthesia into the skin and nerve endings in the area of the procedure

2. **Nerve block:** injection of anesthesia into the major nerves in the area, which will anesthetize the surrounding area

3. **Topical:** anesthesia is painted or sprayed onto the area, skin, or mucous membrane to deaden sensation and relieve pain

SUTURE MATERIALS AND NEEDLES

Suture material is either absorbable or nonabsorbable. Absorbable remains in place until it is absorbed or degraded by the body. It is either catgut, which is made from the intestine of sheep, or a synthetic material such as Vicryl. Nonabsorbable suture is made from silk, nylon, or cotton. The suture material will vary in strength and size dependent on the purpose and place that is sutured. Fine suture is used in areas such as the face or eye surgery. Medium and coarse suture is used for areas that need more support such as arms, legs, and abdomen.

Needles for suture are generally disposable and come with suture material attached. These needles are called atraumatic needles. There is no eye in the needle and the thread is attached. Needles come in different sizes and lengths for use in different areas and for different purposes. The needles may be curved or straight, dependant on the purpose. An instrument called a needleholder may be used for control of curved needles.

Alternatives to sutures include staples, surgical adhesive, and Steri-Strips to hold skin together.

INSTRUMENTS USED FOR MINOR SURGERY

The medical assistant must be familiar with instruments that are commonly used in minor surgical procedures. The type of instruments may vary with the medical specialty and you must know which procedures are commonly performed in your office. By looking at certain identifiable parts of the instruments, you learn to identify frequently used instruments. Handled instruments have ring handles, spring handles, or ratcheted handles. Spring handles are sometimes also called thumb-handled and are found on instruments such as tweezers. Scissors are an example of ring-handled instruments. Ratcheted handles are used to lock an instrument into position, dependant on the thickness of the article being grasped. Instruments can be straight or curved. Some instruments have serrations on the jaws of the instrument. The serrations help to grasp tissue. The jaw of the instrument may also have teeth to assist with grasping. If these teeth are large, they are called rat teeth. If they are small, they are called mouse teeth. Splinter forceps are pointed with a very narrow jaw so it could easily remove a splinter. Instruments are often named for the physician who has designed the instrument or for what the instrument is used for.

Instruments are classified into four categories.

1. *Cutting*: these instruments are used to cut tissue, incise, scrape, puncture, or punch. You will find scissors, scalpels, curettes, drills, punches, chisels, and needles.

   Bandage scissors: blunt tip to remove dressings without damage to skin; come in many different sizes

   Operating scissors: common types are Iris, Metzenbaum, or Mayo—used to cut or dissect tissue and may have straight or curved blades

   Littauer or stitch scissors: used to remove sutures; has a beak or hook used to lift the suture up and cut it

   Scalpel: usually disposable with attached blade but can be a reusable handle with interchangeable blades

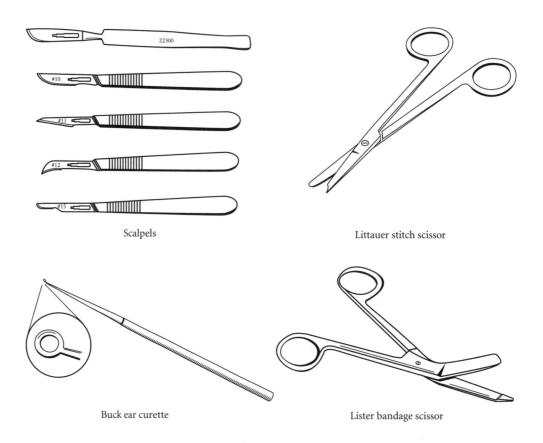

Scalpels

Littauer stitch scissor

Buck ear curette

Lister bandage scissor

Figure 15.1—Surgical Blades and Scissors

2. *Clamping and holding*: used to clamp, hold, and manipulate tissue

   Hemostats: designed to stop bleeding or clamp severed blood vessels; may be serrated, curved, or straight; come in various sizes

   Needle holders: used to hold curved needles to grasp the needle tightly; has serrations or a groove in the center in order to hold the needle

   Dressing forceps: vary in length and usually have serrations but no teeth; used to pick up objects and to inset packing

   Towel forceps: usually have sharp tips to hold surgical draping in place

   Sponge forceps: used to hold dressings or gauze sponges

   Utility forceps: used to transfer or arrange items in a sterile field; come in many different sizes and lengths

   Tissue forceps: different types of forceps used to clamp and hold tissue

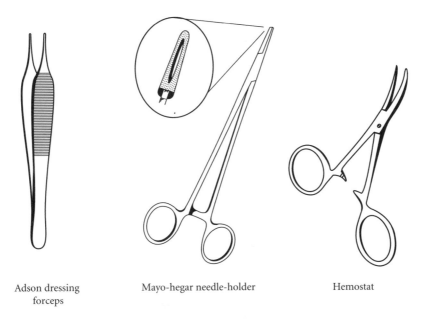

Adson dressing
forceps

Mayo-hegar needle-holder

Hemostat

Figure 15.2—Clamping and Holding Instruments

3. *Retraction*: retractors and skin hooks used to hold tissue away from surgical incisions. The Senn retractor is commonly used in office procedures. The flat end is used as a retractor and the pronged end is used as a skin hook.

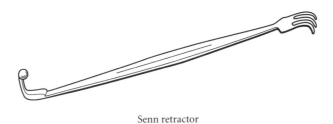

Senn retractor

Figure 15.3—Retractor

4. *Probing and dilating*: used for both surgery and for examinations. Probes can be used to explore a wound or to enter a fistula. Dilators are used to stretch an opening or to open a cavity for examination or prior to inserting another instrument.

    Trocars and obturators: pointed obturator contained within a cannula used to withdraw fluids from cavities or for draining and irrigating with a catheter; specula dilate or open a body orifice or cavity such as the vagina or nasal passage

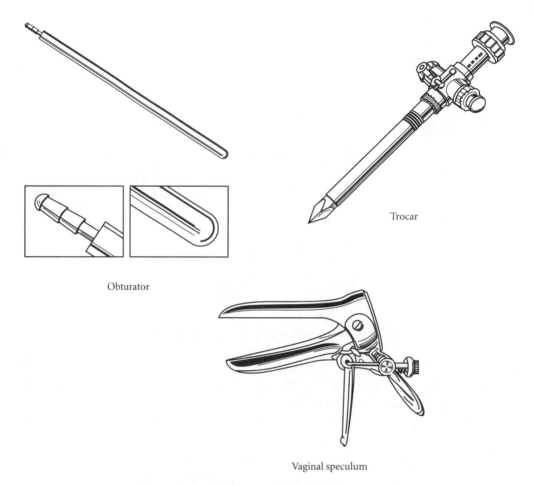

Trocar

Obturator

Vaginal speculum

Figure 15.4—Probing and Dilating Instruments

SPECIAL PROCEDURES

Electrosurgery or electrocautery is the use of an instrument delivering an electrical current to vaporize tissue and to seal blood vessels. Patients receiving treatment with electrocautery must have a grounding pad applied to prevent burns. The grounding pad must be close to the area of the surgery and applied tightly to the skin. The pad should not be applied over areas of bone, areas that are extremely hairy, or areas with metal implants. After use, the skin in the affected area should be checked for burns.

Cryosurgery uses a probe with liquid nitrogen to destroy tissue by freezing it on contact. It is frequently used for removal of skin cancers. It is less invasive than other types of surgery and has fewer complications.

Microsurgery uses magnification by a microscope for small areas. The instruments used are small and delicate. Special training is necessary to assist and care for the microscope and instruments that are used.

Laser surgery is the use of light waves for the thermal vaporization, coagulation, and ablation of tissue. Lasers also are used for photocoagulation therapy. They are used in various medical specialties including ophthalmology. Special training is necessary to use and maintain the laser. There are some safety considerations that must be followed whenever lasers are used. Eye protection must be worn by the patient and all personnel that are in the area of the laser. Sterile normal saline must be kept on hand for irrigation and suction equipment must be available to suction the plume of smoke that is generated by the laser.

Endoscopy procedures are used to visualize hollow body organs or body cavities. The scopes may be rigid, semi-rigid, or flexible. They allow for direct visualization inside the cavity in order to perform diagnosis and treatment procedures. Endoscopes are equipped with cameras, a light source, an irrigator, suction, and monitor.

CARE OF INSTRUMENTS

While disposable instruments should be disposed of according to standard precautions, reusable instruments must be carefully inspected, cleaned, and sterilized for reuse. The first step to clean the instruments is to put on protective gear such as a gown, gloves, and eyewear. The instruments are carefully examined for any damage and then sanitized using a brush and disinfectant soap to remove all debris. Instruments that are delicate and cannot be scrubbed can be cleaned with ultrasonic sanitization. Solution is placed in an ultrasonic cleaning unit and sound waves are used to clean the instruments. After the instruments are cleaned, they then can be wrapped and sterilized.

Wrapping of Instruments

To autoclave instruments, they must be wrapped in autoclave paper or packaged in special peel packs. Heat sensitive indicators are included in the packs to ensure sterile conditions were met. Hinged instruments must be open to allow the steam to penetrate all areas of the instrument. Sharp edges should be wrapped to prevent penetration through the wrapping.

Sterilization

The most common method of sterilization used in the office setting is the autoclave. These units are small and compact and easily used in the outpatient setting. Once materials are wrapped or packaged, they are placed in the autoclave per manufacturer's recommendations. (Standard processing time is 250 degrees at 15 pounds of pressure for 15 to 20 minutes.) Processing and care of the autoclave should be done according to manufacturer's directions to ensure correct operation. Once autoclaved, the items are considered sterile for 28 days, so each item must have the date and time of sterilization clearly visible on the outside of the pack. Indicators placed in the packs and autoclave tape will confirm parameters for sterilization have been met. Other methods of sterilization such as cold sterilization with chemical solutions or gas sterilization are available, but do not have the advantage of the autoclave. Cold sterilization is difficult to confirm and time consuming. Gas sterilization usually is done in a large health care setting, not in the outpatient setting.

ROLE OF THE MEDICAL ASSISTANT

While the physician is responsible for performing the sterile procedure, the medical assistant has many duties related to assisting the physician during the procedure. You will learn what the individual physician prefers for equipment and routine, but having a good understanding of the basics of sterile technique and office surgeries will allow you to assist in any minor procedure. You must be prepared to pass instruments to the physician during the procedure. This should be done in a firm and precise method so that the physician is able to easily grip the instruments. You should make sure that instruments are held so there is no danger of injury to either yourself or the physician. The medical assistant is also is responsible for maintenance of the sterile field. The physician must be notified immediately of any breach of the sterile field. The medical assistant must also be prepared to process specimens that are obtained during the procedure. Suturing of the wound is done at the end of the procedure. You will pass the needleholder and/ or suture material to the physician. Be prepared to cut the suture and swab the area with sterile gauze so the physician has good visualization of the area.

Once the procedure is finished, you will clean and bandage the wound. The area may be rinsed with sterile, normal saline as directed by the physician. A sterile nonadherent dressing should be applied unless ordered otherwise. The patient should be assisted to dress if needed. Instruction for care of the surgical area should be given in writing and a follow-up appointment scheduled prior to the patient leaving the office. The patient must be made aware of the signs and symptoms of infection and informed to call the office if any problems or questions occur. Documentation of the procedure and the instructions should be placed in the patient's chart immediately after the procedure is completed.

SUTURE REMOVAL

Patients will return to the physician's office in 7 to 10 days to have sutures removed. After the physician has examined the surgical site, the medical assistant will remove the sutures. Supplies needed for the procedure include suture removal scissors, dressing forceps, skin antiseptic, gauze sponges, gloves, and Steri-Strips if needed. Any drainage or pus at the suture site may need to be cultured prior to washing the area. If the sutures are dry and intact and ready for removal, you should clean the incision with an antiseptic cleanser. Then you use the forceps to lift the suture and slip the beak of the suture scissors under the stitch and snip it away from the knot. Using the forceps, you will lift the stitch up and toward the incision so that you do not put pressure on the healing area. Place the suture you have removed on a piece of gauze and make sure that the whole suture has been removed. Continue until all are removed. Count the number of sutures that you have removed and make sure that it corresponds to the number of sutures that were placed. Blot any blood from the incision and apply Steri-Strips to the incision. Once again, inform the patient to watch for signs or symptoms of infection and give written directions for care of the area. Document in the patient's chart about what you did, the appearance of the incision, and how the patient tolerated the procedure.

WOUND HEALING AND COMPLICATIONS

Normal wound healing is sometimes called healing by first intention. Normally the tissues come together and heal completely within 21 days following surgical incisions or clean lacerations. Wounds that are jagged, infected, or have a large amount of tissue missing heal by secondary attention. This healing takes place from the bottom of the incision and proceeds at a much slower pace. If the wound is infected or necrotic, it may have to be debrided. Debridement is the surgical removal of necrotic tissue. Wounds will not heal unless this tissue is removed.

The major complication of wound healing is infection at the site of surgery. The patient should be given written instructions on the care of the wound and signs and symptoms of infection and instructed to call immediately with any concerns. The instructions should include how to care for the wound and how often to change the dressing or whether open-wound healing is an option for the patient. Be sure to document the instructions that you give the patient and his response to the instructions. If the wound or the wound care is extensive or the patient is unable to manage due to other health problems, you must make sure that there is a family member or outpatient health care provider to refer the patient to for help with dressing care. If a family member is involved, you must make sure that he or she is instructed. This also must be documented in the patient chart. The patient must also be given a time to return to the office to have the wound checked or to have sutures removed.

CAST CARE

Application of a cast to an extremity may be done in a physician's office. There are several different kinds of casts and all have a different use and care.

1. **Plaster of paris:** impregnated rolls of casting material are moistened in warm water and then rolled onto the extremity, which has been covered by stockinette and padding. This material is easily molded to the extremity and is a wet dressing that gradually hardens. Care must be taken that the cast does not cause any pressure on the skin. This cast is fairly heavy and must be kept dry.

2. **Synthetic or fiberglass cast:** this cast is applied like the plaster of paris cast but is much lighter weight and is fairly waterproof.

3. **Air cast:** a plastic envelope type cast that is inflated and can be easily applied and removed.

Much of the responsibility of the medical assistant in casting is patient education. Instruction should include signs and symptoms of infection, problems with circulation, increase in pain, or drainage from the cast. If the patient experiences any of these symptoms, they should be reported to the office. If the cast is removable, the patient must be instructed on how to reapply the cast and how much movement of the extremity is allowed. Additionally, the patient may need instruction in the use of assistive devices such as a walker, cane, or crutches. Careful documentation is necessary about the type of cast, the initial assessment of the cast, and instructions that are given for home care.

REVIEW QUESTIONS

1. An instrument used to dilate a body orifice is a/an

    (A) speculum

    (B) catheter

    (C) snare

    (D) curette

    (E) extractor

2. Which type of procedure is frequently used for the removal of skin cancers?

    (A) Electrosurgery

    (B) Cryosurgery

    (C) Laser surgery

    (D) Microsurgery

    (E) Endoscopy

3. The order of procedures in preparing the skin for surgery is

    (A) drape, shave, cleanse, rinse, apply antiseptic

    (B) cleanse, rinse, apply antiseptic, shave, drape

    (C) shave, cleanse, rinse, apply antiseptic, drape

    (D) drape, shave, rinse, cleanse, apply antiseptic

    (E) cleanse, shave, rinse, apply antiseptic, drape

4. Which of the following types of anesthesia is NOT used in minor surgical procedures performed in most medical offices?

    (A) Nerve block

    (B) Infiltration

    (C) Local

    (D) General

    (E) Topical

ANSWERS AND EXPLANATIONS

1. **A**

   A speculum dilates a body orifice, such as the vagina. A curette (D) is used for scraping. A catheter (B) drains fluid from a body part. A snare (C) is an instrument used for the removal of an object, usually within a blood vessel. An extractor (E) is used to remove an object from a body part.

2. **B**

   Skin cancers frequently are removed via cryosurgery. In this procedure, a probe with liquid nitrogen destroys tissue by freezing it on contact. Electrosurgery (A) uses an electrical current to vaporize tissue and to seal blood vessels. Laser surgery (C) uses light waves for the thermal vaporization, coagulation, and ablation of tissue. Microsurgery (D) uses a microscope and tiny instruments. Endoscopic procedures (E) are used to visualize areas inside the body such as organs and cavities.

3. **E**

   When preparing skin for surgery, first cleanse the area, then shave if necessary, rinse, apply antiseptic solution, and drape.

4. **D**

   General anesthesia causes unconsciousness and typically is used in major surgery. Nerve blocks (A), infiltration (B), and topical (E) are all types of local anesthesia (C).

Chapter 16: **Emergencies**

Medical emergencies can occur at any time and you must be prepared to identify the emergency and react appropriately. By thinking ahead and having a plan of action, you will be able to respond appropriately to bring about the best possible outcome for the patient. Each office should have a set of emergency protocols and procedures for patient care management during common medical emergencies. You should also have any special plans that are unique to your patient population. The protocols should consider both office-based and home-based emergencies. They should provide the office staff with the treatment and care that your employing physicians recommend in a variety of emergency situations.

For office-based emergencies, it is important to have a "crash cart" or an area stocked with emergency supplies. Supplies should include personal protective equipment including a cardiopulmonary resuscitation (CPR) mask. This breathing device has a one-way valve that prevents contact with body fluid during CPR. A bag-valve-mask (BVM) with or without oxygen may also be available for use in the office. In any emergency, there are general items to keep in mind.

1. Stay calm and do not panic. Reassure the patient and any others in the area that you are in control of the situation. If there is a coworker in the area, send them to notify the doctor and to bring emergency equipment. If the doctor is not in, have someone reach him or her by phone.

2. Quickly assess the situation using CAB (see the cardiopulmonary resuscitation section later in this chapter). Make sure the patient has a patent airway and is breathing. Then make sure there is adequate circulation. If there is no spontaneous respiration, rescue breathing should be started. If there is no carotid pulse, chest compressions must be started. If the patient is breathing and has an adequate pulse, then you can do a more complete assessment to determine what is occurring. When in doubt, call 911 or your local emergency response system.

3. Take steps to ensure that the patient is safe and not in danger of any further injury. Remedy the situation if it is in your ability and training. Otherwise call for assistance. **Remember, you must not do anything that you have not been trained to do, no matter what the situation.** Be able to concisely relate the details of what has happened to the physician or to emergency medical responders.

4. The certified medical assistant should maintain current CPR and first aid training at all times in order to provide the best possible patient care in an emergency situation.

5. Periodically review the policies of the office so that you are familiar with them in an emergency. Make sure that emergency phone numbers of such facilities as local emergency rooms, poison control centers, and ambulance services are posted in a prominent area in the office for easy access.

6. If the emergency is phoned from a patient or patient's family member, follow office policy in suggesting a plan of action. Do not suggest that the patient drive himself to the office or emergency room. If necessary, stay on the line with the patient and have someone else in the office call for emergency assistance to the patient's location. Do not hang up the phone until you are sure that assistance has arrived or until you have spoken to someone else who is with the patient to ensure that medical help is there.

7. Carefully document in the patient's chart the details of the patient's emergency, what care was suggested or delivered, and the outcome of intervention.

HEMORRHAGE

The three types of bleeding are arterial, venous, and capillary. While arterial bleeding is the most serious and life threatening, venous bleeding can also be an emergency situation. Capillary bleeding is usually easily controlled with minor first aid. The goal of treatment is to control the bleeding as soon as possible. Severe bleeding can quickly lead to shock and even death, so timely intervention is necessary. Apply direct pressure to the area. You should use sterile dressing material if available or any clean fabric to hold pressure. If the dressing becomes soaked with blood, apply another dressing over the top and continue to apply pressure. The bleeding area can be elevated higher than the level of the heart if there is not an injury that prevents this. This will help to reduce the pressure of the blood as it moves through the vessels and can reduce bleeding. If these measures do not work, a pressure dressing can be applied by adding an elastic bandage or roller gauze over the bandage Additionally, pressure points can be used to decrease blood flow to the area. Apply pressure over an artery in an area that lays on a bone or a large muscle. Pressure will decrease blood flow into the affected extremity. There are seven pressure areas on each side of the body.

1. **Temporal artery:** located on the side of the head above the ear; compression between the fingers and the facial bones can decrease bleeding in the forehead and the scalp.

2. **Facial artery:** pressure on the facial artery against the jawbone can control bleeding in the facial area.

3. **Carotid artery:** compression of the carotid artery against the neck muscles is used only for severe bleeding in the head. Care must be taken to not compress both carotid arteries. Never use a pressure dressing around the neck.

4. **Subclavian artery:** downward pressure between the fingers and the collar bone can decrease bleeding in the arm and shoulder.

5. **Brachial artery:** compression of the artery against the humerus can control bleeding in the arm and hand.

6. **Radial artery:** compression against the radius can control bleeding in the hand.

7. **Femoral artery:** compression against the pelvic bone can control bleeding in the leg.

Application of a tourniquet is not recommended unless there is no alternative to prevent the loss of life.

Be alert to signs and symptoms of shock with any large amount of bleeding.

BURNS

Burns are classified as first-, second-, or third-degree depending on the thickness of tissue damage.

1. **First-degree burns involve superficial damage only.** The skin is reddened and painful. Treatment is application of cool water or a cool compress to relieve pain. The goal is to prevent infection. Dry dressings can be used if there is the possibility of the skin being irritated. Sunburn is an example of a first-degree burn.

2. **Second-degree burns are also called partial-thickness burns.** You will note blistering of the skin. These blisters should not be broken, nor should tissue be removed from areas where the blister has broken. The goal is to relieve pain and to prevent infection. The burn should be immersed in cool water or covered with a cool compress. The area can be covered loosely with sterile, dry dressings to prevent infection. If the burned patient is a child, the burn is extensive, or is on the hands or feet, it must be closely monitored by the physician.

3. **Third-degree or full-thickness burns are the most serious.** The burn involves all layers of skin and may extend into the muscle and bone. Burn injury to the respiratory tract must be considered and the patient must be monitored very closely for signs and symptoms of shock. Airway assessment is the first priority. Then a careful assessment of the burned area is necessary. Any loose clothing or jewelry in the burned area should be removed, but do not try to remove anything that is stuck to burned tissue. Cover the injured area with sterile cloth if available and apply cool water or sterile, normal saline to the area. If there is no other injury or difficulty breathing, place the patient in a supine position with the head slightly lower than the body. If there are respiratory problems, elevate the head. The patient should be transported to an emergency facility as soon as possible for treatment. Check the vital signs so you can give a concise report to them about the patient's condition. Be alert for changes in the vital signs that may signal that the patient is going into shock. Keep the patient warm and quiet.

CEREBRAL VASCULAR ACCIDENT

A cerebral vascular accident (CVA) is also known as a stroke. Because rapid response and treatment can make a big difference in the patient outcome, it is important for you to understand the signs and symptoms of a CVA. These include the following.

1. Dizziness

2. Mental confusion

3. Difficulty in speaking or difficulty in understanding spoken words

4. Paralysis or weakness on one side of the body

5. Loss of vision or blurred vision in one eye

6. Headache

7. Difficulty in breathing or swallowing

8. Loss of bowel and bladder control

CHEST PAIN

Chest pain is associated with many conditions, but it should be considered cardiac in nature until proven otherwise. The patient should be transferred to an emergency center for assessment. These measures should be taken in the office while waiting for emergency services to transport the patient.

1. Keep the patient quiet, calm, and warm.

2. Notify the physician.

3. Monitor vital signs and record them. If the patient is able to answer questions, ask about previous chest pain and if the patient has nitroglycerin tablets. If the patient has a history of angina and has nitroglycerin with them, you may allow the patient to use these.

4. Apply oxygen if available. Do an EKG if the office is equipped to do this. Send this with the patient when he is transported.

5. Stay with the patient at all times. Monitor his condition continuously. If the patient has had a myocardial infarction, there is a danger of cardiac arrhythmia, which is the leading cause of sudden cardiac death. Be prepared to do CPR if necessary.

6. If an automated defibrillator is available, have it nearby in case it is needed.

CARDIOPULMONARY RESUSCITATION

Cardiopulmonary resuscitation (CPR) is artificial respiration and/or artificial circulation. You should be trained and certified by an accredited agency. Research has shown the early defibrillation is the best treatment for respiratory and cardiac arrest, but CPR is needed to maintain body functions and life support until defibrillation can be accomplished.

Assessment for the need for CPR includes assessing CAB:

C-Circulation

A-Airway

B-Breathing

The 2010 guidelines by the American Heart Association have made changes to simplify the sequences for basic life support in order to make CPR easier for all rescuers to remember and to use. The compression to ventilation ratio for single rescuer CPR is 30:2 for everyone. Rescue breaths should be delivered at the rate of 10 to 12 for adults and 12 to 20 for infants and children.

The American Heart Association's 2010 guidelines changed the order to "CAB" instead of "ABC." Here is a step-by-step guide for the new CPR sequence:

1. Call 911 or ask someone else to do so.

2. Try to get the person to respond; if he/she doesn't, roll the person on his/her back.

3. Start chest compressions. Place the heel of your hand on the center of the victim's chest. Put your other hand on top of the first with your fingers interlaced.

4. Press down so you compress the chest at least 2 inches in adults and children and at least 1.5 inches in infants at a rate of at least 100 per minute. (That's about as fast as the beat of the Bee Gees song "Stayin' Alive.")

5. If you're trained in CPR, open the airway with a head tilt and chin lift to administer breaths.

6. Pinch the victim's nose closed. Take a normal breath, cover the victim's mouth with yours to create an airtight seal, and then give two 1-second breaths as you watch for the chest to rise.

7. Continue compressions and breaths—30 compressions, two breaths—until help arrives.

For sudden collapse in victims of all ages, the single rescuer should notify EMS (emergency medical services) and get the AED (automated external defibrillator), if available, and then begin CPR and use the AED. For unresponsive adult victims with a probable asphyxial arrest, a single rescuer should notify EMS and then should begin CPR. CPR should be continued until EMS arrives to take over. With an infant or child, the single rescuer should complete at least one two-minute cycle of CPR before notifying EMS.

CHOKING

Choking is the partial or complete obstruction of the airway by a foreign body. This is a medical emergency because the patient will lose consciousness and experience cardiac arrest after a period of lack of oxygen to the body. For a conscious patient with an airway obstruction, you should do manual chest or abdominal thrusts to dislodge the obstruction. If the patient becomes unconscious, they must be eased to the floor and manual thrusts continued. Airway assessment should be done and attempts made to remove the obstruction and to ventilate the patient as outlined by the American Heart Association training.

DIABETIC EMERGENCIES

There are two types of diabetic emergencies, hyperglycemia and hypoglycemia Type I. Many people with diabetes do not realize that they have the disease. All diabetics should wear some type of identification to let health care and emergency service workers know that they are diabetic. The diabetic patient may have a medical emergency if their blood sugar levels are too high or too low. It is important to be able to differentiate between these conditions.

	Hypoglycemia (below 60 mg/dL): Insulin Reaction	Hyperglycemia (over 400 mg/dL): Diabetic Coma
Skin	Cold and clammy	Warm and dry
GI system	Nausea, hunger	Thirst, nausea, and vomiting
Breath	No change	Sweet or fruity odor, smell of acetone
Pulse	Normal or rapid	Rapid and weak
Behavior	May be irritable or confused; tremors and restlessness	Fatigue and lethargy, drowsiness
Level of consciousness	May become unresponsive	Disoriented, may go into a coma if not treated
Onset of symptoms	Rapid	Slow onset, may be days

Table 16.1—Hypoglycemia vs. Hyperglycemia

Treatment for Hypoglycemia

1. If the patient is conscious, give simple sugar orally. This could be in the form of orange juice, hard candy, or soda with sugar. If these are not available, any food would be useful. A finger-stick blood glucose level should be taken. Supplement the initial treatment with a snack containing protein, such as milk or soda crackers and peanut butter. If the patient has not responded to initial treatment within 15 to 20 minutes, alert emergency services.

2. If the patient is unconscious, do not attempt to feed him. Call 911 and transport him to a hospital.

Treatment for Hyperglycemia

1. Patients with hyperglycemia should be transported to the nearest hospital for further care to reduce the blood sugar to a safe level.

2. When you are unsure if it is hyper- or hypoglycemia, you always give sugar first.

FRACTURES

A fracture is any break in the bone. There are many different types of fractures and complete diagnosis of the type and extent of the fracture is done by x-ray. A fracture in which the skin is intact is called a closed fracture. If there is a break in the skin, it is called an open fracture.

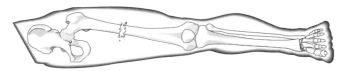

A. Complete: break across entire cross-section of bone

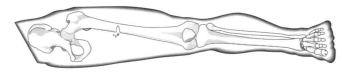

B. Incomplete: break through portion of bone

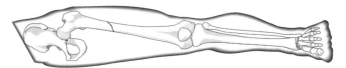

C. Closed: no external communication

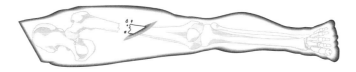

D. Open: extends through skin

Figure 16.1—Fractures

If a patient comes into the office with a suspected fracture, do not attempt to move the area. If the patient has fallen in the office, do not move them until you have received instructions from the physician. Basic steps for first aid of a suspected fracture include:

1. Check the ABCs first (airway, breathing, and circulation).

2. If it is an open fracture, do not attempt to move the bone or any fragments of the bone. Control any severe bleeding and cover with sterile cloth or gauze.

3. Elevate the fractured area if possible.

4. Apply ice to the area.

5. Keep the patient warm and quiet. Monitor vital signs. Look for signs and symptoms of shock.

6. If the patient has fallen in the office and may have a fracture, call for emergency assistance. Once emergency medical personnel arrive, they will take over moving the patient for transport. Be prepared to give information about how the injury occurred and what measures you have taken to assist the patient, and the patient's vital signs.

POISONING

Any ingestion or exposure to a noxious substance must be considered a medical emergency until proven otherwise. If the patient is calling into the office about a substance that he or someone in his household has ingested, try to ascertain what the substance is. Poison control should be consulted and the patient transported for treatment as soon as possible.

SEIZURE

A seizure may or may not be a medical emergency. The patient who has been diagnosed with epilepsy may occasionally have a seizure. A seizure is the result of abnormal brain activity. A patient who has no history of any seizure disorder should be transported by emergency services to a hospital for a complete analysis of the situation. The major goal in response to a seizure is to prevent injury to the patient.

1. Move any items from the patient area that could be dangerous. Provide privacy for the patient.

2. Make sure that the patient's clothing is not restricting circulation.

3. Do not restrain the patient. Do not put anything in the patient's mouth. Monitor the airway for any excessive saliva or vomiting. Roll the patient onto the left side in a continuous motion to allow for drainage of fluids from the mouth.

4. After the seizure is over, the patient will be drowsy and the patient should be allowed to rest for a period of time until they are alert and oriented.

5. If the patient has been diagnosed with epilepsy, the physician should be notified of the seizure. The patient may need to have medications changed or blood levels checked to make sure that medications are in a therapeutic range.

6. Transport the patient to a hospital for treatment.

SHOCK

Shock is a serious condition in which there is a depression of the cardiovascular system. Shock can be caused in several ways, but the signs and symptoms are similar and treatment involves treatment of the underlying cause. Signs and symptoms include decreased blood pressure, a weak and rapid pulse, diaphoresis, weakness, rapid respirations, pale skin, restlessness, and possibly nausea and vomiting. If these symptoms are not recognized and the underlying cause of shock is not treated, the patient may become unconscious and can die.

Hypovolemic shock	Shock due to a decrease in circulating blood in the body system. This can be due to hemorrhage from an injury or into a body cavity. This can also happen due to a third-degree burn over a large part of the body.
Cardiogenic shock	This type of shock is due to the failure of the heart to adequately pump enough blood to supply the body. This is frequently due to a myocardial infarction, congestive heart failure, or electrical conduction problems.
Septic shock	Shock due to a massive bacterial infection in which toxins from the infection are released into the bloodstream.
Neurogenic shock	This type of shock occurs when vasodilatation occurs due to dysfunction or injury to the neurological system.
Anaphylactic shock	Shock due to an allergic reaction from an allergen.

Table 16.2—Types of Shock

First aid for shock requires thorough and rapid assessment. If you can do anything to remedy the cause of shock, such as applying pressure to a bleeding wound, this would be the first measure to take. The patient should be transported to a hospital setting as soon as possible for treatment. Until this can be accomplished, there are some measures that can be taken.

1. Assess the ABCs and address any problems that you discover with the assessment. Oxygen may be necessary if it is available.

2. Position the patient with the lower extremities above the heart level as long as there is no injury that would prevent this.

3. Closely monitor and record the vital signs.

4. Keep the patient warm and quiet and provide emotional support. The patient may be very anxious.

5. Give information to emergency services when they arrive about patient's condition and any treatment that has been provided for the patient.

SYNCOPE

Syncope, or fainting, is the complete or partial loss of consciousness due to decreased circulation to the brain. This can be simple fainting or can be a symptom of a serious medical problem. Simple fainting may be due to a reaction to blood draw, due to the patient not having eaten, or low blood pressure. The patient may complain of feeling weak and dizzy prior to fainting. They may appear to be pale or diaphoretic. The patient may be aware that they are going to faint or may collapse suddenly without warning. First aid measures for fainting include the following.

1. Assist the patient to lie down if she says she is feeling faint. If she falls to the floor, do not move her until she has been checked for injury.

2. Apply a cold cloth to the face or use spirits of ammonia to stimulate consciousness.

3. Assess the ABCs to make sure that the patient has adequate airway and circulation. Monitor the patient's vital signs for any abnormality. Assess level of consciousness. Make notations of these facts for the patient record.

4. Elevate the legs to a higher position than the head if there has been no fall or injury. Make sure that the patient remains in a quiet place for a period of time and keep her warm. Report to the physician if he or she is in the office or seek a nearby physician if available.

5. If the person has a prolonged period of loss of consciousness, repeated episode of syncope, or a physician is not available, call for assistance and transport the patient to a hospital for an evaluation. The episode of syncope may be a symptom of a more serious problem.

WOUNDS

Types of wounds include the following:

Laceration: a tear in the skin or jagged-edged wound

Abrasion: scrape of the surface of the skin or the mucous membrane

Incision: a straight cut made with a cutting instrument

Puncture: an opening in the skin make by a sharp, pointed object such as a nail

Avulsion: forcible tearing of a flap of skin

Contusion: nonpenetrating wound resulting in bleeding beneath the skin and into the tissue

Minor wounds are easily treated in the outpatient setting. The goal of treatment of wounds is to promote healing and prevent infection. Wound treatment measures include the following.

1. Examine the wound for foreign bodies. Superficial wounds can be washed with soap and water.

2. Lacerations and incisions can be irrigated with water or normal saline. If the wounds need to be sutured, prepare the skin for a sterile procedure.

3. Puncture wounds must be explored for debris and washed well to remove microorganisms.

4. Tetanus injection may be necessary if boosters have not been kept up to date.

5. Give the patient written information about how to care for her wound and signs and symptoms of infection, which are:

    *   Redness and swelling

    *   Drainage from the wound

    *   Increase in pain

    *   Fever

    *   Heat and tenderness at the wound site

6. Make sure the patient has a follow-up appointment if sutures need to be removed.

REVIEW QUESTIONS

1. To open the airway of a patient who is discovered lying on the ground, the best method to use would be

   (A) raise the head and support the neck

   (B) head tilt-chin lift

   (C) place hand under neck to support the neck

   (D) jaw thrust maneuver

   (E) tongue thrust-chin lift

2. The most common cause of sudden cardiac death is

   (A) myocardial infarction

   (B) cardiogenic shock

   (C) cardiac arrhythmia

   (D) choking accidents

   (E) drowning

3. Which of the following is true about neurogenic shock?

   (A) It can be caused by a severe allergic reaction.

   (B) It is treated by administration of blood and/or intravenous fluids.

   (C) It may occur after a spinal cord injury.

   (D) It would be treated by administration of antibiotics.

   (E) It would result in hypertension and a slow bounding pulse.

4. With heavy bleeding of the forearm, the FIRST method a medical assistant would use to stop the bleeding would be to

   (A) apply pressure to the wound with a sterile or clean cloth

   (B) apply a tourniquet above the wound

   (C) apply pressure to the brachial artery to decrease blood flow

   (D) apply pressure to the carotid artery

   (E) elevate the arm above the level of the heart

5. According to the 2010 guidelines from the American Heart Association, a single rescuer should use which of the following compressions-to-breaths ratios for all patients except newborns?

   (A) 2:15

   (B) 15:1

   (C) 30:2

   (D) 30:1

   (E) 4:15

6. If a medical assistant suspects that a patient has a fracture of an extremity, it would be appropriate for her to

   (A) attempt to move the extremity to check for range of motion

   (B) schedule the patient for an x-ray later in the day

   (C) splint the extremity from the injury to the joint above it

   (D) hold pressure to the area to prevent bleeding into the tissue

   (E) apply heat to the area to increase circulation

7. If a patient has just had blood drawn and complains of feeling very dizzy, which of the following should the medical assistant do FIRST?

   (A) Reassure him that the blood draw is finished.

   (B) Assist the patient into a supine position and elevate his legs.

   (C) Leave and find the doctor to come in and evaluate the patient.

   (D) Evaluate for hypertension and weakness on one side of the body.

   (E) Check the blood pressure, pulse, and respiratory rate.

ANSWERS AND EXPLANATIONS

1. **D**

   Any patient who may have experienced trauma to the head or the neck and spine should have the airway opened by use of the jaw thrust maneuver. The lower jaw is lifted with both hands and the mandible raised in order to open the airway. Done correctly this does not extend the neck, which can cause further injury. If the patient is known to have no history of trauma, the head tilt-chin lift (B) can be used, which is easier to maintain for an extended period of time.

2. **C.**

   Cardiac arrhythmia is the most common cause of sudden cardiac death. Ventricular fibrillation caused by many different medical causes is most likely to cause sudden cardiac death.

3. **C**

   Neurogenic shock occurs when there is a spinal cord injury or central nervous system injury where there is a dysfunction of the autonomic nervous system. This causes vasodilatation of the circulatory system, which in turn causes the symptoms of shock.

4. **A**

   The first thing the medical assistant would do is apply direct pressure. Then you would use some of the other methods such as elevating the arm above the heart (E), which would slow blood return to the arm. Applying pressure to the brachial artery (C) could decrease blood flow to the area if he were still having a problem with heavy bleeding. A tourniquet (B) would be only used as a last resort to prevent loss of life. Pressure to the carotid artery (D) would not be useful.

5. **C**

   AHA recommendations call for 30 compressions to two breaths for one-rescuer CPR for all patients except newborns. This is to standardize the sequences and make it easier to remember for all rescuers.

6. **C**

   The most appropriate action would be to apply a splint to prevent movement. It would not be appropriate to try to move the extremity (A). That will not give you information about whether the bone is broken and may cause more injury. Pressure would not be held (D) unless it is an open fracture with heavy bleeding. Applying ice would reduce swelling and relieve pain. Increasing circulation in a new fracture by applying heat (E) would not be optimal.

7. **B**

The first thing that should be done is to assist the patient into a safe position and elevate his legs. Most likely, this is syncope due to the blood draw. It would then be appropriate to check the vital signs (E), reassure the patient (A), and have someone else notify the doctor about the situation (C). You should never leave the patient alone especially if they are not in a safe position. Hypertension and weakness on one side of the body would indicate a possible stroke (D). This would be a later assessment if the patient continued to have problems.

Chapter 17: **Emergency Preparedness**

After the trauma of 9/11 and the human and financial suffering rendered by Hurricane Katrina, massive oil spills, and other large-scale disasters, today's health care professionals are well aware of the importance of preparing for a variety of disasters and emergency situations. The time to create a plan that limits risk and protects resources from both natural and man-made catastrophe is in advance. The purpose of this section is to help you consider the essentials of appropriate emergency preparedness for the medical office. An emergency situation can occur due to an urgent or critically ill patient or visitor in the office or as a result of the environment, a man-made disaster, a bioterrorist attack, a public health crisis, or a civil defense issue. As a medical assistant, it is likely that you will be responsible in full or in part for designing, preparing, and executing this plan when and if it is needed. Far from being an unlikely concern, the potential for emergency situations is very real and apparent. In a survey of their member practices, 87 percent of medical office group management association practices felt there was a moderate to strong probability of a disaster affecting their work within the next five years.

After an overview of the essential elements in an emergency plan, consideration will be given to the resources needed in an emergency. The various roles of office staff in protecting the safety and security of patients, facility resources and health information will be reviewed. You should make sure that your workplace has a detailed and well-designed emergency plan to guide your efforts in the event of an emergency event. Your wellbeing and that of your patients could depend on it.

EMERGENCY CARE AND OFFICE PATIENTS

It is highly likely that your practice site will be called upon to render emergency care and treatment to patients while they are in your care. While literature shows that primary care offices handle emergency treatment on a regular basis, it also indicates that the majority of office practices are ill-prepared to manage such occurrences. Some of the reasons for this limitation are the infrequency of emergency management needs in ambulatory practice, the cost and time limits of providing care, and the proximity of hospital emergency rooms. However, with some anticipatory planning and training, medical assistants and medical office staff can work to ensure that

KAPLAN

emergent care needs can be effectively provided in the office. The most common adult medical patient emergencies include asthma attacks, acute psychiatric disturbances, seizures, hypogly-cemic reactions, anaphylaxis, loss of consciousness, shock, poisoning, and cardiac arrest. Given the unique nature of the patient population in your practice or specialty clinic, you should anticipate other risk factors that could become critical or urgent in your setting. Training and preparation in responding to these emergency situations should be one key element of your office emergency preparedness plan. If needed, staff should be trained and certified in basic emergency care, first aid, and cardiopulmonary resuscitation. The practice physicians should determine what supplies and medications to have on hand for emergencies. For example, if your office handles a large number of cardiac patients, you should consider having an auto-matic external defibrillator (AED) on hand. An AED recognizes an atypical cardiac rhythm and, if necessary, delivers a shock or electrical charge to the patient through self-adhesive pads. Newer AEDs have voice and visual prompts and function with a single button. The effectiveness of AEDs and their relatively low cost ($800–$1,500) now account for their availability and use in public places and office buildings.

The specific equipment and supplies to have on hand should also depend on the level of skill and training of the physicians, nurses and other staff. Legally, it is recommended to stock only those supplies with which the staff is skilled and trained to use. Both the American Academy of Pediatrics and the American Academy of Family Physicians have published recommended drug and supply lists for office practices. The distance from the office to emergency care and treatment facilities or a hospital emergency room should also be taken into consideration as you design a response system.

DEVELOPING AN OFFICE EMERGENCY PLAN

Office physicians, nurses, and medical assistants should take responsibility for developing a written plan to follow in the event of an emergency. The plan should detail the steps to follow in a variety of emergencies. A practice emergency occurs whenever an event disrupts or could potentially disrupt the flow of office work for more than 24 hours. Each office staff member should be assigned specific roles and responsibilities in such instances. Guidelines for the stor-age, use, and maintenance of emergency equipment and supplies should be listed. It is also critical that staff assess the level of preparation and test the plan through the use of mock codes or drills. Such testing can ensure patient safety, heighten staff sensitivity, and increase staff awareness of the proper location and use of emergency equipment and supplies.

Components of the Medical Office Emergency Plan

The Institute for Rural Health, along with the Medical Group Management Association, has designed a checklist for offices to use in formulating the details of their emergency plan. A paramount item on the list is *patient safety*. This includes a patient and staff evacuation plan. This plan may vary depending on the presence or absence of electrical power and communica-tion capability. It should be noted who in the office is authorized to trigger or enact the full or partial evacuation of the office. A staff member should be assigned to ensure that all parties are accounted for and have reached a pre-established area of safety. The details of the plan should also specify what office items should be removed and by which personnel. Backup power sources should be identified and support plans for disposition of patients to alternative facilities such as clinics or hospitals should be created. Emergency inventories of stock supplies and emergency supplies should be specified.

Another component of the emergency plan is *employee security and safety*. The plan should include the suggested chain of command and a backup to support loss of key employees. Management staff should be held responsible for tracking their employees and training them in emergency procedures. A central location that is off-site should be agreed upon as a meeting place following an emergency. Preventive vaccinations may be needed at this time in an outbreak or bioterrorist attack. An effort should be made to design and test a communication tree or communication system that can be used if the office phones and computer systems are not functional or out of commission due to weather emergencies.

The *practice capability* of the medical office will be another key area to focus on in an emergency plan. This will include access to patient records and charts and a plan to duplicate and secure off-site data storage and data retrieval files. An office spokesperson should be identified and this person should be comfortable responding to public officials, the press, and the general public about the status of medical care and the practice. If downtime due to the emergency is anticipated, a plan for patient referral for short-term disruptions of care should be stated. Offices may want to establish a contract or agreement for disaster cleanup and office system replacement in the event of a disaster that impacts the physical space and facility. The practice may want to coordinate with the local public health system and define their role in a local community's disaster plan. Key personnel may need to be trained to respond to large-scale disasters and participate in public disaster drills.

A final but significant component of an emergency plan is the *financial survival* of the practice. Cash flow may be disrupted and a backup financial plan may be needed. It may be prudent to locate a safe to hold cash on a temporary basis. Financial records, including up-to-date transaction records, should be stored in secure off-site locations. Personnel who are authorized to access off-site records should be identified and made aware of their duties and responsibilities in a disaster or emergency. A plan for payment of staff wages in full or in part should be considered. It is also critical that the insurance coverage of the office be accessible. Many businesses are covered for interruptions as well as property damage and equipment failure. The office staff needs to know the insurance carrier and should promptly contact the insurer with claim information.

PANDEMICS AND BIOTERRORISM

Recently, the threat of a pandemic of the H1N1 virus led to large-scale immunization and mobilization of governmental and private health care organizations. It was clear from the beginning phases that we were not prepared to handle such a large-scale and potentially fatal disease outbreak. It is likely that in the event of a pandemic, hospitals and emergency clinics would be overtaxed and many members of the general public would seek treatment from the medical practice office. The following 10 suggestions are provided as a guide to caring for patients and the public in the event of an epidemic, outbreak, or suspected act of bioterrorism:

1. Maintain an index of suspicion and know the signs and symptoms associated with the condition or causative agent.

2. Protect yourself and take whatever preventive measures are available and recommended for health care providers.

3. Assess the patients and those who come in for treatment.

4. Decontaminate as appropriate if a causative agent is suspected.

5. Establish a diagnosis and treatment plan.

6. Render prompt treatment according to guidelines from local or national health officials.

7. Practice good infection control and waste disposal.

8. Alert the proper authorities and health department.

9. Assist in the epidemiologic investigation as needed.

10. Maintain proficiency in emergency care and initiation of the office emergency plan.

REVIEW QUESTIONS

1. Which of the following best describes the definition of a disaster situation in a medical practice office?

   (A) An event that disrupts the workflow of the practice for more than 24 hours

   (B) An outbreak of measles in the local high school

   (C) A patient coming to the office with active TB

   (D) The computer system going down

   (E) The physician being called away to a hospital emergency

2. Which medical office staff needs to be considered in preparing an emergency plan?

   (A) The physicians and nurses

   (B) Medical assistants

   (C) Office clerical staff and billers

   (D) All of the above

   (E) Only the physicians

3. To best respond to sudden serious cardiac arrest, what equipment should be on hand in the medical office?

   (A) An AED (automatic electronic defibrillator)

   (B) Oxygen

   (C) Chest tubes

   (D) Suction machine

   (E) IV amigo catheter

4. Which of the following represents the essential components of an emergency preparedness plan for a medical office?

   (A) An office evacuation plan

   (B) A plan for storage of medical records off-site

   (C) An insurance policy on the office and equipment

   (D) An emergency phone communication tree for all staff

   (E) All of the above

5. Which of the following best explains the role of the Federal Emergency Management Agency (FEMA) in a national disaster?

   (A) To fund all insurance claims associated with disasters

   (B) To train your practice staff in managing emergencies

   (C) To provide homeland security to U.S. citizens

   (D) To support U.S. citizens and first responders to prepare for, protect against, respond to, and recover from emergencies and hazards

   (E) None of the above

ANSWERS AND EXPLANATIONS

1. **A**

   A disaster situation in a medical office practice is defined as any event that disrupts the practice's workflow for more than 24 hours. Choice (B) would be correctly identified as a disease outbreak, (C) is an individual patient care situation, (D) is a temporary office situation, and (E) is likely to be a regular occurrence in a medical office.

2. **D**

   Every office staff member should be considered in an effective emergency plan. (E) is incorrect, as it would exclude key roles. (A), (B), and (C) are incorrect because they are not inclusive of all office staff members. So the correct answer is (D), all of the above.

3. **A**

   The correct answer is (A), AED device. (B) would not be effective, as some patients are unable to breathe in during an arrest. (C) is incorrect; chest tubes need to be placed when a lung collapses, not in a cardiac arrest situation. (D) would not be used in a cardiac arrest, as it is used to clear secretions from the mouth and nasal area. (E) is incorrect as well, as it is used to administer medications; it may be used later, but not initially to shock the heart.

4. **E**

   All of the above items represent critical considerations in an emergency preparedness plan. (A), (B), (C), and (D) are incorrect, as they are only component elements of the plan by themselves.

5. **D**

   Choice (D) accurately defines the role of FEMA. (A) is incorrect, as FEMA does not offer assistance with private insurance claims. (B) is incorrect, as it is the responsibility of the medical practice to train staff to manage emergencies. As for (C), while FEMA is a division of the Department of Homeland Security, it does not directly provide security services.

PART FOUR

Practice Test

HOW TO TAKE THE PRACTICE TEST

The following Kaplan-created exam is similar to an actual Certified Medical Assistant exam, and it covers topics included on the Registered Medical Assistant exam. Before taking the practice test, find a quiet space where you can work uninterrupted for four hours.

The test includes three sections: general, administrative, and clinical. Each section contains 100 questions. You have four hours to complete all three sections, but you may complete them in any order. Mark your answers on the answer sheet. Once you finish the exam, refer to the Answers and Explanations section. Remember that the answer explanations can help you pick up important information, even on questions you answered correctly.

Best of luck!

YOUR PRACTICE TEST SCORE

The test included in this book is designed to provide practice answering exam-style questions, along with a review of medical assisting content. Your results on this test indicate where you are now. It is not designed to predict your ability to pass the CMA or RMA exams.

The test has 300 questions total, with 100 questions each in the general, administrative, and clinical sections. Calculate the number of questions you answered correctly in each section. If you answered 70 or more questions correctly in a given section, you have a good understanding of that subject area. If you answered between 60 and 69 questions correctly in a section, you could benefit from further review of that content. If you answered fewer than 59 questions correctly, you need focused study of that content. Examine your incorrect answers to see exactly which areas you should review.

ANSWER SHEET

I. General

1 Ⓐ Ⓑ Ⓒ Ⓓ Ⓔ	26 Ⓐ Ⓑ Ⓒ Ⓓ Ⓔ	51 Ⓐ Ⓑ Ⓒ Ⓓ Ⓔ	76 Ⓐ Ⓑ Ⓒ Ⓓ Ⓔ
2 Ⓐ Ⓑ Ⓒ Ⓓ Ⓔ	27 Ⓐ Ⓑ Ⓒ Ⓓ Ⓔ	52 Ⓐ Ⓑ Ⓒ Ⓓ Ⓔ	77 Ⓐ Ⓑ Ⓒ Ⓓ Ⓔ
3 Ⓐ Ⓑ Ⓒ Ⓓ Ⓔ	28 Ⓐ Ⓑ Ⓒ Ⓓ Ⓔ	53 Ⓐ Ⓑ Ⓒ Ⓓ Ⓔ	78 Ⓐ Ⓑ Ⓒ Ⓓ Ⓔ
4 Ⓐ Ⓑ Ⓒ Ⓓ Ⓔ	29 Ⓐ Ⓑ Ⓒ Ⓓ Ⓔ	54 Ⓐ Ⓑ Ⓒ Ⓓ Ⓔ	79 Ⓐ Ⓑ Ⓒ Ⓓ Ⓔ
5 Ⓐ Ⓑ Ⓒ Ⓓ Ⓔ	30 Ⓐ Ⓑ Ⓒ Ⓓ Ⓔ	55 Ⓐ Ⓑ Ⓒ Ⓓ Ⓔ	80 Ⓐ Ⓑ Ⓒ Ⓓ Ⓔ
6 Ⓐ Ⓑ Ⓒ Ⓓ Ⓔ	31 Ⓐ Ⓑ Ⓒ Ⓓ Ⓔ	56 Ⓐ Ⓑ Ⓒ Ⓓ Ⓔ	81 Ⓐ Ⓑ Ⓒ Ⓓ Ⓔ
7 Ⓐ Ⓑ Ⓒ Ⓓ Ⓔ	32 Ⓐ Ⓑ Ⓒ Ⓓ Ⓔ	57 Ⓐ Ⓑ Ⓒ Ⓓ Ⓔ	82 Ⓐ Ⓑ Ⓒ Ⓓ Ⓔ
8 Ⓐ Ⓑ Ⓒ Ⓓ Ⓔ	33 Ⓐ Ⓑ Ⓒ Ⓓ Ⓔ	58 Ⓐ Ⓑ Ⓒ Ⓓ Ⓔ	83 Ⓐ Ⓑ Ⓒ Ⓓ Ⓔ
9 Ⓐ Ⓑ Ⓒ Ⓓ Ⓔ	34 Ⓐ Ⓑ Ⓒ Ⓓ Ⓔ	59 Ⓐ Ⓑ Ⓒ Ⓓ Ⓔ	84 Ⓐ Ⓑ Ⓒ Ⓓ Ⓔ
10 Ⓐ Ⓑ Ⓒ Ⓓ Ⓔ	35 Ⓐ Ⓑ Ⓒ Ⓓ Ⓔ	60 Ⓐ Ⓑ Ⓒ Ⓓ Ⓔ	85 Ⓐ Ⓑ Ⓒ Ⓓ Ⓔ
11 Ⓐ Ⓑ Ⓒ Ⓓ Ⓔ	36 Ⓐ Ⓑ Ⓒ Ⓓ Ⓔ	61 Ⓐ Ⓑ Ⓒ Ⓓ Ⓔ	86 Ⓐ Ⓑ Ⓒ Ⓓ Ⓔ
12 Ⓐ Ⓑ Ⓒ Ⓓ Ⓔ	37 Ⓐ Ⓑ Ⓒ Ⓓ Ⓔ	62 Ⓐ Ⓑ Ⓒ Ⓓ Ⓔ	87 Ⓐ Ⓑ Ⓒ Ⓓ Ⓔ
13 Ⓐ Ⓑ Ⓒ Ⓓ Ⓔ	38 Ⓐ Ⓑ Ⓒ Ⓓ Ⓔ	63 Ⓐ Ⓑ Ⓒ Ⓓ Ⓔ	88 Ⓐ Ⓑ Ⓒ Ⓓ Ⓔ
14 Ⓐ Ⓑ Ⓒ Ⓓ Ⓔ	39 Ⓐ Ⓑ Ⓒ Ⓓ Ⓔ	64 Ⓐ Ⓑ Ⓒ Ⓓ Ⓔ	89 Ⓐ Ⓑ Ⓒ Ⓓ Ⓔ
15 Ⓐ Ⓑ Ⓒ Ⓓ Ⓔ	40 Ⓐ Ⓑ Ⓒ Ⓓ Ⓔ	65 Ⓐ Ⓑ Ⓒ Ⓓ Ⓔ	90 Ⓐ Ⓑ Ⓒ Ⓓ Ⓔ
16 Ⓐ Ⓑ Ⓒ Ⓓ Ⓔ	41 Ⓐ Ⓑ Ⓒ Ⓓ Ⓔ	66 Ⓐ Ⓑ Ⓒ Ⓓ Ⓔ	91 Ⓐ Ⓑ Ⓒ Ⓓ Ⓔ
17 Ⓐ Ⓑ Ⓒ Ⓓ Ⓔ	42 Ⓐ Ⓑ Ⓒ Ⓓ Ⓔ	67 Ⓐ Ⓑ Ⓒ Ⓓ Ⓔ	92 Ⓐ Ⓑ Ⓒ Ⓓ Ⓔ
18 Ⓐ Ⓑ Ⓒ Ⓓ Ⓔ	43 Ⓐ Ⓑ Ⓒ Ⓓ Ⓔ	68 Ⓐ Ⓑ Ⓒ Ⓓ Ⓔ	93 Ⓐ Ⓑ Ⓒ Ⓓ Ⓔ
19 Ⓐ Ⓑ Ⓒ Ⓓ Ⓔ	44 Ⓐ Ⓑ Ⓒ Ⓓ Ⓔ	69 Ⓐ Ⓑ Ⓒ Ⓓ Ⓔ	94 Ⓐ Ⓑ Ⓒ Ⓓ Ⓔ
20 Ⓐ Ⓑ Ⓒ Ⓓ Ⓔ	45 Ⓐ Ⓑ Ⓒ Ⓓ Ⓔ	70 Ⓐ Ⓑ Ⓒ Ⓓ Ⓔ	95 Ⓐ Ⓑ Ⓒ Ⓓ Ⓔ
21 Ⓐ Ⓑ Ⓒ Ⓓ Ⓔ	46 Ⓐ Ⓑ Ⓒ Ⓓ Ⓔ	71 Ⓐ Ⓑ Ⓒ Ⓓ Ⓔ	96 Ⓐ Ⓑ Ⓒ Ⓓ Ⓔ
22 Ⓐ Ⓑ Ⓒ Ⓓ Ⓔ	47 Ⓐ Ⓑ Ⓒ Ⓓ Ⓔ	72 Ⓐ Ⓑ Ⓒ Ⓓ Ⓔ	97 Ⓐ Ⓑ Ⓒ Ⓓ Ⓔ
23 Ⓐ Ⓑ Ⓒ Ⓓ Ⓔ	48 Ⓐ Ⓑ Ⓒ Ⓓ Ⓔ	73 Ⓐ Ⓑ Ⓒ Ⓓ Ⓔ	98 Ⓐ Ⓑ Ⓒ Ⓓ Ⓔ
24 Ⓐ Ⓑ Ⓒ Ⓓ Ⓔ	49 Ⓐ Ⓑ Ⓒ Ⓓ Ⓔ	74 Ⓐ Ⓑ Ⓒ Ⓓ Ⓔ	99 Ⓐ Ⓑ Ⓒ Ⓓ Ⓔ
25 Ⓐ Ⓑ Ⓒ Ⓓ Ⓔ	50 Ⓐ Ⓑ Ⓒ Ⓓ Ⓔ	75 Ⓐ Ⓑ Ⓒ Ⓓ Ⓔ	100 Ⓐ Ⓑ Ⓒ Ⓓ Ⓔ

II. Administrative

101 Ⓐ Ⓑ Ⓒ Ⓓ Ⓔ	126 Ⓐ Ⓑ Ⓒ Ⓓ Ⓔ	151 Ⓐ Ⓑ Ⓒ Ⓓ Ⓔ	176 Ⓐ Ⓑ Ⓒ Ⓓ Ⓔ
102 Ⓐ Ⓑ Ⓒ Ⓓ Ⓔ	127 Ⓐ Ⓑ Ⓒ Ⓓ Ⓔ	152 Ⓐ Ⓑ Ⓒ Ⓓ Ⓔ	177 Ⓐ Ⓑ Ⓒ Ⓓ Ⓔ
103 Ⓐ Ⓑ Ⓒ Ⓓ Ⓔ	128 Ⓐ Ⓑ Ⓒ Ⓓ Ⓔ	153 Ⓐ Ⓑ Ⓒ Ⓓ Ⓔ	178 Ⓐ Ⓑ Ⓒ Ⓓ Ⓔ
104 Ⓐ Ⓑ Ⓒ Ⓓ Ⓔ	129 Ⓐ Ⓑ Ⓒ Ⓓ Ⓔ	154 Ⓐ Ⓑ Ⓒ Ⓓ Ⓔ	179 Ⓐ Ⓑ Ⓒ Ⓓ Ⓔ
105 Ⓐ Ⓑ Ⓒ Ⓓ Ⓔ	130 Ⓐ Ⓑ Ⓒ Ⓓ Ⓔ	155 Ⓐ Ⓑ Ⓒ Ⓓ Ⓔ	180 Ⓐ Ⓑ Ⓒ Ⓓ Ⓔ
106 Ⓐ Ⓑ Ⓒ Ⓓ Ⓔ	131 Ⓐ Ⓑ Ⓒ Ⓓ Ⓔ	156 Ⓐ Ⓑ Ⓒ Ⓓ Ⓔ	181 Ⓐ Ⓑ Ⓒ Ⓓ Ⓔ
107 Ⓐ Ⓑ Ⓒ Ⓓ Ⓔ	132 Ⓐ Ⓑ Ⓒ Ⓓ Ⓔ	157 Ⓐ Ⓑ Ⓒ Ⓓ Ⓔ	182 Ⓐ Ⓑ Ⓒ Ⓓ Ⓔ
108 Ⓐ Ⓑ Ⓒ Ⓓ Ⓔ	133 Ⓐ Ⓑ Ⓒ Ⓓ Ⓔ	158 Ⓐ Ⓑ Ⓒ Ⓓ Ⓔ	183 Ⓐ Ⓑ Ⓒ Ⓓ Ⓔ
109 Ⓐ Ⓑ Ⓒ Ⓓ Ⓔ	134 Ⓐ Ⓑ Ⓒ Ⓓ Ⓔ	159 Ⓐ Ⓑ Ⓒ Ⓓ Ⓔ	184 Ⓐ Ⓑ Ⓒ Ⓓ Ⓔ
110 Ⓐ Ⓑ Ⓒ Ⓓ Ⓔ	135 Ⓐ Ⓑ Ⓒ Ⓓ Ⓔ	160 Ⓐ Ⓑ Ⓒ Ⓓ Ⓔ	185 Ⓐ Ⓑ Ⓒ Ⓓ Ⓔ
111 Ⓐ Ⓑ Ⓒ Ⓓ Ⓔ	136 Ⓐ Ⓑ Ⓒ Ⓓ Ⓔ	161 Ⓐ Ⓑ Ⓒ Ⓓ Ⓔ	186 Ⓐ Ⓑ Ⓒ Ⓓ Ⓔ
112 Ⓐ Ⓑ Ⓒ Ⓓ Ⓔ	137 Ⓐ Ⓑ Ⓒ Ⓓ Ⓔ	162 Ⓐ Ⓑ Ⓒ Ⓓ Ⓔ	187 Ⓐ Ⓑ Ⓒ Ⓓ Ⓔ
113 Ⓐ Ⓑ Ⓒ Ⓓ Ⓔ	138 Ⓐ Ⓑ Ⓒ Ⓓ Ⓔ	163 Ⓐ Ⓑ Ⓒ Ⓓ Ⓔ	188 Ⓐ Ⓑ Ⓒ Ⓓ Ⓔ
114 Ⓐ Ⓑ Ⓒ Ⓓ Ⓔ	139 Ⓐ Ⓑ Ⓒ Ⓓ Ⓔ	164 Ⓐ Ⓑ Ⓒ Ⓓ Ⓔ	189 Ⓐ Ⓑ Ⓒ Ⓓ Ⓔ
115 Ⓐ Ⓑ Ⓒ Ⓓ Ⓔ	140 Ⓐ Ⓑ Ⓒ Ⓓ Ⓔ	165 Ⓐ Ⓑ Ⓒ Ⓓ Ⓔ	190 Ⓐ Ⓑ Ⓒ Ⓓ Ⓔ
116 Ⓐ Ⓑ Ⓒ Ⓓ Ⓔ	141 Ⓐ Ⓑ Ⓒ Ⓓ Ⓔ	166 Ⓐ Ⓑ Ⓒ Ⓓ Ⓔ	191 Ⓐ Ⓑ Ⓒ Ⓓ Ⓔ
117 Ⓐ Ⓑ Ⓒ Ⓓ Ⓔ	142 Ⓐ Ⓑ Ⓒ Ⓓ Ⓔ	167 Ⓐ Ⓑ Ⓒ Ⓓ Ⓔ	192 Ⓐ Ⓑ Ⓒ Ⓓ Ⓔ
118 Ⓐ Ⓑ Ⓒ Ⓓ Ⓔ	143 Ⓐ Ⓑ Ⓒ Ⓓ Ⓔ	168 Ⓐ Ⓑ Ⓒ Ⓓ Ⓔ	193 Ⓐ Ⓑ Ⓒ Ⓓ Ⓔ
119 Ⓐ Ⓑ Ⓒ Ⓓ Ⓔ	144 Ⓐ Ⓑ Ⓒ Ⓓ Ⓔ	169 Ⓐ Ⓑ Ⓒ Ⓓ Ⓔ	194 Ⓐ Ⓑ Ⓒ Ⓓ Ⓔ
120 Ⓐ Ⓑ Ⓒ Ⓓ Ⓔ	145 Ⓐ Ⓑ Ⓒ Ⓓ Ⓔ	170 Ⓐ Ⓑ Ⓒ Ⓓ Ⓔ	195 Ⓐ Ⓑ Ⓒ Ⓓ Ⓔ
121 Ⓐ Ⓑ Ⓒ Ⓓ Ⓔ	146 Ⓐ Ⓑ Ⓒ Ⓓ Ⓔ	171 Ⓐ Ⓑ Ⓒ Ⓓ Ⓔ	196 Ⓐ Ⓑ Ⓒ Ⓓ Ⓔ
122 Ⓐ Ⓑ Ⓒ Ⓓ Ⓔ	147 Ⓐ Ⓑ Ⓒ Ⓓ Ⓔ	172 Ⓐ Ⓑ Ⓒ Ⓓ Ⓔ	197 Ⓐ Ⓑ Ⓒ Ⓓ Ⓔ
123 Ⓐ Ⓑ Ⓒ Ⓓ Ⓔ	148 Ⓐ Ⓑ Ⓒ Ⓓ Ⓔ	173 Ⓐ Ⓑ Ⓒ Ⓓ Ⓔ	198 Ⓐ Ⓑ Ⓒ Ⓓ Ⓔ
124 Ⓐ Ⓑ Ⓒ Ⓓ Ⓔ	149 Ⓐ Ⓑ Ⓒ Ⓓ Ⓔ	174 Ⓐ Ⓑ Ⓒ Ⓓ Ⓔ	199 Ⓐ Ⓑ Ⓒ Ⓓ Ⓔ
125 Ⓐ Ⓑ Ⓒ Ⓓ Ⓔ	150 Ⓐ Ⓑ Ⓒ Ⓓ Ⓔ	175 Ⓐ Ⓑ Ⓒ Ⓓ Ⓔ	200 Ⓐ Ⓑ Ⓒ Ⓓ Ⓔ

III. Clinical

201 Ⓐ Ⓑ Ⓒ Ⓓ Ⓔ	226 Ⓐ Ⓑ Ⓒ Ⓓ Ⓔ	251 Ⓐ Ⓑ Ⓒ Ⓓ Ⓔ	276 Ⓐ Ⓑ Ⓒ Ⓓ Ⓔ
202 Ⓐ Ⓑ Ⓒ Ⓓ Ⓔ	227 Ⓐ Ⓑ Ⓒ Ⓓ Ⓔ	252 Ⓐ Ⓑ Ⓒ Ⓓ Ⓔ	277 Ⓐ Ⓑ Ⓒ Ⓓ Ⓔ
203 Ⓐ Ⓑ Ⓒ Ⓓ Ⓔ	228 Ⓐ Ⓑ Ⓒ Ⓓ Ⓔ	253 Ⓐ Ⓑ Ⓒ Ⓓ Ⓔ	278 Ⓐ Ⓑ Ⓒ Ⓓ Ⓔ
204 Ⓐ Ⓑ Ⓒ Ⓓ Ⓔ	229 Ⓐ Ⓑ Ⓒ Ⓓ Ⓔ	254 Ⓐ Ⓑ Ⓒ Ⓓ Ⓔ	279 Ⓐ Ⓑ Ⓒ Ⓓ Ⓔ
205 Ⓐ Ⓑ Ⓒ Ⓓ Ⓔ	230 Ⓐ Ⓑ Ⓒ Ⓓ Ⓔ	255 Ⓐ Ⓑ Ⓒ Ⓓ Ⓔ	280 Ⓐ Ⓑ Ⓒ Ⓓ Ⓔ
206 Ⓐ Ⓑ Ⓒ Ⓓ Ⓔ	231 Ⓐ Ⓑ Ⓒ Ⓓ Ⓔ	256 Ⓐ Ⓑ Ⓒ Ⓓ Ⓔ	281 Ⓐ Ⓑ Ⓒ Ⓓ Ⓔ
207 Ⓐ Ⓑ Ⓒ Ⓓ Ⓔ	232 Ⓐ Ⓑ Ⓒ Ⓓ Ⓔ	257 Ⓐ Ⓑ Ⓒ Ⓓ Ⓔ	282 Ⓐ Ⓑ Ⓒ Ⓓ Ⓔ
208 Ⓐ Ⓑ Ⓒ Ⓓ Ⓔ	233 Ⓐ Ⓑ Ⓒ Ⓓ Ⓔ	258 Ⓐ Ⓑ Ⓒ Ⓓ Ⓔ	283 Ⓐ Ⓑ Ⓒ Ⓓ Ⓔ
209 Ⓐ Ⓑ Ⓒ Ⓓ Ⓔ	234 Ⓐ Ⓑ Ⓒ Ⓓ Ⓔ	259 Ⓐ Ⓑ Ⓒ Ⓓ Ⓔ	284 Ⓐ Ⓑ Ⓒ Ⓓ Ⓔ
210 Ⓐ Ⓑ Ⓒ Ⓓ Ⓔ	235 Ⓐ Ⓑ Ⓒ Ⓓ Ⓔ	260 Ⓐ Ⓑ Ⓒ Ⓓ Ⓔ	285 Ⓐ Ⓑ Ⓒ Ⓓ Ⓔ
211 Ⓐ Ⓑ Ⓒ Ⓓ Ⓔ	236 Ⓐ Ⓑ Ⓒ Ⓓ Ⓔ	261 Ⓐ Ⓑ Ⓒ Ⓓ Ⓔ	286 Ⓐ Ⓑ Ⓒ Ⓓ Ⓔ
212 Ⓐ Ⓑ Ⓒ Ⓓ Ⓔ	237 Ⓐ Ⓑ Ⓒ Ⓓ Ⓔ	262 Ⓐ Ⓑ Ⓒ Ⓓ Ⓔ	287 Ⓐ Ⓑ Ⓒ Ⓓ Ⓔ
213 Ⓐ Ⓑ Ⓒ Ⓓ Ⓔ	238 Ⓐ Ⓑ Ⓒ Ⓓ Ⓔ	263 Ⓐ Ⓑ Ⓒ Ⓓ Ⓔ	288 Ⓐ Ⓑ Ⓒ Ⓓ Ⓔ
214 Ⓐ Ⓑ Ⓒ Ⓓ Ⓔ	239 Ⓐ Ⓑ Ⓒ Ⓓ Ⓔ	264 Ⓐ Ⓑ Ⓒ Ⓓ Ⓔ	289 Ⓐ Ⓑ Ⓒ Ⓓ Ⓔ
215 Ⓐ Ⓑ Ⓒ Ⓓ Ⓔ	240 Ⓐ Ⓑ Ⓒ Ⓓ Ⓔ	265 Ⓐ Ⓑ Ⓒ Ⓓ Ⓔ	290 Ⓐ Ⓑ Ⓒ Ⓓ Ⓔ
216 Ⓐ Ⓑ Ⓒ Ⓓ Ⓔ	241 Ⓐ Ⓑ Ⓒ Ⓓ Ⓔ	266 Ⓐ Ⓑ Ⓒ Ⓓ Ⓔ	291 Ⓐ Ⓑ Ⓒ Ⓓ Ⓔ
217 Ⓐ Ⓑ Ⓒ Ⓓ Ⓔ	242 Ⓐ Ⓑ Ⓒ Ⓓ Ⓔ	267 Ⓐ Ⓑ Ⓒ Ⓓ Ⓔ	292 Ⓐ Ⓑ Ⓒ Ⓓ Ⓔ
218 Ⓐ Ⓑ Ⓒ Ⓓ Ⓔ	243 Ⓐ Ⓑ Ⓒ Ⓓ Ⓔ	268 Ⓐ Ⓑ Ⓒ Ⓓ Ⓔ	293 Ⓐ Ⓑ Ⓒ Ⓓ Ⓔ
219 Ⓐ Ⓑ Ⓒ Ⓓ Ⓔ	244 Ⓐ Ⓑ Ⓒ Ⓓ Ⓔ	269 Ⓐ Ⓑ Ⓒ Ⓓ Ⓔ	294 Ⓐ Ⓑ Ⓒ Ⓓ Ⓔ
220 Ⓐ Ⓑ Ⓒ Ⓓ Ⓔ	245 Ⓐ Ⓑ Ⓒ Ⓓ Ⓔ	270 Ⓐ Ⓑ Ⓒ Ⓓ Ⓔ	295 Ⓐ Ⓑ Ⓒ Ⓓ Ⓔ
221 Ⓐ Ⓑ Ⓒ Ⓓ Ⓔ	246 Ⓐ Ⓑ Ⓒ Ⓓ Ⓔ	271 Ⓐ Ⓑ Ⓒ Ⓓ Ⓔ	296 Ⓐ Ⓑ Ⓒ Ⓓ Ⓔ
222 Ⓐ Ⓑ Ⓒ Ⓓ Ⓔ	247 Ⓐ Ⓑ Ⓒ Ⓓ Ⓔ	272 Ⓐ Ⓑ Ⓒ Ⓓ Ⓔ	297 Ⓐ Ⓑ Ⓒ Ⓓ Ⓔ
223 Ⓐ Ⓑ Ⓒ Ⓓ Ⓔ	248 Ⓐ Ⓑ Ⓒ Ⓓ Ⓔ	273 Ⓐ Ⓑ Ⓒ Ⓓ Ⓔ	298 Ⓐ Ⓑ Ⓒ Ⓓ Ⓔ
224 Ⓐ Ⓑ Ⓒ Ⓓ Ⓔ	249 Ⓐ Ⓑ Ⓒ Ⓓ Ⓔ	274 Ⓐ Ⓑ Ⓒ Ⓓ Ⓔ	299 Ⓐ Ⓑ Ⓒ Ⓓ Ⓔ
225 Ⓐ Ⓑ Ⓒ Ⓓ Ⓔ	250 Ⓐ Ⓑ Ⓒ Ⓓ Ⓔ	275 Ⓐ Ⓑ Ⓒ Ⓓ Ⓔ	300 Ⓐ Ⓑ Ⓒ Ⓓ Ⓔ

Practice Test

Time: 4 hours

Part I–General

DIRECTIONS (Questions 1–100): All of the following questions and incomplete statements are followed by five answer choices. For each question, select the single answer that best answers the question or completes the statement. Fill in the corresponding circle on your answer sheet.

1. The combining form *hepat/o* refers to the

   (A) stomach
   (B) intestine
   (C) pancreas
   (D) liver
   (E) gallbladder

2. Sarcasm, repression, and denial are examples of which psychological mechanism used to deal with stressful situations?

   (A) Grief
   (B) Unconscious mind
   (C) Defense mechanisms
   (D) Ego
   (E) Self-actualization

3. The function of the optic nerve is

   (A) hearing
   (B) seeing
   (C) smelling
   (D) tasting
   (E) touching

4. Your coworker tells you that her next-door neighbor has just come in for a health exam. She asks you to give her the health history form to review it. Which of the following actions is appropriate?

   (A) Give her the record to review.
   (B) Tell the office manager.
   (C) Remind her that the patient record is protected health information.
   (D) Ask the patient if you can show her the record.
   (E) Leave the chart on the work desk so she can read it after you leave.

5. Which condition is treated with use of the DASH diet?

   (A) High blood pressure
   (B) Diarrhea
   (C) Ulcers
   (D) Muscle weakness
   (E) Cancer

6. Sworn testimony given outside of court is called

   (A) subpoena
   (B) deposition
   (C) standard of care
   (D) evidence
   (E) verdict

7. In order for a case of negligence to be valid, all of the "four D's" must be present EXCEPT

    (A) a duty must be owed

    (B) a duty must be breeched

    (C) a desire to harm must exist

    (D) damages must have occurred

    (E) damages must be directly related to act

8. According to Piaget, at what developmental stage would a child be expected to understand the differences in size and weights of a group of objects?

    (A) Sensorimotor

    (B) Preoperational

    (C) Formal operations

    (D) Concrete operations

    (E) Self-actualization

9. The prefix meaning "many" is

    (A) *semi-*

    (B) *macro-*

    (C) *pseudo-*

    (D) *poly-*

    (E) *dia-*

10. Myelomeningocele means

    (A) swelling of the brain

    (B) hardening of the bone marrow

    (C) herniation of the spinal cord and covering on the spinal cord

    (D) formation of brain and spinal cord

    (E) drooping of the testicles and scrotum

11. Oranges, bananas, broccoli, and tomatoes are rich sources of which of the following minerals?

    (A) Calcium

    (B) Vitamin C

    (C) Vitamin K

    (D) Potassium

    (E) Iron

12. Which of the following is not a type of body tissue?

    (A) Epithelial

    (B) Connective

    (C) Respiratory

    (D) Muscle

    (E) Nervous

13. Confidential information can be disclosed in all of the following cases EXCEPT

    (A) the patient requests the information be released

    (B) the patient's power of attorney for health care signs a release of information

    (C) the physician feels it is necessary for the public's welfare

    (D) someone is in imminent danger if the information is withheld

    (E) the patient is mentally ill and out of touch with reality

14. A terminally ill patient says that he is angry and feels that his illness could have been treated successfully by a "better doctor." Which of the following would be an appropriate response to this comment?

    (A) Say "Nonsense, the doctor is wonderful!"

    (B) Say nothing, but call an attorney.

    (C) Say "I understand that you are angry right now."

    (D) Nod in agreement and say nothing.

    (E) Tell the patient that you will speak to the doctor.

15. If AC interference occurs on an EKG tracing, what is the likely cause?

    (A) The electrodes are too tight.

    (B) The electrodes are incorrectly placed.

    (C) One of the electrodes is not completely attached.

    (D) The patient sneezed or coughed.

    (E) There is electrical interference from within the room.

16. Which of the following terms refers to sewing or stitching of veins?

    (A) Venostenosis

    (B) Phlebosclerosis

    (C) Vasoplasty

    (D) Venopexy

    (E) Phleborrhaphy

17. It is a hectic day in the office and the physician is backed up in seeing patients who have been in the waiting room. Mr. Hall approaches the reception desk and pounds his fist and starts yelling that his time is valuable and that he has waited long enough. All of the following steps are appropriate ways to handle the first stages of an encounter with an angry patient EXCEPT

    (A) ask the patient to come into the next room and politely explain the delay and apologize

    (B) lower the volume and tone of your own voice when speaking to Mr. Hall

    (C) listen to his statement, nod, and let him know that you too find it unpleasant to have delays

    (D) apologize and give him a coupon for free coffee in the lobby coffee shop

    (E) tell him that you will need to call the security guard and have him removed from the office if he does not calm down

18. Which of the following vitamins is used for clotting?

    (A) Vitamin A

    (B) Vitamin B_6

    (C) Vitamin B_{12}

    (D) Vitamin C

    (E) Vitamin K

19. Within the cell, the organelle responsible for the production of energy is the

    (A) lysosome

    (B) Golgi body

    (C) endoplasmic reticulum

    (D) nucleus

    (E) mitochondria

20. The word root for "tumor" is

    (A) *onc/o*

    (B) *-oma*

    (C) *onc*

    (D) *carcin/o*

    (E) *carcin*

21. Which of the following thought leaders in the field of psychology believed that repressed memories created emotional conflict and possible mental disorders later in life?

    (A) Elisabeth Kübler-Ross

    (B) Jean Piaget

    (C) Erick Erickson

    (D) Sigmund Freud

    (E) Abraham Maslow

22. When the plaintiff is found to be in some part responsible for injury and the health care giver is NOT held responsible, it is called

    (A) assumed risk

    (B) contributory risk

    (C) comparative risk

    (D) technical defense

    (E) intervening cause

23. Which of the following terms would describe an infestation of gallstones?

    (A) Cholecystitis

    (B) Cholecystosis

    (C) Cholecystolithiasis

    (D) Cholelithiasis

    (E) Cholecystectomy

24. A medical assistant is working with an obese child on a weight reduction program. When his patient loses five pounds at her follow-up appointment, he gives her a movie ticket. Which psychological principle is the medical assistant using in this case?

    (A) Reinforcement

    (B) Cognitive therapy

    (C) Health promotion

    (D) Latency theory

    (E) Fight versus flight

25. Which of the following vitamins is NOT fat soluble?

    (A) Vitamin A
    (B) Vitamin C
    (C) Vitamin D
    (D) Vitamin K
    (E) Vitamin E

26. A defense based on assigning portions of the responsibility for damages to both plaintiff and defendant is called a

    (A) technical defense
    (B) defense of denial
    (C) contributory defense
    (D) comparative defense
    (E) assumed risk

27. Which of the following body systems is responsible for hearing?

    (A) Skeletal
    (B) Endocrine
    (C) Nervous
    (D) Integumentary
    (E) Respiratory

28. During this period of development, young children experience the world only through what they can experience with their senses. At the early part of this stage, they may not be able to differentiate between themselves and the rest of the world. Piaget termed this period

    (A) the preoperational stage
    (B) the latency stage
    (C) the stage of formal operations
    (D) the sensorimotor stage
    (E) infancy

29. Which of the following anatomical locations contains the patella?

    (A) Arm
    (B) Foot
    (C) Torso
    (D) Leg
    (E) Head

30. Which of the following specialists would treat ARDS, SOB, and COPD?

    (A) Nephrologist
    (B) Gastroenterologist
    (C) Pulmonologist
    (D) Cardiologist
    (E) Hospitalist

31. Which of the following gives a choice to those over 18 years of age to determine the disposition of their body or body parts?

    (A) The Uniform Anatomical Gift Act
    (B) The living will
    (C) The power of attorney for health care
    (D) ERISA
    (E) *Res ipsa loquitur*

32. Which of the following terms refers to blood in the urine?

    (A) Hematemesis
    (B) Uremia
    (C) Hematuria
    (D) Anemia
    (E) Enuresis

33. Perspiration is produced by the

    (A) ceruminous glands
    (B) sudoriferous glands
    (C) parathyroid glands
    (D) sebaceous glands
    (E) adrenal glands

34. Which of the following formed elements is responsible for blood clotting?

    (A) Erythrocytes
    (B) Leukocytes
    (C) Thrombocytes
    (D) Neutrophils
    (E) Eosinophils

35. Which of the following would NOT be an unintentional tort when done by a medical assistant?

    (A) Giving the wrong medicine in an injection

    (B) Improperly cleaning a surgical site

    (C) Showing photos of a surgery without patient consent

    (D) Not drawing a blood test the physician ordered

    (E) Suturing a laceration for a patient

36. The prefix meaning "beyond" is

    (A) *mal-*

    (B) *ambi-*

    (C) *meta-*

    (D) *retro-*

    (E) *multi-*

37. A court mandate to bring a portion of the medical record to court is called

    (A) *respondeat superior*

    (B) *res ipsa loquitur*

    (C) *subpoena duces tecum*

    (D) *res judicata*

    (E) *caveat emptor*

38. A medical assistant is providing instruction on care of sutures to a young mother whose child has been injured in a fall. She is distracted and tells the medical assistant that she and her child have not eaten for two days because their public aid check is late. Which of the hierarchy of needs is preventing this mother from considering the patient teaching that is being presented to her?

    (A) Self-esteem

    (B) Safety and security

    (C) Physiological needs

    (D) Love and belonging

    (E) Self-actualization

39. Pathogens that thrive in the presence of oxygen are called

    (A) microorganisms

    (B) spores

    (C) aerobes

    (D) anaerobes

    (E) protists

40. Which of the following suffixes is NOT an adjective ending meaning "pertaining to"?

    (A) *-ic*

    (B) *-ac*

    (C) *-al*

    (D) *-ity*

    (E) *-ous*

41. The physician can terminate the care of a patient in all of the following situations EXCEPT when

    (A) the patient does not pay the bills

    (B) the patient is noncompliant with treatment recommendations

    (C) the patient uses abusive language with staff

    (D) the patient misses repeated appointments

    (E) the patient states that she is seeing another doctor

42. Which of the following prefixes means "near"?

    (A) *peri-*

    (B) *para-*

    (C) *-para*

    (D) *-oma*

    (E) *meta-*

43. Which type of fracture is a bone that is broken into pieces?

    (A) Compound

    (B) Pathological

    (C) Impacted

    (D) Comminuted

    (E) Open

44. Which of the following is considered high in antioxidants?

    (A) Liver and organ meats

    (B) Dark green and yellow vegetables

    (C) Citrus fruits

    (D) Root vegetables like turnips and potatoes

    (E) Dairy products

KAPLAN

45. A plane that cuts the body parallel to the horizon is called a/an

   (A) transverse plane
   (B) sagittal plane
   (C) frontal plane
   (D) coronal plane
   (E) midsagittal plane

46. Which of the following specialists would a person see for IBS, PUD, or pyloric stenosis?

   (A) Cardiologist
   (B) Gastroenterologist
   (C) Urologist
   (D) Pulmonologist
   (E) Nephrologist

47. The major site where carbohydrates are broken down is the

   (A) colon
   (B) stomach
   (C) mouth
   (D) large intestine
   (E) small intestine

48. Crimes that are committed against another person or property and are punished with fines are called

   (A) felonies
   (B) misdemeanors
   (C) treason
   (D) torts
   (E) negligence

49. Which of the following words is CORRECTLY spelled?

   (A) Opthalmologist
   (B) Hemorrhoid
   (C) Colesterol
   (D) Anasthesia
   (E) Migrain

50. The pancreas is located in which body cavity?

   (A) Thoracic
   (B) Abdominal
   (C) Pelvic
   (D) Spinal
   (E) Cranial

51. Which of the following patients CANNOT consent to his/her own care?

   (A) A married 17-year-old female needing cough syrup
   (B) An unmarried 18-year-old needing birth control pills
   (C) A 17-year-old Marine needing acne medicine
   (D) A 17-year-old with a 6-inch laceration of the leg
   (E) A confused 83-year-old with no guardian who wants a tummy tuck

52. All of the following are parenteral routes of medication administration EXCEPT

   (A) IV
   (B) IM
   (C) PO
   (D) subQ
   (E) intradermal

53. Which of the following words is MISSPELLED?

   (A) Menstration
   (B) Glaucoma
   (C) Accommodation
   (D) Hemorrhoid
   (E) Circumcision

54. Which item should a patient on a low-sodium diet select for a snack?

   (A) Jumbo dill pickle
   (B) Ham sandwich
   (C) Cornflakes and whole milk
   (D) Banana
   (E) Baked pretzel sticks

55. Which of the following is the pacemaker for the heart?

    (A) Bundle of His
    (B) AV node
    (C) Bundle branch
    (D) SA node
    (E) Purkinje fibers

56. Which of the following is NOT a purpose of the medical record?

    (A) Research tool
    (B) Communication tool for health care team
    (C) Verification record of physician skill level
    (D) Legal record
    (E) Personal record of health treatment

57. The length of time in which a person can file a lawsuit is called

    (A) statute of limitations
    (B) doctrine of informed consent
    (C) mandatory reporting
    (D) HIPAA
    (E) COBRA

58. The medical assistant draws blood for a patient's pregnancy test and she leaves the office. Later that day, the laboratory delivers the results and they are positive. The medical assistant phones the patient to give her the news but she is not at home. Which of the following actions should the medical assistant take?

    (A) Send her a follow-up appointment card.
    (B) Leave the good news on her home answering machine.
    (C) Leave a name and number and ask her to call the office.
    (D) Try to remember to call her back later in the day.
    (E) Tell her to come back to the office.

59. Which of the following words describes bone pain?

    (A) Chondromalacia
    (B) Osteochondritis
    (C) Chrondralgia
    (D) Osteolysis
    (E) Osteodynia

60. Which of the following is NOT a good source of calcium?

    (A) Milk
    (B) Sardines
    (C) Canned salmon
    (D) Cauliflower
    (E) Cheese

61. The abbreviation that indicates a patient should take the medication before a meal is

    (A) NPO
    (B) NOS
    (C) PRN
    (D) PC
    (E) AC

62. Which of the following phrases describes the amount of evidence required to convict in a civil case?

    (A) Evidence beyond a reasonable doubt
    (B) 100 percent of proof
    (C) A preponderance of evidence
    (D) Evidence beyond the shadow of a doubt
    (E) Only minimal evidence

63. Which mineral helps prevent dental cavities?

    (A) Calcium
    (B) Potassium
    (C) Iron
    (D) Fluoride
    (E) Iodine

64. Which of the following blood types can give to all other blood types?

    (A) Type A
    (B) Type B
    (C) Type O
    (D) Type AB
    (E) Type ABO

65. A patient who is instructed to take 10 mL of a medication would be able to use which of the following household equivalents?

    (A) $\frac{1}{2}$ pint

    (B) $\frac{1}{2}$ teaspoon

    (C) 2 teaspoons

    (D) 2 tablespoons

    (E) 60 drops

66. When a physical exam has been performed and the physician documents PERRLA, what part(s) of the body is this term referring to?

    (A) Eyes

    (B) Ears

    (C) Throat

    (D) Heart

    (E) Abdomen

67. Which of the following words is NOT a correctly spelled medical term?

    (A) Scrotum

    (B) Prostrate

    (C) Testicle

    (D) Foreskin

    (E) Circumcision

68. Which of the following is descriptive of arteries?

    (A) Thick, elastic, return blood to heart

    (B) Thin, fragile, carry blood away from heart

    (C) Thin, elastic, return blood to heart

    (D) Thin, elastic, carry blood away from heart

    (E) Thick, elastic, carry blood away from heart

69. Torticollis or wryneck is a spasm of which muscle?

    (A) Gastocnemius

    (B) Sternocleidomastoid

    (C) Rectus abdominus

    (D) Deltoid

    (E) Sartorius

70. Laws that protect consumers from harassing phone calls for collection are part of the

    (A) Fair Credit Reporting Act

    (B) Equal Credit Opportunity Act

    (C) Consumer Protection Act

    (D) Fair Labor Standards Act

    (E) Fair Debt Collection Act

71. Bones are joined to muscles by

    (A) ligaments

    (B) periosteum

    (C) cartilage

    (D) meninges

    (E) tendons

72. "Multipara" means

    (A) near many

    (B) many nearby

    (C) many pregnancies

    (D) many live births

    (E) many pairs

73. Which of the following does NOT describe Schedule IV drugs?

    (A) Physician must sign a triplicate prescription

    (B) Can be refilled five times over six months

    (C) Can be called in to pharmacy over phone

    (D) Frequently abused

    (E) Must be stored in locking cabinet for administration

74. Which region is referred to when charting a notation about the area near the navel?

    (A) Suprapubic

    (B) Epigastric

    (C) Umbilical

    (D) Hypochondriac

    (E) Lumbar

75. Which term did Freud use to describe the area of the mind that determined a person's basic identity?

    (A) Ego

    (B) Id

    (C) Superego

    (D) Unconscious mind

    (E) Subconscious mind

76. Which of the following words means "without menstrual flow"?

    (A) Nullipara

    (B) Amenorrhea

    (C) Oligomenorrhea

    (D) Dysmenorrhea

    (E) Nulligravida

77. Which of the following food items would NOT be consumed by a lacto-vegetarian?

    (A) Rice

    (B) Eggs

    (C) Beans

    (D) Milk

    (E) Corn

78. The act that protects patient rights including the right to agree to or refuse medical treatment is the

    (A) Patient Self-Determination Act of 1990

    (B) Consumer Protection Act of 1971

    (C) Civil Rights Act of 1964

    (D) HIPAA Act

    (E) Americans with Disabilities Act

79. The disease in which blood accumulates due to a tear in the meningeal layer is

    (A) Concussion

    (B) Subdural hematoma

    (C) Intracerebral hematoma

    (D) Epilepsy

    (E) Hydrocephalus

80. The abbreviation for potassium is

    (A) P

    (B) Fe

    (C) K

    (D) Au

    (E) Pm

81. Which of the following is NOT an early warning symptom of cancer?

    (A) Sore that does not heal

    (B) Pain and weight loss

    (C) Unexplained bleeding

    (D) Chronic cough or hoarseness

    (E) Lump or mass

82. Which of the following practitioners would treat patients for ADHD, PTSD, and bipolar disorder?

    (A) Psychiatrist

    (B) Hematologist

    (C) Gynecologist

    (D) Rheumatologist

    (E) Pulmonologist

83. All of the following are duties performed by the public health department EXCEPT

    (A) collecting data on communicable diseases

    (B) recording vital statistics of animal bites and injuries

    (C) predicting and managing epidemics

    (D) managing Medicare and Medicaid

    (E) tracking births, deaths, and stillborns

84. Which of the following waves represents relaxation of the ventricles?

    (A) P wave

    (B) Q wave

    (C) QRS wave

    (D) T wave

    (E) U wave

KAPLAN

85. The term "carcinogenic" means

    (A) formation of tumors
    (B) pertaining to the formation of tumors
    (C) formation of cancer
    (D) pertaining to cancer
    (E) study of tumors

86. The disease where the coating on the axon begins to disintegrate and slows neural transmissions is called

    (A) multiple sclerosis
    (B) myasthenia gravis
    (C) amyotrophic lateral sclerosis
    (D) cerebral palsy
    (E) Parkinson's disease

87. Erythema may be caused by all of the following EXCEPT

    (A) sunburn
    (B) carbon monoxide poisoning
    (C) dermatitis
    (D) bile problems
    (E) blushing

88. Which of the following terms means "the process of using an instrument to record data of electrical activity of the heart"?

    (A) electrocardiography
    (B) electrocardiograph
    (C) electrocardiogram
    (D) echocardiogram
    (E) echocardiography

89. If an elderly patient refuses an antibiotic injection, but the medical assistant holds the patient down "for her own good" and gives it anyway,

    (A) it is legal
    (B) it is an example of assault
    (C) it is legal, but immoral
    (D) it is an example of battery
    (E) it is an example of invasion of privacy

90. A papule with clear fluid is called a

    (A) pustule
    (B) vesicle
    (C) macule
    (D) nevus
    (E) nodule

91. Which abbreviation would be unlikely to appear on a chart in a gynecologist's office?

    (A) TAH
    (B) LMP
    (C) LOC
    (D) PID
    (E) STD

92. The person accused of a crime or illegal act is the

    (A) plaintiff
    (B) defendant
    (C) jury
    (D) bench
    (E) agent

93. The disease where uric acid collects in the joint and crystallizes is called

    (A) bursitis
    (B) arthritis
    (C) kyphosis
    (D) scoliosis
    (E) gout

94. One state accepting the licensure requirements of another state to enable a health care worker to practice is called

    (A) certification
    (B) revocation
    (C) registration
    (D) reciprocity
    (E) licensure

95. A patient with cryptorchidism, balantitis, or hematuria would likely see a/an

    (A) epidemiologist
    (B) pulmonologist
    (C) urologist
    (D) gynecologist
    (E) hematologist

96. Which of the following is NOT an action of the sympathetic nervous system?

    (A) Increased blood pressure
    (B) Increased pulse
    (C) Release of glucose
    (D) Decrease of respiration
    (E) Decreased libido

97. Which of the following is NOT true about a legal contract?

    (A) There is a consideration.
    (B) It is always written and witnessed.
    (C) The parties must be of legal capacity.
    (D) The contract is for a specific good or service.
    (E) The contract must be accepted by both parties.

98. A procedure such as a CABG or EKG is likely to be done by a/an

    (A) neurologist
    (B) rheumatologist
    (C) nephrologist
    (D) urologist
    (E) cardiologist

99. Intentional misrepresentation of facts and figures is called

    (A) negligence
    (B) slander
    (C) defamation
    (D) libel
    (E) fraud

100. A dying patient tells the medical assistant that if she survives, she will give the rest of her life to caring for children. What stage of Kübler-Ross's model of grief is this patient currently in?

    (A) Denial
    (B) Acceptance
    (C) Bargaining
    (D) Anger
    (E) Detachment

Part II—Administrative

DIRECTIONS (Questions 101–200): All of the following questions and incomplete statements are followed by five answer choices. For each question, select the single answer that best answers the question or completes the statement. Fill in the corresponding circle on your answer sheet.

101. The practice of one insurance company working with other insurance plans to determine the amount each will pay when a patient has more than one insurance plan is referred to as

    (A) capitation
    (B) coinsurance
    (C) third-party payment
    (D) assignment of benefits
    (E) coordination of benefits

102. The recorded financial transactions in a bookkeeping or accounting system are called

    (A) ledger
    (B) superbill
    (C) posting
    (D) trial balance
    (E) deductions

103. Which appointment scheduling technique determines the number of patients to be seen each hour by dividing the hour by the length of the average visit?

    (A) Double booking
    (B) Cluster
    (C) Time specified
    (D) Wave
    (E) Advance

104. Which of the following filing steps includes ensuring that the appropriate people have taken action on a document before filing it?

    (A) Releasing
    (B) Indexing
    (C) Conditioning
    (D) Storing
    (E) Sorting

105. Another name for a reminder file is a/an

    (A) tickler file
    (B) supplemental file
    (C) retained file
    (D) inactive file
    (E) active file

106. Which of the following is NOT a true statement about the Health Information Technology for Economic and Clinical Health (HITECH) Act of 2009?

    (A) The act establishes financial incentives for adoption of electronic health records (EHRs).
    (B) The act establishes a single EHR software system that all health care providers must use.
    (C) Health care providers must show "meaningful use" of EHRs systems to receive incentive payments.
    (D) A goal of using EHRs is to improve Americans' health.
    (E) More than half of U.S. physicians have adopted EHRs.

107. The portion of salary held back from payroll checks for paying government taxes is known as the

    (A) W-4 form
    (B) Federal Unemployment Tax Act
    (C) withholding
    (D) annual tax return
    (E) FICA

108. In a letter written in block format, the salutation is followed by a

    (A) comma
    (B) dash
    (C) colon
    (D) period
    (E) semicolon

109. Which of the following concerns have providers raised about the use of EHRs and the required data entry they must complete?

    (A) It is impersonal.
    (B) It interferes with communication with the patient during an encounter.
    (C) It is busy work.
    (D) They prefer handwritten notes.
    (E) Electronic records are confusing.

110. Which of the following are the dimensions of the envelope size most frequently used in office correspondence?

    (A) 4 inches × 9 inches

    (B) $3\frac{1}{2}$ inches × $8\frac{1}{2}$ inches

    (C) $4\frac{1}{2}$ inches × $9\frac{1}{2}$ inches

    (D) $5\frac{1}{2}$ inches × $9\frac{1}{2}$ inches

    (E) $10\frac{1}{2}$ inches × $10\frac{1}{2}$ inches

111. Account aging receivable

    (A) means that the physician must collect the receivable on time

    (B) is not necessary in a single-physician office

    (C) is a tool to show the status of each account

    (D) involves writing off accounts that are over one year past due

    (E) involves writing off accounts that are over five years past due

112. A system used in emergency centers but not used in private practices is

    (A) modified-wave scheduling

    (B) double-booking scheduling

    (C) open-hours scheduling

    (D) cluster scheduling

    (E) time-specified scheduling

113. Appointments that are anticipated to require more time should be scheduled

    (A) at the beginning of the hour

    (B) never

    (C) at the end of the hour

    (D) with another patient's 10-minute time slot

    (E) during a 10-minute slot

114. For a tickler file to work effectively, it must be

    (A) kept in file folders

    (B) located in a secure area

    (C) checked frequently

    (D) organized into weekly files

    (E) kept in a separate area of the office

115. "Write-it-once" is a bookkeeping system also known as

    (A) single-entry

    (B) pegboard

    (C) double-entry

    (D) disbursement

    (E) balance sheet

116. Which of the following activities should be integrated in an effective EHR?

    (A) Patient scheduling of appointments

    (B) Patient billing

    (C) Inventory use of supplies

    (D) Medical and procedural coding

    (E) All of the above

117. A spreadsheet is a type of

    (A) worksheet

    (B) hardware

    (C) patient list

    (D) cover letter

    (E) work grid

118. First-class mail is classified as

    (A) only postcards

    (B) newspapers only

    (C) items weighing 13 ounces or more

    (D) items weighing 13 ounces or less

    (E) all bulk mail

119. In written communication, no matter what form is used, the most important issue to take into consideration is

    (A) lack of body language

    (B) the speed of the document transmitted

    (C) formatting

    (D) legal and ethical issues

    (E) grammar

120. Which of the following does NOT refer to a managed care organizational model?

    (A) Integrated delivery system

    (B) Health maintenance organization

    (C) Preferred provider organization

    (D) Double-entry system

    (E) Utilization review organization

121. The federal government is currently offering incentives to support what aspect of implementation of EHRs?

    (A) System selection among vendors

    (B) Planning for EHR implementation

    (C) Staffing and staff training

    (D) Cost of purchase or lease of a system

    (E) Patient use of a system

122. Which of the following represents an important way to maintain the security and integrity of an electronic health record?

    (A) A password secured sign-on credential for each user in a facility

    (B) Limited access to anyone but the physician providers

    (C) Single sign-on credentials for the practice office team

    (D) Keeping the data entry device or computer out of sight of patients

    (E) None of the above

123. When revising the policies and procedures manual, the medical assistant needs to FIRST

    (A) talk to fellow employees

    (B) chose a color for the manual

    (C) decide on a format

    (D) buy paper for the manual

    (E) talk to the physician

124. Leaving large, unused gaps in the physician's schedule is

    (A) underbooking

    (B) overbooking

    (C) clustering

    (D) wave

    (E) advance

125. The correct order of filing units for Anise K. Strong-Morse (Mrs. Adam H. Morse) is

    (A) Anise K. Strong-Morse

    (B) Strong-Morse, Anise K.

    (C) Morse, Mrs. Adam H.

    (D) Morse, Anise, Strong

    (E) Strong, Mrs. Adam H.

126. What should the medical assistant do if a patient misses an appointment?

    (A) Document the no-show in the appointment book and in the patient's chart.

    (B) Notify the patient that she will be charged for the appointment.

    (C) Refuse to reschedule an appointment for the patient.

    (D) Schedule another appointment for the patient but patient must confirm.

    (E) Erase the appointment from the appointment book.

127. Referrals to outside physicians or specialists must be entered into the

    (A) appointment book

    (B) data entry

    (C) medical records

    (D) claim report

    (E) tickler file

128. Which of the following is a trial balance?

    (A) A daily summary

    (B) A way of checking the accuracy of accounts

    (C) An accounting system

    (D) Accrual accounting

    (E) Bookkeeping

129. A new patient must provide all of the following information EXCEPT

    (A) Social Security Number

    (B) income

    (C) marital status

    (D) occupation

    (E) age

130. For a medical office to run smoothly, each employee must

    (A) help write the policies and procedures manual

    (B) know where the policies and procedures manual is kept

    (C) read the policies and procedures manual

    (D) give patients copies of the policies and procedures manual

    (E) have a personal copy of the policies and procedures manual

131. Which insurance carriers would the medical assistant enter into the database?

    (A) All insurance carriers

    (B) Each insurance carrier that the physician accepts

    (C) Medicare and Medicaid only

    (D) The most popular insurance carriers

    (E) The insurance that the physician offers his employees

132. Checks and cash from a medical practice should be deposited in the bank

    (A) daily

    (B) biweekly

    (C) weekly

    (D) monthly

    (E) semimonthly

133. The type of scheduling where patients arrive at their own convenience is

    (A) open hours

    (B) time specified

    (C) wave

    (D) double booking

    (E) clustering

134. Which of the following is NOT a true statement about workers' compensation?

    (A) A qualifying illness or injury originates on the job.

    (B) An illness or injury unrelated to one's job cannot be seen under workers' compensation insurance.

    (C) Short-term, long-term, or permanent disability benefits may apply.

    (D) The individual with a qualifying illness or injury can go to the doctor of his/her choice.

    (E) The individual with a qualifying illness or injury receives no bills for medical expenses specifically related to the illness or injury.

135. SOAP refers to

    (A) a method of documentation used in medical records

    (B) a filing system used in medical offices

    (C) a procedure for making medical appointments

    (D) a protocol for answering patient phone calls

    (E) a bookkeeping system used in medical offices

136. When transcribing material from recorded dictation, what should the medical assistant do if a word is unclear?

    (A) Leave a blank space and write a note to the physician.

    (B) Guess which word the physician intended and insert it.

    (C) Stop transcribing until the physician is available to clarify the word.

    (D) Reword the sentence so the word is no longer needed.

    (E) Mark the space with an "X" and ask the physician later.

137. Cycle billing is a system of billing

    (A) completed every fourth month

    (B) done by computer

    (C) completed by the first of the month

    (D) in which accounts are divided alphabetically for billing purpose

    (E) completed by the 25th of the month

138. The term "software" means

    (A) portable hardware

    (B) a set of instructions

    (C) the input device

    (D) palmtop

    (E) tower case

139. It would be appropriate to send which of the following to a patient via email?

    (A) Diagnosis

    (B) Lab test results

    (C) Follow-up information

    (D) Appointment request

    (E) List of medications

140. When the medical assistant makes an appointment, to ensure he has the correct information, he should

    (A) say "Thank you" before hanging up

    (B) tell the caller "Have a nice day"

    (C) ask the caller to repeat the information

    (D) repeat the name and phone number back to the caller

    (E) say "Good-bye" and hang up

141. Which of the following items facilitates communication in the medical office?

    (A) Tickler file

    (B) Patient's medical records

    (C) Data entry

    (D) Appointment book

    (E) Policies and procedures manual

142. How often should the policy and procedures manual be updated?

    (A) Every month

    (B) Every six months

    (C) Every year

    (D) Every two years

    (E) Every five years

143. When preparing business correspondence, the first step is to

    (A) start writing

    (B) organize key points to be addressed

    (C) use language that is easy to understand

    (D) compose a rough draft

    (E) choose a letter format

144. The unethical practice of deliberately coding a patient encounter incorrectly in order to increase reimbursement is called

    (A) dirty claims

    (B) EOB

    (C) bundling

    (D) superbilling

    (E) upcoding

145. Before scheduling an appointment with a specialist, the medical assistant must

    (A) obtain an order from the physician for the exact procedure to be performed

    (B) talk with the patient to find convenient appointment times

    (C) ask the patient if she would rather schedule the appointment

    (D) determine the day and time the procedure must be performed

    (E) determine who will be with the patient at the time of procedure

146. The process of converting descriptions of diseases, injuries, and procedures into numerical designations is termed

    (A) coding

    (B) claims

    (C) subrogation

    (D) superbill

    (E) charge slip

147. Medicare is a federally funded entitlement insurance program for

    (A) children of veterans who died of service-related disabilities

    (B) the blind who are at least 40 years of age

    (C) individuals who are financially indigent

    (D) anyone over 62 years of age

    (E) individuals age 65 and older who are retired and receive Social Security benefits

148. Which of the following choices describes time-specified scheduling?

    (A) Patients arrive at the top of the hour.

    (B) Appointments are double booked.

    (C) One appointment is made for every hour.

    (D) Patients are scheduled all day long at regular specified intervals.

    (E) Patients are seen on a first-come, first-seen basis.

149. Which of the following actions should the medical assistant take if a medical record is misplaced?

    (A) Say nothing.

    (B) Proceed as if the chart can be located.

    (C) Duplicate the information.

    (D) Try to recreate the original file.

    (E) Start a new file.

150. Which postal class would the medical assistant use to send a monthly newsletter to all patients in the practice?

    (A) Third-class

    (B) First-class

    (C) Second-class

    (D) Bulk mail

    (E) Priority mail

151. The term "debit" means

    (A) total

    (B) subtract

    (C) charge

    (D) subtotal

    (E) balance

152. The body of an email communication should

    (A) provide all available background information on the topic

    (B) be written in italic using bold and color for emphasis

    (C) be brief and to the point

    (D) be written in capital letters

    (E) be written without any capital letters

153. Under which of the following systems are two patients scheduled for the same appointment time?

    (A) Modified wave

    (B) Double booking

    (C) Wave scheduling

    (D) Open scheduling

    (E) Modified scheduling

154. Referrals are given to which of the following patients?

    (A) All patients who need to see a specialist

    (B) PPO insurance patients who need to see a specialist

    (C) HMO insurance patients who need to see a specialist

    (D) Only POS insurance patients who need to see a specialist

    (E) Uninsured patients who need to see a specialist

155. The MOST important use of computers in the medical office is to

    (A) schedule appointments

    (B) verify appointments

    (C) diagnose patients

    (D) take vital signs

    (E) locate files

156. The billing schedule is often determined by

    (A) the number of physicians in the group

    (B) the size of the medical practice

    (C) what types of physicians are in the medical office

    (D) how many employees do the billing

    (E) when the physician wants the billing cycle to take place

157. All money owed by the practice to other businesses is called

    (A) accounts payable

    (B) accounts receivable

    (C) charges

    (D) debits

    (E) owner's equity

158. All of the following documents should be shredded prior to disposal EXCEPT

    (A) appointment list

    (B) patient lab results

    (C) patient referral

    (D) photocopy of patient insurance card

    (E) unmarked HCFA-1500 form

159. Flexible office hours occur most often

    (A) in group practices

    (B) in hospitals

    (C) in specialists' offices

    (D) in primary care physicians' offices

    (E) in single-physician practices

160. POMR is the abbreviation for

    (A) problem-oriented medical record

    (B) patient-orientated medical record

    (C) problem-orientated medical record

    (D) patient-oriented medical report

    (E) program-oriented medical record

161. Petty cash may be used

    (A) for paying minor incidental expenses

    (B) for paying an invoice for supplies ordered

    (C) for paying the electric bill for the medical facility

    (D) only by the physician

    (E) only in emergencies

162. After opening the mail, a medical assistant should

    (A) date-stamp the letter

    (B) put it aside until the patients are gone

    (C) give it to the physician immediately

    (D) read the mail for importance

    (E) put it in a folder to deliver later

163. When removing a medical chart from the file cabinet, which of the following items should the medical assistant put in its place?

    (A) A sticky note
    (B) An empty folder
    (C) Another patient's chart
    (D) A process note with the medical assistant's name
    (E) An outguide

164. When a patient has to cancel an appointment, the medical assistant should

    (A) say "Thank you" and hang up
    (B) try to reschedule the appointment
    (C) ask the patient to call back
    (D) remind the patient of the importance of appointments
    (E) ask the physician if it is okay for the patient to cancel

165. Which of the following items is a collection of records created and stored on a computer?

    (A) Scanner
    (B) Internet
    (C) Cursor
    (D) Database
    (E) Hard copy

166. The motherboard of a computer is

    (A) the main circuit board
    (B) the flash drive
    (C) the hard disk drive
    (D) the operating system
    (E) the memory

167. The patient pays a copayment

    (A) after seeing the physician
    (B) upon receiving a bill from the medical office
    (C) before being seen by the physician
    (D) in advance of the visit to the medical office
    (E) while in the exam room

168. Which of the following is the most secure way to mail something through the United States Postal Service?

    (A) Certified mail
    (B) Insured mail
    (C) Registered mail
    (D) First-class mail
    (E) Priority mail

169. The pegboard system provides control over

    (A) payments and charges
    (B) charge slips
    (C) collections, payments, and charges
    (D) third-party payments
    (E) collections only

170. Which of the following is an accurate statement about the implementation of the new ICD-10 coding system?

    (A) it only applies to hospitals
    (B) it is likely to be overturned
    (C) it is taking effect in October 2014
    (D) it is optional for all providers
    (E) medical assistants do not need to prepare for this; only billers need to prepare

171. If the medical office has a patient who is always late for appointments, the best time to try to book this patient is

    (A) at the beginning of the day
    (B) in the middle of the day
    (C) right after lunch
    (D) never (do not schedule)
    (E) at the end of the day

172. Wave scheduling works best when used in which of the following types of offices?

    (A) Urgent care facilities
    (B) Specialist offices
    (C) Two-physician practices
    (D) One-physician practices
    (E) Large medical facilities

173. Which of the following systems divides the patients of a practice into groups and bills each group at a different time of the month?

    (A) Past due

    (B) Account aging

    (C) Cycle billing

    (D) Wave scheduling

    (E) Monthly billing

174. How frequently should the medical assistant renew on-call repair service contracts?

    (A) Every three months

    (B) Every six months

    (C) Every year

    (D) Every two years

    (E) Every five years

175. The ICD-9 and ICD-10 systems of classifying diseases into categories were devised by what organization?

    (A) HCFA (Health Care Financing Administration)

    (B) AMA (American Medical Association)

    (C) AHIMA (American Health Information Management Association)

    (D) WHO (World Health Organization)

    (E) IRS (Internal Revenue Service)

176. Which of the following terms refers to the actual daily recording of the accounts or business transactions of the medical office?

    (A) Day sheets

    (B) Charges

    (C) Account receivable

    (D) Bookkeeping

    (E) Pegboard

177. The physical components of a computer system include all of the following EXCEPT

    (A) hardware

    (B) software

    (C) keyboard

    (D) mouse

    (E) printer

178. Which is the easiest and least expensive type of billing for a health service facility?

    (A) Cycle billing

    (B) Ledger card billing

    (C) Computerized mailed statement

    (D) Superbill at time of visit

    (E) Telephone system

179. It is recommended that records of appointments be kept for

    (A) two years

    (B) three years

    (C) one year

    (D) five years

    (E) ten years

180. A charge slip is also known as a/an

    (A) CMS1500

    (B) Claim

    (C) Subrogation

    (D) HCPCS

    (E) Superbill

181. When scheduling, the medical assistant should ask the patient the purpose of the visit

    (A) so the doctor can prepare

    (B) to determine how much time is needed for the appointment

    (C) to determine what supplies are needed for the visit

    (D) to make sure that there is enough room on the progress note

    (E) so the medical assistant can try to double book

182. Which of the following BEST describes the intent of the move to the ICD-10-CM system in the United States?

    (A) To add complexity to the delivery of health care

    (B) To improve the specificity and efficiency of medical coding and billing

    (C) To add more codes to the list of available ways to name a disease

    (D) To use the same system that other countries on the globe use

    (E) To require electronic records and bills

KAPLAN

183. The claim form that is accepted by most insurance carriers is a/an

    (A) claim register
    (B) superbill
    (C) CMS1500
    (D) diagnosis codes
    (E) modifiers

184. The information entered on claims is called

    (A) demographic information
    (B) health history information
    (C) chief complaint
    (D) DRG
    (E) medical information

185. Which of the following represents a change that ICD-10 makes to the structure of the coding format currently in use?

    (A) Codes will contain seven digits versus five.
    (B) Codes will no longer be in alphabetical order within a chapter.
    (C) There will be no reference to the anatomic site involved in a disease, condition, or injury.
    (D) All codes will contain only numbers.
    (E) E and V codes will continue to be used for special circumstances.

186. Which of the following is NOT a section of the CPT book?

    (A) Evaluation and management
    (B) Anesthesia
    (C) Pathology and lab
    (D) Surgery
    (E) Gynecology

187. Which of the following types of incoming mail should the medical assistant attend to first?

    (A) Priority mail
    (B) Registered mail
    (C) Insurance payment
    (D) Physician's personal mail
    (E) Airmail

188. Which of the following statements is NOT true about a typical purchasing procedure in a medical office?

    (A) An authorized person should be in charge of purchasing
    (B) Receipts of goods should be recorded
    (C) High-quality goods should be ordered at the lowest price
    (D) Shipments should be checked against packing slips
    (E) Every employee can order supplies and write a check from petty cash

189. Lack of payment is usually not considered serious until after

    (A) 120 days
    (B) 45 days
    (C) 60 days
    (D) 90 days
    (E) 30 days

190. Which of the following methods is used to correct an error in a patient's chart?

    (A) Cover the error with correction fluid
    (B) Try to write over the error
    (C) Draw a single line through the error and make the correction above the error
    (D) Use red ink to write the correction in the margin
    (E) Rewrite the process note

191. Which type of check is frequently used for payroll because it itemizes the purposes of the check and deductions?

    (A) Bank draft
    (B) Voucher check
    (C) Limited check
    (D) Certified check
    (E) Cashier's check

192. It will be most difficult to collect past due accounts from

    (A) those who just forgot their bill
    (B) someone who is unwilling to pay
    (C) a person having financial hardships
    (D) someone who has no insurance
    (E) everyone who owes money

193. Which of the following systems bills all accounts at the same time each month?

    (A) Past due
    (B) Account aging
    (C) Cycle billing
    (D) Wave scheduling
    (E) Monthly billing

194. The medical assistant should ensure the physician has room for which of the following each day?

    (A) Wave scheduling
    (B) Double booking
    (C) Open-hours scheduling
    (D) Emergency booking
    (E) Pharmaceutical booking

195. In which of the following locations should medical file drawers be labeled?

    (A) Inside the drawer
    (B) On the side of the drawer
    (C) In a separate listing in the tickler file
    (D) On the outside of the drawer
    (E) In the office database

196. The ICD-10 procedure codes are to be used exclusively in what setting?

    (A) The emergency room
    (B) Hospitals
    (C) Physician offices
    (D) Pharmacies
    (E) Psychiatric long-term care homes

197. Which of the following documents is the record of a professional meeting?

    (A) Minutes
    (B) Agenda
    (C) Bylaws
    (D) Itinerary
    (E) Resolution

198. Which of the following should NOT be included in a job description?

    (A) Supervisor's title
    (B) Job duties
    (C) Job specifications
    (D) Job summary
    (E) Address of office

199. A physical inventory of office equipment should be taken

    (A) every year
    (B) every two years
    (C) every three years
    (D) every five years
    (E) every ten years

200. Examining a document for damage before filing it is an example of which of the following filing steps?

    (A) Conditioning
    (B) Storing
    (C) Releasing
    (D) Sorting
    (E) Indexing

Part III—Clinical

DIRECTIONS (Questions 201–300): All of the following questions and incomplete statements are followed by five answer choices. For each question, select the single answer that best answers the question or completes the statement. Fill in the corresponding circle on your answer sheet.

201. Sterilization means that

    (A) all organisms have been removed from an object

    (B) all pathogenic organisms have been removed from an object

    (C) debris has been removed from and object with soap and water

    (D) the object has been placed in boiling water

    (E) the object has been subjected to ultrasonic cleaning

202. Which of the following actions should the medical assistant take to ensure disposable thermometers are ready for an exam?

    (A) Make sure they have been autoclaved within 28 days

    (B) Ensure the expiration dates have not passed

    (C) Swab the tips with alcohol

    (D) Place probe covers on them

    (E) Store them in a locked cabinet

203. What information will not be found in the medical record of a patient?

    (A) If the patient admits to any illegal drug use

    (B) Personal opinion of the medical staff

    (C) Legal history of the patient

    (D) Direct quotations from the patient

    (E) Medication history

204. Using a tape measure to evaluate the head and chest circumference of an infant is called

    (A) auscultation

    (B) mensuration

    (C) palpation

    (D) percussion

    (E) observation

205. What is the maximum time allotted for a collected blood sample to sit in a serum separator tube before being centrifuged?

    (A) 1 minute

    (B) 5 minutes

    (C) 15 minutes

    (D) 30 minutes

    (E) 60 minutes

206. A medical assistant is giving a DPT injection to a six-month-old infant. The assistant would give the injection at which of the following sites?

    (A) Upper outer quadrant of the gluteus muscle

    (B) Deltoid muscle

    (C) Vastus lateralis

    (D) Subcutaneous tissue of the thigh

    (E) Gluteus medius

207. If the physician is going to do a Pap smear, the medical assistant should have which the following equipment available?

    (A) Curette and dilator

    (B) Speculum and water soluble lubricant

    (C) Suture removal tray

    (D) Hemocult card

    (E) Sterile gloves and a light source

208. Emergency treatment for a second-degree burn would include

    (A) bandaging tightly

    (B) breaking any blisters seen

    (C) applying a clean, cool, wet cloth to the area

    (D) scrubbing the site with antiseptic soap

    (E) applying an emollient cream

209. Evaluation of the spinal column is accomplished easily from which of the following positions?

    (A) Knee-chest

    (B) Prone

    (C) Supine

    (D) Lithotomy

    (E) Trendelenburg

210. To respect the patient's privacy while obtaining information about her history, you should

    (A) ask the patient to fill out a form rather than asking the questions in an interview

    (B) ask the patient to specify people who can give information about her

    (C) take the patient to a quiet and private area to obtain the history

    (D) let the doctor ask any questions that you feel the patient may be sensitive about

    (E) inform the patient that she is not required to answer any questions that she does not want to

211. Which of the following terms is defined as the concentration at which a substance in the blood, not normally excreted by the kidney, begins to appear in the urine?

    (A) Supernatant

    (B) Refractive index

    (C) Renal threshold

    (D) Micturition

    (E) Aliquot

212. The patient is having occult blood in the stool caused by a medication that he is taking. Which of the following medications would you suspect?

    (A) Lisinopril

    (B) Coumadin

    (C) Prozac

    (D) Hydrocholothiazide

    (E) Ativan

213. A fomite is

    (A) an animal or insect that can transmit disease

    (B) a method of removing pathogens used on objects

    (C) an inanimate object that can harbor pathogens

    (D) a sexually transmitted disease

    (E) a method of sanitization used on objects that cannot be scrubbed

214. To correctly treat an adult with a foreign body airway obstruction, the medical assistant should first

    (A) open the patient's mouth and attempt to remove any foreign body that can be seen

    (B) lower the victim to the floor and start to perform abdominal thrusts

    (C) with the left hand, check the pulse at the left carotid artery

    (D) ask the patient if he can speak

    (E) place your hands around the victim from behind palms against abdomen and thrust upward

215. The Ishihara test is used to diagnose

    (A) myopia

    (B) hyperopia

    (C) presbyopia

    (D) color blindness

    (E) need for reading glasses

216. A nonsterile item is accidentally added to a sterile field being prepared for the suture of a skin laceration. Once the medical assistant discovers this, he should

    (A) report it to the physician

    (B) remove it at once

    (C) leave it on the sterile field but cover it with a sterile towel

    (D) replace the item with a similar sterile one

    (E) redo the sterile field and resterilize any instruments

217. The process used to wash and remove tissue from medical instruments is called

    (A) asepsis

    (B) disinfection

    (C) sanitization

    (D) sterilization

    (E) boiling

218. Which of the following is the maximum amount of time a tourniquet should remain on the patient's arm during the performance of a routine venipuncture?

    (A) 30 seconds

    (B) 60 seconds

    (C) 2 minutes

    (D) 3 minutes

    (E) 5 minutes

KAPLAN

219. In a large-scale national disaster or disease outbreak, which of the following considerations should be taken into account by a medical practice office?

    (A) Some patients will come to the office for care due to overcrowded emergency rooms.

    (B) The practice may need to administer vaccinations or immunizations to their patients.

    (C) Open lines of communication with local public health officials and participation in a coordinated plan.

    (D) None of the above

    (E) All of the above

220. Employment, use of tobacco and alcohol, and exercise habits are listed in which of the following sections of the patient's chart?

    (A) Social history

    (B) Chief complaint

    (C) Review of systems

    (D) Medical history

    (E) Family history

221. If your patient is being treated for a severe upper respiratory infection, which of the following medications would you NOT expect to see ordered?

    (A) Amoxicillin

    (B) Albuterol

    (C) Robitussin

    (D) Hydrochlorothiazide

    (E) Cipro

222. The microscope condenser is responsible for

    (A) collecting and concentrating light rays

    (B) holding and moving the slide

    (C) controlling the amount of light focused on an object

    (D) coarse and fine adjustment for object focus

    (E) evaporating water from the slide

223. You should suspect that a patient might possibly be having a heart attack if she is complaining of

    (A) blurred or double vision

    (B) severe headache

    (C) pain in the shoulder or jaw

    (D) difficulty understanding spoken words

    (E) weakness on one side of the body

224. When drawing multiple tubes of blood via venipuncture, what is the correct order of draw based on colored stoppers?

    (A) Lavender, red, green, yellow

    (B) Red, yellow, lavender, green

    (C) Green, yellow, lavender, red

    (D) Gray, yellow, red, blue

    (E) Yellow, red, lavender, green

225. Which of the following is a CLIA-waived (low complexity) test?

    (A) Microscopic examination of urine

    (B) Gram stain

    (C) Blood chemistry

    (D) Pregnancy test

    (E) Pap smear

226. Normal respiratory rate for an adult is

    (A) 8–12 breaths per minute

    (B) 8–16 breaths per minute

    (C) 12–20 breaths per minute

    (D) 12–26 breaths per minute

    (E) 20–26 breaths per minute

227. After drying and removing packs from the autoclave, the FIRST thing that you should do is

    (A) place the newly sterilized packs under the older ones in the storage area

    (B) discard all outdated packs

    (C) check the indicators to make sure it has changed color

    (D) mark packs with your initials and the date sterilized

    (E) seal in a plastic bag to ensure sterility

228. Which of the following medications would NOT be ordered for an elderly patient with cardiovascular disease?

    (A) Lanoxin

    (B) Lasix

    (C) Potassium chloride

    (D) Lisinopril

    (E) Prozac

229. To be prepared for an office emergency, the medical assistant should

(A) keep policies for emergencies nearby for reference

(B) ask a more experienced person in the office to handle any emergency

(C) review the office policies and be aware of location of emergency supplies

(D) call 911 immediately

(E) make a list of emergency phone numbers to place close to the telephone

230. Examples of a bandage include

(A) Steri-Strips

(B) Telfa

(C) Tubular gauze

(D) 4 × 4 gauze

(E) Clear IV site

231. Which one of the following tests is used to determine the best antibiotic to treat a condition?

(A) Blood agar

(B) Culturing

(C) Morphology

(D) Liquid culture medium

(E) Sensitivity

232. A "blind" weight is done on a patient by

(A) not writing the weight in the patient's chart

(B) asking the patient to weigh himself at home and report it when he comes to the office

(C) weighing the patient in the wheelchair and then subtracting the weight of the chair

(D) shielding the readout so the patient is not aware of what the reading is

(E) taking the weight at the appointment

233. An effective way to handle patient emergencies in a medical practice office is to take which of the following steps in advance?

(A) Ask very sick patients to go to the hospital emergency room.

(B) Identify the at-risk situations that are most likely to occur, given the patient population seen in the office, and prepare to provide care for these situations.

(C) Make sure that a doctor is consistently available.

(D) Have a first aid kit in the office.

(E) Post the phone number for poison control.

234. In the event of a large-scale act of bioterrorism, which of the following steps would NOT be an approach to be used by a medical office practice?

(A) coordination and communication with local public health officials

(B) providing vaccines and/or immunizations

(C) knowing the signs and symptoms related to a disease outbreak

(D) sending patients to the emergency room for diagnosis

(E) practicing proper infection control and waste disposal of contaminated material

235. Snellen testing results give information about

(A) Blood sugar results

(B) Visual acuity

(C) Ability to hear vibratory sound

(D) Blood pressure

(E) Colorblindness

236. Which of the following emergency situations should receive the first priority?

(A) Bleeding from a laceration of the forearm

(B) Occluded airway

(C) Open fracture of the femur

(D) Mid-sternal chest pain

(E) Grand mal seizure

237. The medical assistant's role in obtaining informed consent is

(A) explaining the benefits and risks of the procedure

(B) making sure that the patient understands and has no questions

(C) answering all questions that the patient has about the procedure

(D) witnessing the signature of the patient

(E) explaining alternative treatments to the patient

238. To remove sutures, the medical assistant should have a tray with instruments that should include

(A) Kelly hemostat

(B) Mayo scissors

(C) Senn retractor

(D) Littauer scissors

(E) bandage scissors

239. When there is an unidentified clear liquid on the floor of the exam room after a patient has left the room, the medical assistant should

    (A) go and ask the patient if they are aware of what the liquid is

    (B) clean up the spill with a disposable paper towel and place in the biohazard garbage

    (C) put up a wet floor sign and ask a housekeeper to clean up the area

    (D) put on disposable gloves and clean up with a paper towel and put in the biohazard garbage

    (E) put on sterile gloves and clean up the spill with disposable paper towels

240. A viral infection

    (A) cannot be transmitted by droplets

    (B) will always resolve in 7 to 10 days

    (C) does not respond to antibiotic treatment

    (D) causes tuberculosis

    (E) can always be prevented by vaccination

241. Factors that affect the action of drugs include all EXCEPT

    (A) body weight

    (B) use of generic medication

    (C) sex

    (D) age

    (E) disease processes

242. When checking supplies in the office, the medical assistant notices that the hemostats in the cupboard were autoclaved 28 days ago. He would

    (A) check to see if the packages are intact and without damage

    (B) count to see if there are enough available for the amount of expected procedures

    (C) place the packages back in the autoclave and run the appropriate cycle to re-sterilize using the autoclave

    (D) unwrap and repackage items and run through the appropriate cycle to sterilize using the autoclave

    (E) re-date the packages for an additional 28 days

243. Symptoms of insulin shock include

    (A) fruity or acetone smell to the breath and a decreased blood sugar reading

    (B) tremulousness and an elevated blood sugar reading

    (C) diaphoresis and a fruity smell to the breath with an increased blood sugar reading

    (D) confusion, tachycardia, and an elevated blood sugar reading

    (E) diaphoresis, tremulousness, confusion, and decreased blood sugar reading

244. Which of the following steps helps ensure smooth operation in the medical office during a patient emergency?

    (A) adhering to a pre-established plan and protocols for managing the emergency

    (B) avoiding setting up appointments for seriously ill patients

    (C) arranging for close proximity to the local emergency room

    (D) clearing the office out during a patient emergency

    (E) having an AED device on hand

245. Prior to administration of a local anesthesia, the medical assistant should

    (A) administer a test dose to make sure the patient does not have an allergic reaction

    (B) ask the patient what local anesthesia they have had in the past and use the same medication

    (C) carefully take an allergy history from the patient prior to the procedure

    (D) make sure that the patient has brought someone along to drive them home after the procedure

    (E) look in the patient's chart to see if the patient has had a minor surgery procedure done prior

246. The knee-chest position is used for

    (A) procotological exams

    (B) vaginal exams

    (C) exam of the chest and upper torso

    (D) patients who have difficulty breathing

    (E) for treatment of hypotension

247. Which of the following positions should the patient be in for a vaginal exam?

    (A) Prone

    (B) Lithotomy

    (C) Sims's

    (D) Fowler's

    (E) Semi-Fowler's

248. The FIRST thing a medical assistant should do when she comes across an adult who is not breathing is

    (A) give two rescue breaths and then start chest compressions

    (B) roll the person onto the left side, keeping the neck and body in alignment

    (C) check for a carotid pulse on the side closest to the assistant

    (D) look into the mouth to see if there is an object obstructing the airway

    (E) reposition the airway and check again for spontaneous respirations

249. When checking the sterile supplies in the office, the medical assistant should

    (A) unwrap and resterilize any sterile packs that are older than 21 days

    (B) examine sterile packs and discard any that are damaged

    (C) arrange sterile packs so that the ones that will expire last are used first

    (D) seal sterile packs that are expired in plastic in order to extend the time they may be used

    (E) discard sterile packs that have been taken into patient rooms but not used

250. Sterile technique must be used when

    (A) placing sutures in a new laceration

    (B) removing sutures from a healed laceration

    (C) performing a Pap smear

    (D) performing a rectal exam in order to do a hemoccult

    (E) cleaning the skin prior to placement of sutures

251. Which of the following measures is a normal specific gravity of urine?

    (A) 1.000

    (B) 1.025

    (C) 1.050

    (D) 1.125

    (E) 1.275

252. Which of the following is a disposable glass or plastic tube used for hematocrit determination?

    (A) Microcollection tube

    (B) Capillary tube

    (C) Reagent tube

    (D) Serum separator tube

    (E) Evacuated glass tube

253. Which of the following medications would most likely NOT be ordered for a 52-year-old postmenopausal woman?

    (A) Premarin

    (B) Provera

    (C) Aricept

    (D) Calcium citrate

    (E) Multivitamin

254. The ratio for making a disinfectant from bleach and water is

    (A) 1:5

    (B) 1:10

    (C) 1:20

    (D) 10:1

    (E) 1:100

255. To screen for hearing acuity or bone conduction of sound, the medical assistant would use a/an

    (A) otoscope

    (B) ophthalmoscope

    (C) tuning fork

    (D) Snellen test

    (E) reflex hammer

256. Which of the following is NOT considered proper patient instruction for obtaining a clean-catch mid-stream urine specimen?

    (A) Have the patient remove undergarments.

    (B) Make sure not to touch the inside of the container.

    (C) Continue to hold the labia apart and void a small amount into the toilet.

    (D) Clean the urinary meatus from back to front.

    (E) The specimen container should not touch any part of the body.

257. If a medical assistant discovers a known diabetic patient who is disoriented and confused, the first thing she should do is

    (A) check the vital signs

    (B) give a form of glucose to the patient

    (C) draw a blood glucose or accucheck

    (D) check for spontaneous respirations

    (E) ask him what symptoms he is having

258. A procedure that a medical assistant would not expect to take part in when doing minor surgeries in the office is

    (A) suture of lacerations

    (B) biopsy of the lung

    (C) cyst removal

    (D) biopsy of a skin lesion

    (E) incision and drainage of a wound

259. Heart sounds that are heard when the blood pressure is being measured are called the

    (A) Korotkoff sounds

    (B) Rinne sounds

    (C) Snellen sounds

    (D) Isharhar sounds

    (E) Jeager sounds

260. The popliteal pulse is located

    (A) on the thumb side of the wrist

    (B) behind the knee

    (C) on the dorsal surface of the foot

    (D) at the apex of the heart

    (E) at the inner aspect of the leg in the groin

261. The most important thing to do to prevent transfer of infectious material is

    (A) use biohazard bags

    (B) dispose of sharps in a rigid container

    (C) wash your hands

    (D) disinfect patient care equipment between uses

    (E) wear gloves when exposed to body fluids

262. Which of the following types of urine specimen contains the greatest concentration of dissolved substances?

    (A) Random

    (B) First-voided morning

    (C) Clean-catch midstream

    (D) 24-hour

    (E) Second-voided

263. When moving a heavy object one should

    (A) bend from the waist to lift the object

    (B) ask for help if you try to lift the object but feel it is too heavy

    (C) make sure that the object is at least 5 inches away from the body

    (D) assess the object prior to trying to lift it and ask for help if needed

    (E) lift heavy objects only if they are stored at waist level or higher

264. When removing paper that is soiled with biohazardous waste from the exam table, the medical assistant should do which of the following before cleaning the table with disinfectant and pulling down unused paper?

    (A) Use sterile gloves.

    (B) Roll the paper inward and toward the body working from the end of the exam table.

    (C) Gather the soiled paper in gloved hands and discard.

    (D) Using unsterile gloves, roll the paper down toward the body and discard.

    (E) Roll the paper inward and away from the body, discard, and change gloves.

265. In an infant, you should check the pulse in which of the following arteries in an emergency situation?

    (A) Carotid

    (B) Radial

    (C) Brachial

    (D) Femoral

    (E) Temporal

266. The generic name for Lipitor is

    (A) atenolol

    (B) altorvastatin calcium

    (C) clopidogrel bisulfate

    (D) furosemide

    (E) amlodipine

267. After a patient has had a grand mal seizure, one would expect the patient to be

    (A) confused and drowsy

    (B) excited and hyperactive

    (C) hypotensive with a decreased pulse

    (D) in need of airway management

    (E) needing immediate transport to the hospital

268. The most appropriate position for a patient with respiratory problems is

    (A) Trendelenburg

    (B) Fowler's

    (C) lithotomy

    (D) dorsal recumbent

    (E) prone

269. Which of the following is NOT a normal vein for phlebotomy?

    (A) Cubital vein

    (B) Brachial vein

    (C) Hepatic vein

    (D) Cephalic vein

    (E) Basilic vein

270. Which of the following situations would be of least concern when involved in a sterile procedure?

    (A) Talking over the sterile field

    (B) A member of the sterile team having his or her hair loose

    (C) A nonsterile person entering the room

    (D) Adding nonsterile items to the sterile field

    (E) A tear in the glove of a member of the sterile team

271. Draping is done primarily for

    (A) convenience of the doctor

    (B) keeping the patient warm

    (C) patient privacy

    (D) convenience of the medical assistant

    (E) facilitating the specific exam

272. To take the blood pressure correctly, the medical assistant should

    (A) use any blood pressure cuff that is available as long as it fits the patient's arm

    (B) have the arm at or near the level of the heart

    (C) pump up the cuff until she is unable to hear the pulse anymore

    (D) release the air from the cuff rapidly in order to decrease patient discomfort

    (E) position the cuff so that the artery marker is at the level of the elbow

273. A person who has difficulty breathing and experiences swelling of the respiratory tract following a bee sting may have

    (A) a myocardial infarction

    (B) anaphylactic shock

    (C) obstructive airway disease

    (D) cardiogenic shock

    (E) an asthma attack

274. Which of the following is NOT a true statement regarding tuberculin testing?

    (A) A small amount of tubercle bacillus is administered intradermally.
    (B) The results are read in 48–72 hours.
    (C) Induration is a positive indicator of disease.
    (D) A person who has been vaccinated with BCG will test positive.
    (E) Follow-up testing for a positive test includes chest x-ray.

275. Which one of the following is NOT a proper procedure for performing the Multistix 10 reagent strip test?

    (A) Immediately recap the testing strip bottle.
    (B) Do not touch the strip with your fingers.
    (C) Hold the strip in a vertical position.
    (D) Completely immerse the strip in the specimen.
    (E) Discolored strips should be discarded.

276. Major depression is most commonly treated with

    (A) Xanax
    (B) Ativan
    (C) Zoloft
    (D) Buspar
    (E) Serax

277. Which of the following instruments would NOT be needed when preparing for a cyst removal?

    (A) Scalpel
    (B) Needle holder
    (C) Senn retractor
    (D) Dressing forceps
    (E) Speculum

278. To encourage an elderly patient to give information while taking the patient history, the medical assistant should

    (A) ask questions that can be answered with "yes" or "no" answers
    (B) interview a family member instead of the patient
    (C) speak loudly because the patient is likely to be hard of hearing
    (D) inform the patient in the beginning that there is only a short time to perform this history
    (E) ask open-ended questions

279. Urine or serum pregnancy tests are utilized to detect the presence of which of the following?

    (A) Antidiuretic hormone (ADH)
    (B) Human growth hormone (hGH)
    (C) Heterphile antibody
    (D) Human chorionic gonadotropin hormone (hCG)
    (E) Phenylketonuria

280. The correct position to place a patient who has fainted is

    (A) prone
    (B) Trendelenburg
    (C) lithotomy
    (D) supine
    (E) Fowler's

281. If a medical assistant is giving a 75-pound child a dose of antibiotic using Clark's Law, which of the following would she administer if the usual adult dose is 500 mg?

    (A) 500 mg
    (B) 250 mg
    (C) 200 mg
    (D) 125 mg
    (E) 375 mg

282. When performing an EKG on a patient, if the tracing on the paper is not what is expected, the FIRST thing that should be checked is

    (A) placement of the electrodes
    (B) the status of the patient
    (C) electrical interference
    (D) machine settings
    (E) patient movement

283. When performing a surgical hand scrub, make sure to

    (A) wash for 60 seconds
    (B) hold fingers lower than the wrists
    (C) dry hands with paper toweling
    (D) hold fingers higher than the elbows
    (E) dry hands before turning off the water faucet

284. Lyme disease, if untreated, can progress into a/an

    (A) viral infection

    (B) contagious disease

    (C) chronic infection

    (D) acute infection

    (E) nonpathogenic condition

285. Initial treatment for a sprained ankle would include

    (A) application of a heating pad in 20-minute intervals for the first 48 hours

    (B) exercise the ankle in order to prevent stiffness

    (C) application of ice in 20-minute intervals for the first 48 hours

    (D) massage the ankle with pain relief ointment as needed

    (E) application of an air cast to the lower extremity

286. Which of the following reagent strip panels would show an abnormal finding if a person is suffering from a bacterial urinary tract infection?

    (A) (+) glucose

    (B) (+) nitrites

    (C) (+) ketones

    (D) (+) bilirubin

    (E) (+) protein

287. To palpate the pulse in an adult, the usual procedure would be to

    (A) listen with a stethoscope at the apex of the heart

    (B) feel at the inner aspect of the thumb side of the wrist with the first two fingers

    (C) use the thumb of the dominant hand to feel the temple area of the skull

    (D) locate it between the larynx and the sternocleido-mastoid muscle in the side of the neck

    (E) press deeply below the inguinal ligament in the groin

288. In order to have a method of checking to see if an autoclaved item is sterile, the medical assistant should

    (A) place indicator strips in the packs and envelopes and use autoclave tape to secure the packs

    (B) set the timer on the autoclave to run for 30 minutes to make sure that the items are sterilized

    (C) open one pack and check the indicator strip for sterilization after each autoclave batch is run

    (D) leave an open flap in the packs to view the indicator strip to make sure that it is sterile

    (E) open the autoclave prior to the drying cycle in order to make sure that the indicators and tape have indicated that the item is sterile

289. In which of the following radiographic positions is the patient lying on his back?

    (A) Prone

    (B) Supine

    (C) Oblique

    (D) Lateral

    (E) Posteroanterior

290. Which of the following values is considered a desirable cholesterol level?

    (A) 0 mg/dl

    (B) 180 mg/dl

    (C) 230 mg/dl

    (D) 250 mg/dl

    (E) 300 mg/dl

291. Using sterile instruments to perform a breast biopsy is an example of

    (A) surgical asepsis

    (B) sterilization

    (C) medical asepsis

    (D) personal protective equipment

    (E) sanitization

292. Wearing a mask, gown, and gloves when working with a patient is an example of using

    (A) barrier method
    (B) standard procedure
    (C) personal protective equipment
    (D) body substance isolation
    (E) surgical asepsis

293. Applying an elastic or ACE wrap to a sprained ankle is an example of

    (A) bandaging
    (B) applying a dressing
    (C) splinting
    (D) casting
    (E) treating a wound

294. Which one of the following is the correct angle for a needle to enter the vein for venipuncture?

    (A) 5 degrees
    (B) 15 degrees
    (C) 30 degrees
    (D) 45 degrees
    (E) 90 degrees

295. Which of the following is a Gram-positive cocci that grows in clusters?

    (A) *Staphylococcus aureus*
    (B) *Neisseria meningitidis*
    (C) *Mycobacterium tuberculosis*
    (D) *Escherichia coli*
    (E) *Streptococcus pneumoniae*

296. A scraping of the superficial layer of skin is called a/an

    (A) abrasion
    (B) avulsion
    (C) laceration
    (D) incision
    (E) contusion

297. When preparing the skin for a minor surgical procedure, the medical assistant should

    (A) wash the skin with antiseptic soap in an up and down motion and using friction
    (B) wash the skin with antiseptic soap from the inner area to the outer in a circular motion
    (C) wash the skin with alcohol and air dry
    (D) wash the skin with antiseptic soap after applying sterile gloves and gown
    (E) wash the skin with a disinfectant solution from the inner area to the outer in a circular motion

298. Which one of the following diseases is confirmed by a positive VDRL and RPR?

    (A) Hepatitis
    (B) Mononucleosis
    (C) Syphilis
    (D) Rheumatoid arthritis
    (E) Systemic lupus erythematosus

299. If the medical assistant notices a small tear in her sterile glove during a procedure, she should

    (A) put a piece of sterile tape over the hole in the glove
    (B) alert the physician that she is not able to assist any longer
    (C) ask a coworker to put on sterile gloves and take over for her
    (D) continue the procedure but do not pick up sterile objects with that hand
    (E) step away from the procedure and replace her gloves with new ones

300. Which of the following statements is TRUE?

    (A) A spirometer is used to measure the relative humidity of exhaled air.
    (B) The specific gravity of urine is part of the microscopic examination of urine.
    (C) The erythrocyte sedimentation rate is a means of identifying how fast blood clots.
    (D) Hematocrit is expressed in mm/sec.
    (E) Hemoglobin measures the oxygen-carrying capacity of blood and is expressed in g/dl.

ANSWER KEY

I. General

1.	D	26.	D	51.	D	76.	B
2.	C	27.	C	52.	C	77.	B
3.	B	28.	D	53.	A	78.	A
4.	C	29.	D	54.	D	79.	B
5.	A	30.	C	55.	D	80.	C
6.	B	31.	A	56.	C	81.	B
7.	C	32.	C	57.	A	82.	A
8.	D	33.	B	58.	C	83.	D
9.	D	34.	C	59.	E	84.	D
10.	C	35.	C	60.	D	85.	D
11.	D	36.	C	61.	E	86.	A
12.	C	37.	C	62.	C	87.	D
13.	E	38.	C	63.	D	88.	A
14.	C	39.	C	64.	C	89.	D
15.	E	40.	D	65.	C	90.	B
16.	E	41.	C	66.	A	91.	C
17.	E	42.	B	67.	B	92.	B
18.	E	43.	D	68.	E	93.	E
19.	E	44.	B	69.	B	94.	D
20.	C	45.	A	70.	E	95.	C
21.	D	46.	B	71.	E	96.	D
22.	B	47.	C	72.	D	97.	B
23.	D	48.	D	73.	A	98.	E
24.	A	49.	B	74.	C	99.	E
25.	B	50.	B	75.	A	100.	C

II. Administrative

101. E
102. C
103. D
104. A
105. A
106. B
107. C
108. C
109. B
110. C
111. C
112. C
113. A
114. C
115. B
116. E
117. A
118. D
119. D
120. D
121. D
122. A
123. E
124. A
125. B
126. A
127. C
128. B
129. B
130. C
131. B
132. A
133. A
134. D
135. A
136. A
137. D
138. B
139. D
140. D
141. E
142. C
143. B
144. E
145. A
146. A
147. E
148. D
149. D

150. C
151. C
152. C
153. B
154. C
155. A
156. B
157. A
158. E
159. A
160. A
161. A
162. A
163. E
164. B
165. D
166. A
167. C
168. C
169. C
170. C
171. A
172. E
173. C
174. C
175. D
176. D
177. B
178. D
179. B
180. E
181. B
182. B
183. C
184. E
185. A
186. E
187. B
188. E
189. D
190. C
191. B
192. B
193. E
194. D
195. D
196. B
197. A
198. E
199. A
200. A

III. Clinical

201. A
202. B
203. B
204. B
205. D
206. C
207. B
208. C
209. B
210. C
211. C
212. B
213. C
214. D
215. D
216. E
217. C
218. B
219. E
220. A
221. D
222. A
223. C
224. E
225. D
226. C
227. C
228. E
229. C
230. C
231. E
232. D
233. B
234. D
235. B
236. B
237. B
238. D
239. D
240. C
241. B
242. D
243. E
244. A
245. C
246. A
247. B
248. E
249. B

250. A
251. B
252. B
253. C
254. B
255. C
256. D
257. B
258. B
259. A
260. B
261. C
262. B
263. D
264. E
265. C
266. B
267. A
268. B
269. C
270. C
271. C
272. B
273. B
274. C
275. C
276. C
277. E
278. E
279. D
280. B
281. B
282. B
283. D
284. C
285. C
286. B
287. B
288. A
289. B
290. B
291. A
292. C
293. A
294. B
295. A
296. A
297. B
298. C
299. E
300. E

ANSWERS AND EXPLANATIONS

Part I—General

1. D

Hepat/o means liver. Stomach (A) is *gastr/o*, intestine (B) is *enter/o*, pancreas (C) is *pancreat/o*, gallbladder (E) is *cholecyst/o*.

2. C

Defense mechanisms assist us with circumstances that are difficult for the mind to cope with. Grief (A) is a process that people experience during a time of loss. The unconscious mind (B) is the term Freud used to describe repressed thoughts and feelings. Freud defined the ego (D) as the conscious mind containing our thoughts and feelings. Maslow defined self-actualization (E) as the attainment of the peak of one's capabilities in life.

3. B

The optic nerve carries visual stimulation to the brain. The vestibular cochlear nerve deals with hearing (A). The olfactory nerve carries stimulation for smell to the brain (C). The nerve pathway for taste (D) is the lingual nerve. Touch (E) is carried by pressure receptors in the skin.

4. C

Medical assistants are expected to comply with rules and regulations that protect individual health information. Unless your coworker has a legitimate reason in the course of care or treatment, the patient record is off limits, and you need to make sure the information remains confidential and secure in your office setting. None of the other actions supports your obligation in regard to patient privacy.

5. A

The DASH diet lowers blood pressure significantly. The BRAT diet is for diarrhea (B). The bland diet is used with digestive disorders (C). Antioxidant diets help prevent cancer (E). High protein diets assist with muscle strength (D).

6. B

A deposition is sworn testimony given outside of the courtroom. A subpoena (A) is a legal directive to come to court to testify. Standard of care (C) refers to the expectation that a level of care will be given that is equal to what a reasonable, prudent person with the same training would offer. Evidence (D) is proof submitted supporting a plaintiff. A verdict (E) is the final decision.

7. C

Intent has nothing to do with malpractice or negligence. Negligence occurs when a heath care provider has a *duty* toward a patient, is *derelict* in performing that duty and *damages* occur *directly* because of it. When all four D's are present, negligence exists.

8. D

The ability to recognize and categorize objects by size and weight is part of the period of concrete operations. Children ages 7 to 11 are normally in this stage of cognitive development. Self-actualization (E) is not one of Piaget's stages.

9. D

Poly- means many. *Semi-* (A) means half, *macro-* (B) means large, *pseudo-* (C) means false, and *dia-* (E) means through.

10. C

Begin by dividing the word into word parts: *myel/o/mening/o/cele. Cele* means herniation. *Myel/o* means bone marrow or spinal cord. *Mening/o* means meninges or covering on the brain and spinal cord. When we look over the options, we want one close to "herniation of the spinal cord and meninges."

11. D

Potassium is the correct answer. Calcium (A) is found in dairy products, sardines, and canned salmon. Vitamin C (B) and vitamin K (C) are vitamins, not minerals. Iron (E) is found in red meats, dried fruit, and organ meat.

12. C

There are four types of body tissue: epithelial, connective, nervous, and muscular.

13. **E**

All of the following are true except (E). A patient owns the information in the chart and may request to have it disclosed and the physician cannot refuse (A). Having a power of attorney for health care gives all the powers normally given to a patient to the designee (B). Any member of the health care team can release information without permission if another person is in imminent, life-threatening danger (D). For example, the patient who storms out of the office brandishing a knife saying that he is going to kill his girlfriend. The last answer is incorrect because the mentally ill do not lose any rights and even if a person is not in touch with reality; they are entitled to confidentiality unless the guardian or power of attorney signs a release of information.

14. **C**

This patient is experiencing the anger stage of grieving. Kübler-Ross pointed out in her study of terminally ill patients that anger is often displaced on health professionals and that the anger should not be taken personally. In this response, you are supporting the patient's feelings and acknowledging his issue. None of the other responses would be appropriate to this patient's remark.

15. **E**

There is electrical interference from within the room. This type of interference results from any extraneous electrical source, such as lights or computers, and also from excessive current running through the walls. There will be even, sharp peaks on the tracing. When electrodes are too tight (A) or not attached completely (C), the result is a wandering baseline, in which the tracing does not continue in a straight line across the graph paper. Incorrect placement of the electrodes (B) produces artifacts in the tracing that can mimic serious conditions such as ischemia or gross arrhythmia. If the patient moves in any way (D), interference referred to as "somatic tremors" occurs, and uneven, rounded peaks will appear on the tracing.

16. **E**

Orrhaphy means sewing or stitching. Phlebo means vein. Venostenosis (A) means narrowing of veins. Phlebosclerosis (B) means hardening of veins. Vasoplasty (C) means surgical repair of vessel. Venopexy (D) means surgical repair of veins.

17. **E**

Threatening him with calling security should be your last and least preferred strategy for managing the patient's anger. It is reasonable to attempt to defuse Mr. Hall's anger and offer him empathy (C) and a sincere apology (A) even when you are not responsible for the delay. By lowering your own voice (B), he is likely to follow your lead and lower his. In some instances, service recovery with an unhappy patient can occur if you offer a small and tangible token of apology for a problem or delay in service (D).

18. **E**

Vitamin K is the clotting vitamin. Vitamin A (A) is used for skin and night vision. Vitamin B_6 (B) and B_{12} (C) have a role in the nervous system. Vitamin C (D) assists with immunity.

19. **E**

The mighty mitochondria is responsible for the production of energy in the cell. The Golgi body (B) transports mucous. The endoplasmic reticulum (C) transports ribosomes. The nucleus (D) is the "command center" and responsible for DNA production in the cell. Lysosomes (A) are the waste-removing organelles in the cell.

20. **C**

Onc is a word root that means tumor. *Onc/o* (A) is incorrect because it is a combining form. Because it is a suffix, *-oma* (B) is incorrect. Carcin (E) and *carcin/o* (D) deal with cancer.

21. **D**

Sigmund Freud's psychoanalytic theories held that people experienced problems because of repressed memories and thoughts from childhood. Kübler-Ross (A) is associated with the grieving process. Maslow (E) developed the hierarchy of needs, and Piaget (B) and Erickson (C) are developmental theorists.

22. **B**

    Defendants are not held liable for damages when contributory risk is the defense because the patient was in part responsible for the injury. In assumed risk (A), the patient willingly accepts the risk. In comparative risk (C), both the plaintiff and defendant are assigned a portion of the responsibility for the injury. A technical defense (D) is based on a point of law being violated. An intervening cause (E) is an extraneous variable that came into existence altering the course of events.

23. **D**

    Start by looking for a suffix meaning infestation of stones: lithiasis. Either choice (C) or choice (D) will be correct. *Chole* means gall and *lithiasis* means infestation of stones. Together they mean infestation of gallstones making (D) the correct choice. Cholecystolithiasis (C) means infestation of gallbladder stones which is close but not the best answer. Cholecystitis (A) means inflammation of the gallbladder. Cholecystosis (B) means a condition of the gall bladder. Cholecystectomy is a surgical removal of the gallbladder.

24. **A**

    By rewarding the child for losing weight, the medical assistant is reinforcing the behavior of weight loss.

25. **B**

    Vitamin C is the only water-soluble vitamin listed. Excess is excreted from the body in the urine. Vitamins A, D, K, and E are fat-soluble and can build up to a toxin level in the body.

26. **D**

    A comparative defense assigns portions of the responsibility for damages to both plaintiff and defendant. A technical defense (A) is based on errors in the legal system. Denial (B) is not an affirmative defense. Contributory defense (C) means a defendant cannot be found guilty of negligence if the patient is in any part responsible. Assumed risk (E) is when the patient willingly takes on a risk.

27. **C**

    The senses are part of the nervous system because they pick up information and deliver it to the brain for a response.

28. **D**

    The stage described in this question is the sensorimotor stage. In this stage, from birth until about age two, children learn what they take in from hearing, touching, smelling, and seeing. They have limited motor skills.

29. **D**

    The patella is the kneecap of the leg.

30. **C**

    ARDS is the abbreviation for adult respiratory distress syndrome. SOB is an abbreviation for shortness of breath. COPD is chronic obstructive pulmonary disease. These are all respiratory diseases and should be handled by a physician who specializes in respiratory disease, a pulmonologist. A nephrologist (A) is a physician who specializes in kidney disease. A gastroenterologist (B) treats gastrointestinal diseases. A cardiologist (D) treats the heart and cardiac diseases. A hospitalist (E) sees persons who are inpatients in the hospital.

31. **A**

    The Uniform Anatomical Gift Act allows those over 18 years of age to make decisions about disposal of their body or body parts for medical education, research, or transplantation. A living will (B) authorizes the continuation or withdrawal of life support if the person is too sick to voice an opinion. A power of attorney for health care (C) is the designation of another person to serve as agent in making all decisions, including surgical or life-threatening decisions, when the patient is unable to voice an opinion. ERISA (D) is a federal act designed to protect retirement fund and pensions. *Res ipsa loquitor* (E) is a circumstance where the responsibility for a situation is grossly obvious.

32. **C**

    In the word hematuria, *-uria* is the suffix meaning condition of urine. The prefix *hemat-* means blood. Uremia (B) is not correct. Remember, you begin translating at the back of the word. Uremia is a condition of the blood.

33. **B**

    Sudoriferous glands produce perspiration. Ceruminous glands (A) produce earwax. Parathyroid glands (C) are endocrine glands imbedded in the thyroid gland. Sebaceous glands (D) produce sebum to moisturize the skin and scalp. Adrenal glands (E) produce glucocorticosteroids that involve immunity.

KAPLAN

34. C

Thrombocytes are called platelets. They are the initial patch to prevent blood loss when a vessel is injured. Erythrocytes (A) carry oxygen and nutrients. Leukocytes (B) fight invaders/infection. Neutrophils (D) and eosinophils (E) are specific types of white blood cells.

35. C

Showing photos of a surgery without patient consent is an intentional tort. Intentional torts include assault, battery, slander, libel, invasion of privacy, fraud, and false imprisonment. Showing photos without permission (C) is invasion of privacy. Giving the wrong medication (A) is misfeasance, improperly cleaning a surgical site (B) is misfeasance, not drawing an ordered lab (D) is nonfeasance and suturing a laceration (E) is malfeasance. These are all unintentional torts.

36. C

Meta- (C) means beyond. *Mal-* (A) means bad, *ambi-* (B) means both, *retro-* (D) means behind, and *multi-* (E) means many.

37. C

Subpoena duces tecum means "come and bring records." *Respondeat superior* (A) involves the responsibility of the employer for the employee's actions. *Res ipsa loquitur* (B) translates literally to mean "the thing speaks for itself." It is used when an error is grossly obvious and blame is directed at one person. *Res judicata* (D) means "a matter decided by judgment." *Caveat emptor* (E) means "buyer beware" and has nothing to do with law.

38. C

Food, water, oxygen, and shelter are fundamental needs that must be met before this mother can attend to the safety and security needs of her child. The other stages are all higher-ranking items on Maslow's Hierarchy of Needs. The mother would be more likely to attend to the instruction if she had food available.

39. C

Most pathogenic organisms are aerobic, meaning that they require oxygen to survive. An example of an aerobe is Streptococcus, which causes strep throat. Pathogens that are able to thrive with minimal or no oxygen are anaerobes (D); one example is tetanus. Microorganisms (A) are microscopic living creatures and can be pathogenic or nonpathogenic, aerobic or anaerobic. Spores (B) are encapsulated, inactive bacteria that are difficult to destroy. Protists (E) are a varied group of mostly single-celled microorganisms; some are pathogenic (such as Plasmodium falciparum, which causes malaria) and others are nonpathogenic (such as algae).

40. D

The suffix *-ity* means condition.

41. C

The physician can terminate care of a patient if the patient is noncompliant with treatment (B), misses appointments (D), does not pay her bills (A), or sees another physician (E). However, abusive language (C) is insufficient cause to break a contract.

42. B

Prefixes come at the beginning of a word. That eliminates *-para* (C) and *-oma* (D). *Meta* (E) means beyond, *peri-* (A) means around and *para-* (B) means near.

43. D

A bone broken into pieces is a comminuted fracture. A compound (A) or open (E) fracture has broken the skin. A pathological fracture (B) is the secondary result of another disease. An impacted fracture (C) is the jamming of one bone into another.

44. B

Dark green, orange, and yellow vegetables are high in antioxidants. Liver and organ meats (A) are high in iron. Citrus fruit (C) is high in vitamin C. Root vegetables (D) have no special significance. Dairy products (E) are rich in vitamin D and calcium.

45. A

A transverse plane cuts through the body parallel to the horizon. A sagittal cut (B) goes through the midline. A frontal (C) or coronal (D) plane divides the body into a front and back half. The midsagittal (E) plane divides the body into right and left halves.

46. B

IBS is the abbreviation for irritable bowel syndrome. PUD is the abbreviation for peptic ulcer disease. Pyloric stenosis involves the stomach and small intestine. These diseases would be treated by a physician who specializes in the stomach and intestine and disease of the gastrointestinal tract: a gastroenterologist.

47. C

Digestion begins in the mouth with the breakdown of carbohydrates by amylase.

48. D

Torts are crimes against another person or property. Misdemeanors (B) are crimes against the state punishable by incarceration in jail for less than a year. Felonies (A) are serious crimes, such as burglary, that are punished by incarceration in prison for more than a year. Treason (C) is a crime against the state and negligence (E) occurs when a professional is derelict in performing a duty and damages occur directly because of it.

49. B

Hemorrhoid is spelled correctly.

50. B

The pancreas is a digestive organ and is located in the abdominal cavity. The thoracic cavity (A) holds the lungs and heart. The pelvic cavity (C) holds the organs of reproduction and some of the organs related to the urinary system. The spinal cavity (D) contains the spinal cord and the cranial cavity (E) contains the cranium.

51. D

Minors cannot make their own health care decisions unless it involves reproductive care, substance abuse, or psychiatric treatment. The only exceptions are when the minor is emancipated by marriage, is self-supporting, or is enlisted in the military. Elderly persons who have not been designated as incompetent or have no guardian may make their own medical choices despite confusion.

52. C

PO (from the Latin *per os*), meaning "by mouth," is not a parenteral route of medication administration. Parenteral refers to the introduction of a substance into the body via a route other than the alimentary canal (digestive tract). Intravenous, or IV, administration (A) is infusion into the vein; IM, or intramuscular (B), is injection into the muscle; subQ, or subcutaneous (D), is injection under the skin; intradermal (E) is injection just under the epidermis, or outer layer of skin.

53. A

Menstruation is the correct spelling. None of the other answer choices is misspelled.

54. D

A banana is low in sodium. High-sodium foods are processed items like packaged cheese and salty items like chips, pretzels, and snack foods. Pickled and smoked items like ham are high in sodium.

55. D

The SA node is the pacemaker of the heart. The impulse travels to the AV node (B) where it slows. It separates at the bundle of His (A) and travels down the left or right bundle branches (C). The impulse travels to the purkinje fibers (E) that are imbedded in the walls of the atria, causing them to contract.

56. C

The medical chart has four purposes. It is a research tool, a communication tool among health team members, legal record, and record of personal health.

57. A

The length of time after an event in which a person can file a lawsuit is called statute of limitations. Doctrine of informed consent (B) means making certain the patient is aware of all details about any procedure, alternative choices, potential complications and side effects, consequences of refusing treatment, etc. Mandatory reporting (C) refers to the obligation of medical assistants to report child or elder abuse. HIPAA (D) refers to regulations for confidentiality in reporting health information. COBRA (E) refers to federal regulations regarding continuation of health insurance after leaving a job.

58. C

Laboratory results are protected health information that should only be given directly to the patient. Leaving the information on an answering machine is a violation of patient confidentiality. None of the other items is as effective as asking her to call the office back.

59. E

Either *-dynia* or *-algia* is the suffix meaning pain. That means the correct choice is either (C) or (E). *Chrondr/o* means cartilage and *oste/o* means bone. This makes the correct choice osteodynia (E). Chondromalacia (A) is softening of cartilage. Osteochrondritis (B) is inflammation of bone and cartilage. Chrondralgia (C) is pain in cartilage. Osteolysis (D) is destruction of bone.

60. D

Cauliflower is not a source of calcium. Milk, sardines, canned salmon, and cheese are rich in calcium.

61. E

AC (from the Latin *ante cibum*) means "before a meal." The abbreviation PC (D) (*post cibum*) indicates "after meals." NPO (A) (*nil per os*) means "nothing by mouth" and is used when a patient should have nothing to eat or drink prior to a test, exam, or procedure. NOS (B) stands for "not otherwise specified" and is used to code encounters. PRN (C) (*pro re nata*) means "as needed."

62. C

In civil cases, only a preponderance of evidence is sufficient to prove guilt. In criminal cases, there must be overwhelming evidence beyond a reasonable doubt.

63. D

Fluoride is added to water and toothpaste to prevent dental decay (cavities). Calcium (A) builds bones and teeth. Potassium (B) keeps heart contraction regular. Iron (C) prevents anemia and iodine (E) prevents goiters.

64. C

Type O can donate to all blood types and is called the universal donor. Type A (A) can donate to type A or type AB. Type B (B) can donate to type B or type AB. Type AB (D) can donate to only AB blood type. ABO (E) refers to the overall blood typing group and is not an actual blood type.

65. C

The household equivalent of 10 mL is 2 teaspoons. One teaspoon equals approximately 5 mL; it is also equivalent to 60 drops (E)—too little of the medication. A half-teaspoon (B) equals approximately 2.5 mL—too little of the medication. There are 3 teaspoons or 15 mL in a tablespoon, so 2 tablespoons (D) equals 30 mL—too much of the medication. A half-pint (A) equals 8 ounces, which is equivalent to 240 mL—too much of the medication.

66. A

The abbreviation PERRLA refers to eyes and stands for "pupils equal, round, and reactive to light and accommodation." It indicates that the pupils are normal; it has no bearing on physical exam results for the ears (B), throat (C), heart (D), or abdomen (E). The eye examination may involve using a penlight or flashlight to observe the dilation and constriction of the pupil.

67. B

Prostrate is not a medical term. The correct term is prostate.

68. E

Arteries are thick, elastic, and carry blood away from the heart. Veins are thin, fragile, and return blood to the heart.

69. B

The sternocleidomastoid muscle originates at the back of the head and inserts into the sternum. A severe spasm prevents moving or turning of the head. The gastocnemius (A) is a calf muscle that often spasms and give the patient a "charley horse." The rectus abdominus (C) is the "six pack" muscle of the abdomen. The deltoid (D) is the muscle of the upper arm that we use for injection. The sartorius (E) involves the "tailor muscle." Sitting on the floor, putting the soles of the feet together, and pressing down on the knees stretches the sartorius.

70. E

The Fair Debt Collection Act is a regulation to protect debtors from collectors calling at work, leaving incriminating messages, or calling at inconvenient hours to harass the debtor. The Fair Credit Reporting Act (A) allows persons to see their credit record and the information given to potential lenders. The Equal Credit Opportunity Act (B) prohibits discrimination against extending credit based on race, sex, gender, religion, or marital status. The Consumer Protection Act of 1971 (C) protects the patient's finances by regulating the lending of funds. Fair Labor Standards Act (D) regulates the minimum wage and controls the number of hours worked.

71. E

Tendons join muscle to bone. Ligaments (A) join bone to bone. Perisoteum (B) is the protective covering on the outside of a long bone. Cartilage (C) is a semi-hard, fibrous connective tissue. The meninges (D) are a three-layer covering over the brain and spinal cord.

72. D

The suffix *-para* means only live births. The prefix *multi-* means many.

73. A

Only schedule II drugs must be ordered in writing on a triplicate form, signed by the physician, filled within a time limit, and no refills given. Schedule IV drugs are frequently abused (D), but have a lower potential for abuse. Drugs like Xanax, Ativan, and Valium are in this category. They must be locked in a secure place (E), but they can be called in over the phone (C) and may be refilled up to five times in six months (B) if the doctor thinks this appropriate.

74. C

The umbilical or gastric region surrounds the navel. The epigastric region (B) is above the navel. The suprapubic region (A) is below the navel and above the pubic bone. The hypochondriac regions (D) are in the area of the false ribs. The lumbar regions (E) are in the lower back.

75. A

The ego is the part of the conscious mind that contains our thoughts and behaviors.

76. B

Menstrual flow is menorrhea. That means the correct choice is (B), (C), or (D). The prefix for without is *a-* or *an-*. That makes amenorrhea (B) correct. Nullipara (A) would be translated as no live births. Oligomenorrhea (C) translates to scanty menstrual flow. Dysmenorrhea (D) means painful menstruation. Nulligravida (E) means no pregnancies.

77. B

Eggs are not eaten by a lacto-vegetarian. Lacto-vegetarians eat only plant-based items and dairy foods such as milk and cheese.

78. A

The Patient Self-Determination Act allows patients to control their own lives and make informed decisions about what medical care they do or do not want. The Consumer Protection Act of 1971 (B) protects the patient's finances by regulating the lending of funds. The Civil Rights Act of 1964 (C) prohibits discrimination based on race, religion, color, sex, or national origin. The HIPAA Act (D) is recent legislation to protect individual health information. The Americans with Disabilities Act (E) protects those with physical, mental, or emotional handicaps from discrimination.

79. B

A subdural hematoma is a bleed under the layers of tissue covering the brain, but the bleeding does not go into the brain itself. An intracerebral hematoma (C) is bleeding into the brain tissue itself. A concussion (A) is a head injury in which the brain has a temporary injury (bruising and bleeding) due to a blow. Epilepsy (D) is irregular electrical activity of the brain that may result in seizure. Hydrocephalus (E) is an increase in fluid pressure because ventricles in the brain do not drain properly.

80. C

K is the abbreviation for potassium.

81. B

Pain and weight loss are advanced symptoms of cancer. Early warning symptoms allow treatment and increase survival rates. The seven early warning symptoms are: a sore that does not heal, a lump or mass, unexplained bleeding, a mole that has changed shape or color, chronic cough or hoarseness, change in bowel or bladder habits, and persistent indigestion.

KAPLAN

82. A

ADHD is the abbreviation for attention-deficit hyper-activity disorder. PTSD is the abbreviation for post-traumatic stress disorder. Bipolar disorder is a mental illness. Stress, attention disorders, and mental illness are treated by a psychiatrist.

83. D

The duties of the public health department include recording of vital statistics such as births, deaths, communicable diseases, animal bites, gunshot and knife wounds, epidemic control, and research. Medicare is managed by the federal government and Medicaid is managed by the state.

84. D

The T wave indicates the relaxation of the ventricles. The P wave (A) shows the contraction of the atria, and the QRS complex (C) indicates the contraction of the ventricles and the relaxation of the atria. A U wave (E) is not always seen on an EKG and may indicate hypokalemia. The Q wave (B) is a componenet of the QRS complex, showing the depolarization of the ventricles of the heart.

85. D

Carcinogenic means pertaining to the formation of cancer. The suffix -ic means pertaining to, *carcin/o* means cancer, and *gen/* means formation. Formation of tumors (A) would be oncogenesis. Pertaining to the formation of tumors (B) would be oncogenic. The study of tumors (E) is oncology.

86. A

Multiple sclerosis involves the appearance of bare spots on the myelin sheath (demyelization of the axon). Myasthenia gravis (B) involves extreme fatigue of muscles with the slightest exertion. Amyotrophic lateral sclerosis (C) is a progressive degeneration of voluntary motor neurons. Cerebral palsy (D) is a disorder of balance and movement often caused by anoxia during the birth process. Parkinson's disease (E) is a disease of dopamine deficiency that affects gait. It often is accompanied by "pill-rolling" movements of the fingers.

87. D

(A), (B), (C), and (E) correctly describe reasons for erythema (redness of the skin). Bile problems (D) would likely result in jaundice (yellowing of the skin and mucus membranes).

88. A

Begin by dividing the word into parts and look at the ending.

(A) electr/o/cardi/o/graphy

(B) electr/o/cardi/o/graph

(C) electr/o/cardi/o/gram

(D) ech/o/cardi/o/gram

(E) ech/o/cardi/o/graphy

Only two endings mean "the process of using an instrument to record data."

(A) electr/o/cardi/o/graphy

(E) ech/o/cardi/o/graphy

When we look at the beginning of the word, only electrocardiography (A) involves electrical activity. Echocardiography (E) involves reflected sound (ech/o/cardi/o/graphy). Looking at the entire word, electrocardiography does mean "the process of using an instrument to record data of the electrical activity in the heart."

89. D

Battery is illegal touching. It is an intentional tort. Assault is the mere threat of illegal touching.

90. B

A vesicle is a papule with clear fluid; for example, a blister or chicken pox lesion. A pustule (A) is a papule filled with white or yellow pus. A macule (C) is a flat lesion and although visible, it cannot be felt. A nevus (D) is a mole. A nodule (E) is a large, hard knot or tumor.

91. C

One of these abbreviations does not belong with the others. Start by figuring out the meaning of each. TAH is total abdominal hysterectomy. LMP is last menstrual period. LOC is level of consciousness. PID is pelvic inflammatory disease. STD is sexually transmitted disease. The one that does not seem to fall under the area of women's health where a gynecologist would specialize is the LOC (C).

92. B

The person accused of a crime is the defendant. The plaintiff (A) offers a complaint. The jury (C) is a group of peers who try a case. Bench (D) refers to a judge trying a case. An agent (E) is someone representing another, such as the medical assistant representing the physician.

93. E

Gout (E) is an accumulation of uric acid crystals in joints. Bursitis (A) is an enlarged sac between joints that fills with fluid to provide extra protection to the joint. Arthritis (B) is inflammation of a joint causing pain and stiffness. Kyphosis (C) is an exaggerated curvature to the thoracic spine. Scoliosis (D) is a deviation of the spine to the side.

94. D

Reciprocity allows a person licensed in one state to practice in another. Revocation is canceling a license to practice.

95. C

Recognizing the word parts help us to know what body area is involved. Translating the end first, *-ism* is a condition. The beginning of the word is *crypt/o*, which means hidden, and the middle of the word is *orchid/o* or testicles. Cryptorchidism is a condition of hidden testicles. Balanitis is inflammation of the glans penis. Hematuria is a condition of blood in the urine. These conditions would be treated by a doctor who specializes in male reproductive organs and urinary problems, a urologist.

96. D

Respiration would increase under the effect of the sympathetic nervous system as the body prepares for "fight or flight." Muscles require glucose and oxygen for energy.

97. B

A contract can be written or oral. All contracts involve a good or service for a consideration that is accepted by two parties of legal capacity.

98. E

CABG is coronary artery bypass graft and an EKG is an electrocardiogram. Both would involve the heart and require the services of a physician who specializes in the heart, a cardiologist.

99. E

Negligence (A) is failure to perform at the reasonable standard of care. Defamation of character (C) is malicious misrepresentation of facts to harm another. Slander (B) is defamation of character through spoken words and libel (D) is defamation of character through written words.

100. C

The scenario described in the question is an example of bargaining. In this state of the grief process, patients seek to negotiate with a higher power and resolve their illness.

Part II—Administrative

101. E

Coordination of benefits is undertaken when the patient has more than one insurance plan: After the primary carrier has made payment based on its plan, the secondary carrier determines its own amount of payment based on the balance. Capitation (A) means that the insurance carrier pays a set fee per patient regardless of degree of injury or illness. Coinsurance (B) requires the insured patient to pay for portion of a medical bill, while the insurance carrier pays the remainder. A third-party payment (C) is one made by an insurance carrier, government-funded program, or other payer that is not the patient. In assignment of benefits (D), a patient authorizes the health insurance carrier to make payment for a covered procedure directly to his/her health-care provider rather than to himself/herself.

102. C

Posting is the process of copying or recording an amount from one record, such as a journal, onto another record, such as a ledger or from a day sheet onto a ledger card. A ledger (A) is a record of charges, payments, and adjustments for individual patients or families. A superbill (B) is a combination charge slip, statement, and insurance reporting form. A trial balance (D) is a method of checking the accuracy of accounts. It should be done once a month. Deducting (E) refers to when money is subtracted or deducted from an employee pay to cover taxes, insurance, and possible other expenses.

103. D

The goal of using wave is to keep the office on track. To determine how many patients to be seen in an hour, divide the hour by the length of the average visit.

104. A

Inspecting and releasing means ensuring that the appropriate people have taken action on a document. Before the document is filed, a release mark should be noted on it.

105. A

"Tickler file" and "reminder file" are two names for the file that holds work that has to be completed. A supplemental file (B) is a file that holds papers that are needed in addition to main papers. A retained file (C) may be a file that retains or holds specific information. An inactive file (D) holds paperwork from patients that are no longer part of the medical practice. An active file (E) may hold information on patients that are currently using the medical office.

106. B

The HITECH Act of 2009 does not dictate any single electronic health record (EHR) software system, and many software and hardware vendors have entered the market for EHRs. The act establishes financial incentives for EHR adoption (A) to promote the goal of improving Americans' health (D), and it requires health care providers to demonstrate "meaningful use" of EHRs (C). As of 2013, 78 percent of U.S. physicians had adopted an EHR system (E).

107. C

Withholding is the amount of salary held out of payroll checks for the purpose of paying government taxes or for employees' benefits. To determine the amount of money to be withheld from each paycheck, each new employee must complete a W-4 (A). The Federal Unemployment Tax Act (B) requires employers to pay a percentage of each employee's income, up to a specified dollar amount, to fund an account used to pay employees who have been laid off. All employees file an annual tax return (D). FICA (E) governs the Social Security system.

108. C

In block format the salutation is followed by a colon.

109. B

A common concern among clinical providers is that the simultaneous entry of patient information during an examination places a barrier between themselves and the patient. Often the computer station is across the room from the exam table and the clinician has their back turned to the patient as they are talking. While some clinicians do not like keyboarding aspects the communication issue is the most common issue being raised.

110. C

The standard size business envelope is No. 10, $4\frac{1}{2}$ inches by $9\frac{1}{2}$ inches.

111. C

Account aging is the method of identifying how long an account is overdue. Collecting the receivable on time (A) is the best way to keep accounts accurate but this is not always feasible. Account aging is necessary in all physician offices regardless of size (B). Account aging shows how the account is aging; it does not allow the account to be written off (D and E).

112. C

Open-hours scheduling is when patients come at their own convenience. Modified-wave (A) can be used in different ways. One way is to schedule in 15-minute slots, regardless of appointment type. Double-booking (B) is used when two patients are scheduled at the same time. Cluster scheduling (D) groups similar appointments together during the day. Time-specified scheduling (E) assumes a steady stream of patients all day long.

113. A

Scheduling these appointments at the beginning of the hour will allow time for catching up. The less time-consuming appointments can be given 10-minute time slots. Ten-minute time slots (B) may not be enough for all patients. Scheduling these appointments at the end of the hour (C) will not allow the doctor to catch up. Scheduling an appointment at the same time as another patient's 10-minute slot (D) will not give the time needed for the appointment. Ten-minute appointments (E) would be used for follow-up care.

114. C

For the tickler file to be most effective, it has to be checked frequently; so all paperwork is quickly put in patients' charts. A tickler file is kept in a folder (A), but it still has to be checked frequently. If the tickler file is locked in a secure area (B), it may not get checked as needed. Tickler files should be cleaned out every week, not left in weekly files (D). Keeping the tickler file in a separate area of the office (E) may cause it to be overlooked.

115. B

A pegboard system usually includes a lightweight board with pegs on the left or right edges and is sometimes called a "one-write" system. Single-entry (A) is the oldest bookkeeping system, requiring only one entry for each transaction. It is the easiest system to use. The double-entry system (C) requires more skills and is more time consuming. Disbursement (D) is the payments of funds, whether in cash, or by check. A balance sheet (E) is the financial statement for a specific date or period that indicates the total assets, liabilities, and capital of the business.

116. E

All aspects of the flow and provision of care in a practice office or health care setting will be part of a well-integrated EHR system. This includes not only the clinical systems but billing and scheduling aspects as well.

117. A

A spreadsheet is a worksheet that is used to see many types of information at once. Hardware (B) refers to a computer's physical components. A patient list (C) is created by the medical office. A cover letter (D) is used to send to introduce you or the medical office to the reader. A work grid (E) shows what time employees are in.

118. D

The U.S. Postal Service defines first-class mail as all items weighing 13 ounces or less.

119. D

Written communication, such as letters, memos, and email, must take into consideration legal and ethical issues. Body language (A) is useful when speaking directly to someone, but cannot be viewed in written communication. The speed of the document (B) has no bearing on the written communication. Formatting (C) is important in written communication, but is not as important as legal and ethical issues. Grammar (E) is important in written communication, but is not as important as legal and ethical issues.

120. D

A double-entry system is a bookkeeping system. When the practice charges for a medical service, the patient's account is debited and the appropriate account for the practice is credited. All the other options are commonly used models for managed care organizations.

121. D

The federal government is proposing a "meaningful use" program that would reimburse medical offices for some costs related to implementation of EHRs. The other items are important sets in implementation but they are not eligible for funding at this time.

122. A

A key strategy to secure a computer network is the use of password protected log-ons. In this way, only approved staff members can access health records in a particular locaton. A single sign-on could be used by any individual; it would defeat the purpose of the system to only allow access to physician providers and it would be a logistical problem to keep the computer station out of the patient care and office areas of the facility.

123. E

Always consult the physician when determining the policy and procedures of an office. Talking to fellow employees (A) will not determine what the physician wants for the office. Choosing a color of the manual (B) would not be the first step in preparing the manual. Deciding on the format (C) can be done after the wishes of the physician are established. Buying paper for the manual (D) would not be the first step.

124. A

Leaving gaps in a doctor's schedule will cause the doctor and staff to have excess time that could be used for patients. Overbooking (B) occurs when more patients are scheduled than open appointment slots. Clustering (C) is grouping similar appointments together during the day. Wave scheduling (D) is scheduling a set number of patients per hour, all of whom will arrive at the top of the hour. Advance scheduling (E) is scheduling appointments weeks or months in advance.

125. B

In the alphabetical filing system, the patient's last name is unit 1, first name is unit 2, and middle name (or initial) is unit 3. Hyphenated names are treated as one unit.

126. **A**

Documenting the no-show information is necessary because the medical chart is a legal document and this information is important for the health of the patient. Doctors' offices can request payment for missed appointments, but patients should be notified of this practice when they first become a patient (B). Refusing to reschedule an appointment is not good customer relations (C). Rescheduling is a good idea while the patient is on the phone, but telling the patient that they have to confirm is not good customer relations (D). Erasing an appointment is not an option (E). The appointment book must be treated as a legal document.

127. **C**

A copy or duplicate of a referral has to go into a patient's medical chart.

128. **B**

Trial balance is a method used to check the accuracy of accounts. A daily summary (A) is used to record charges and payments in the physician's office. An accounting system (C) is used to record, classify, and summarize financial transactions. Accrual accounting (D) is recording income when it is earned and expenses when they are incurred. Bookkeeping (E) is the recording of the accounting processes. Bookkeeping records income, charges, and disbursements.

129. **B**

A new patient does not need to provide information regarding income. All of the other information is required.

130. **C**

For the office to run smoothly, all employees must read the policy and procedures manual. All employees can help write the manual (A), but all old and new employees *must* read the manual. Knowing where the manual is kept is a great idea (B), but it needs to be read also. It is not necessary to give patients a copy of the manual (D). It is not necessary for each employee to have a personal copy of the manual (E).

131. **B**

Physicians do not accept all insurance. The database would contain the names of the insurance that the physician accepts. Since the physician usually does not accept all insurance, all insurance would not be listed (A). The database would contain all the insurance that physician accepts, not just Medicare and Medicaid (C). Only the insurance carriers that the physician accepts would be entered, not the most popular ones (D). The medical insurance that a physician offers his employees (E) would not be entered into the patient database.

132. **A**

All checks and cash should be deposited on a daily basis so that no money is lying around the office. It is easier to keep track of the money in a bank account.

133. **A**

Open-hours scheduling is the system in which patients arrive at their own convenience with the understanding that they will be seen on a first-come, first-seen basis, unless it is an emergency.

134. **D**

The individual cannot choose which doctor he or she goes to. When a report is made to the employer, the employer directs the individual where to go for treatment. This may or may not be the individual's primary care physician. The other four choices (A, B, C, and E) are true statements about workers' compensation.

135. **A**

SOAP is a standard method of documentation used in medical records. It stands for Subjective, Objective, Assessment, and Plan.

136. **A**

When a word is unclear during transcription, leave a blank space and write a note to the physician specifying the location of the space in the document. The medical assistant should never guess while transcribing dictation (B). The medical assistant should continue transcribing the rest of the dictation and wait to ask the physician about the confusing word (C). The medical assistant should never reword sections of dictation without first consulting the physician (D). It is better to leave a blank space rather than an "X" (E).

137. D

Using cycle billing, all accounts are divided alphabetically into groups, with each group billed at a different time. No billing cycle is completed every fourth month (A). This can be done by computer (B), but a medical assistant has to go into the computer to divide the bills alphabetically. A monthly billing system is mailed out by the 25th of the month in order to receive payment on the 1st of the month (C and E).

138. B

Software is a set of instructions, or a program, that tells the computer what to do. Portable hardware (A) is not a term used for computers. Input devices (C) are used to enter data into the computer. A palmtop computer (D) is very light and the size of your palm. The system unit of many newer desktop models is housed in a tower case (E).

139. D

An appointment request is information that can be sent through email. This information is not confidential. Diagnosis (A) is confidential information and should not be sent by email. Lab test results (B) also are confidential and cannot be sent by email. Follow-up information (C) should not be discussed by email. The physician should speak with the patient directly. A list of medications (E) can tell a reader why the patient has seen the physician, so this information is confidential.

140. D

The medical assistant should repeat the patient's name and phone number back to the caller to reduce errors.

141. E

The policy and procedures manual is the most important communication tool for all employees in a medical office. A tickler file (A) is used to keep track of papers that have to be filed. A patient's medical records (B) are never used as a communication tool. Data entry (C) is used to store raw facts in the doctor's office. The appointment book (D) is used to keep track of appointments.

142. C

It is important to update the policies and procedures on a yearly basis.

143. B

Organizing the key points before you write up a rough draft will help put your thoughts in order. It allows you to make sure that all the information is included. To just start writing without any thought as to what has to be included (A) will cause you to make many mistakes and will reflect poorly on you. Once you begin writing the rough draft, using language that is easy to understand (C) improves the communication. Anyone reading will know what the subject is. Composing a rough draft (D) would be the next step after organizing your thoughts. Choosing a letter format (E) would be done when you are ready to write.

144. E

CPT codes are based on the level of service provided. When the code is manipulated to a higher level, or upcoded, it dishonestly claims a higher level of payment due. Dirty claims (A) are those with mistakes or omissions; they must be corrected and resubmitted to be paid. An EOB, or Explanation of Benefits (B), is the statement an insurance carrier provides to patients to explain the outcome of medical payment requests. Bundling (C) refers to an insurance carrier's combining two or more CPT codes under one, usually less costly, "umbrella" code. Superbilling (D) is preparing the patient encounter form, also called a superbill or charge slip.

145. A

For the medical assistant to schedule the proper procedure with the right specialist, he must have the exact procedure to be performed. Though finding out what would be a good time to schedule an appointment for the patient (B), it is not necessary. The patient could not schedule the appointment herself (C), as she would not have all the appropriate information. Determining the day and time the procedure must be performed (D) is not necessary. Determining who will be with the patient at the time of the procedure before making an appointment is not necessary (E).

146. A

Coding is the basis for information on the claim form. A claim (B) is a demand for payment. Subrogation (C) is the right of an insurer to collect monies. A superbill (D) is the bill the patient receives from the physician at the time of service delineating the visit, tests, diagnosis, charges, and when to return. A charge slip form (E) is used to record services supplied, and charges and payments for those services; it functions as a billing form for insurance reimbursement.

147. E

Individuals age 65 and older who are retired and receive Social Security benefits qualify for Medicare, as do those retired from the railroad or civil service. The minimum age for the general population is 65, not 62 (D). Children of veterans who died of service-related disabilities (A) qualify for medical coverage through the Civilian Health and Medical Program of the Department of Veterans Affairs (CHAMPVA). There is no age restriction to Medicare for blind individuals (B), and the finically indigent (C) are eligible for Medicaid benefits, not Medicare.

148. D

Time-specified is the type of scheduling that is recognized by the regular time intervals in the appointment schedule.

149. D

If after 48 hours the medical chart cannot be found, it is best to recreate the original file. Saying nothing is not an option (A). Proceeding as if the file can be located will only make it likely that more information will be lost (B). Duplicating the information (C) may not be possible. Starting a new blank chart without trying to recreate information will leave gaps in the medical history of the patient (E).

150. C

Authorized newsletters and periodicals ship via second-class mail. Third-class (A), also known as bulk mail (D), includes books, catalogs, and other printed material weighing less than 16 ounces. First-class (B) includes correspondence, billing statements, and other letters weighing 13 ounces or less. Priority mail (E) may be used for items weighing more than 13 ounces. It allows them to arrive more quickly.

151. C

A debit is an amount usually representing things acquired for the intended use or benefit of a business. A debit is also called a charge; debits are incurred when the practice pays for something, such as medical supplies. The total (A) is the entire amount owed, collected, or accrued on the daily summary. You would subtract (B) or remove an amount from the total when a payment is made. The subtotal (D) is the amount before taxes are added. The balance (E) is the amount owed after payments are deducted and taxes added.

152. C

Email has to be short and to the point. Email is set up to be read quickly. Additional background information can be communicated later (A). Writing in italic can be harder to read. Not all email systems pick up formatting such as bold, italics, and color (B), so the recipient may not see it. Writing in capitals is equivalent to shouting in an email and may be harder to read (B). It is more professional to use capital letters in email just as you would in a business letter (E).

153. B

Double booking is commonly used in scheduling appointments when the patients only need to see the physician for a short time.

154. C

HMO insurance requires a referral to see a specialist. The primary care physician must create the referral for insurance purposes.

155. A

Computers have many uses in the medical office, but a main one is scheduling appointments. Verifying appointments (B) is not possible on the computer. Diagnosing patients (C) is the physician's job. The medical assistant or physician takes the vital signs of a patient (D). Most medical offices still use paper files, and a member of the office staff would be responsible for locating them (E).

156. B

The size of the medical practice always determines which billing cycle is used. The size of the practice, rather than the number of physicians (A), determines the billing cycle. The type of medicine that the physicians practice (C) is not a factor. The amount of employees who do the billing (D) does not matter. The physician will prefer a billing cycle that fits the practice size (E).

157. A

Accounts payable refers to all money owed by the practice to other businesses. Accounts receivable (B) is the money owed to the practice. Charges (C) are the items billed to patients; debits (D) is an accounting term used to describe money paid out by the practice; and owner's equity (E) is the profit made after taxes and expenses.

158. E

HCFA-1500 is the "universal" claim form accepted by most insurance carriers. If left blank, this form contains no sensitive patient or medical office information and can be disposed of without shredding. The appointment list (A), patient lab results (C), patient referral, and patient insurance card (D) should all be shredded before disposal to maintain confidentiality.

159. A

When a practice has flexible office hours, it stays open at unusual hours on certain days in addition to normal business hours. This occurs most frequently in group practices.

160. A

The problem-oriented medical record is used to document a patient's information according to the problem the patient is having.

161. A

Petty cash in a physician's office is used to pay for minor things needed by the staff. Paying an invoice for supplies ordered (B) would not come out of petty cash. Petty cash would not have a large amount of money in it. The electric bill (C) would be paid with the monthly bills and taken out of the medical office account. The petty cash would be available to authorized employees to use (D). Petty cash should be used not only in an emergency but also as needed (E).

162. A

It is necessary to date-stamp each piece of mail when it is opened so the mail can be answered or addressed in a timely manner. Putting the mail aside until the patients are gone for the day (B) is a way for mail to get lost. The mail should be given to the physician immediately (C), but after it has been stamped with the current date. It is not the job of the medical assistant to read the physician's mail (D). The mail should be delivered immediately to the physician after being stamped, not set aside to be delivered later (E).

163. E

An outguide can be used to identify who has the medical record. It can be plastic or paper and is available in a variety of colors.

164. B

Rescheduling the appointment while the patient is on the telephone will save both the medical assistant and the patient time. Saying "thank you" is polite (A), but it is best to ask the patient if he would like to reschedule. Asking the patient to call back to reschedule an appointment (C) is not an effective way to run an office. Appointments are important (D) but there are times when an emergency does come up. The physician cannot make a patient keep an appointment (E).

165. D

A database is a collection of records created and stored on a computer. A scanner (E) is used to scan documents to forward in email. The Internet (B) is an electronic communication network. The cursor (C) is a symbol used to mark one's place on the computer screen. "Hard copy" means any printed material.

166. A

The main circuit board is the motherboard, which controls the other components in the system. A flash drive (B) is used to copy and transfer information. The hard disk drive (C) is where information is stored permanently for later retrieval. The operating system (D) is the main software system that the computer uses. Memory (E) is information stored for later use.

167. C

Copayments are collected when the patient checks in to see the physician, unless other arrangements have been made prior to the appointment. Collecting a copayment after the patient sees the physician (A) is not ideal because the patient may be able to leave without paying. Bills are only sent out if the patient has an outstanding balance (B). Patients do not need to pay in advance before coming to the medical office (D). The patient should not pay while in the exam room (E).

168. C

Registered mail is the most secure service offered by the post office. Registered mail provides insurance coverage for valuable items and is controlled from the point of mailing to the point of delivery. Certified mail (A) offers a guarantee that the item has been mailed and received by the correct party by requiring the mail carrier to obtain a signature on delivery. Insured mail (B) is for any piece of domestic mail for damage or loss. First-class mail (D) is classification by the weight of 13 ounces or less. Priority (E) is the classification for mail that weighs 70 pounds or less.

KAPLAN

169. C

The pegboard system provides an overview of collections, payments, and charges through use of a day sheet that is easy to read. The pegboard not only includes payments and charges (A), but collections as well. A charge slip (B) is a piece of paper that identifies what charges have been made. A third-party check (D) is written by an unknown party to a payee. "Collections only" (E) is collecting on delinquent accounts.

170. C

As of the printing of this book, the new system is scheduled to take effect in October 2014. Answer (A) is incorrect because the coding system will change for all providers as it relates to the classification of diseases, illnesses and injuries. (B) is incorrect because the legislation and rule making for the ICD-10 implementation has been enacted. (D) is incorrect because the system is NOT optional, it is mandatory. (E) is incorrect because medical assistants will need to be familiar with the new system to complete documentation and medical record information for office patients.

171. A

The beginning of the day would be the best time to schedule. If the patient is late, it will not disrupt the end of the day's schedule. Middle of the day (B) would disrupt the afternoon schedule. Right after lunch (C) could cause the afternoon to back up. Never scheduling a patient (D) is not appropriate and does not support a customer service approach. Scheduling the patient at the end of the day (E) could delay closing the office on time.

172. E

Wave scheduling works best in large facilities where there are enough personnel to give service to several patients at once.

173. C

In the cycle billing system, all accounts are divided alphabetically into groups, and each group billed at a different time. Past due (A) is when services are rendered and a balance is owed but has not been paid in the past 30 days. Account aging (B) is a method used to determine how long an account is overdue. Wave scheduling (D) is a method of scheduling appointments and is not related to billing. Monthly billing (E) is the method that sends all bills out at the same time each month, usually around the 25th of the month.

174. C

If the medical office has contracted with a repair service to fix office machines whenever necessary, the medical assistant should renew the agreement annually.

175. D

The World Health Organization developed the International Classification of Disease system for use in describing and tracking diseases across the globe. (A) is incorrect; HCFA was the former name of the Centers for Medicare and Medicaid, a branch of the U.S. government that is accountable for oversight of Medicare and Medicaid entitlement programs. (B) is incorrect, as it is the professional association for U.S. physicians. (C) is incorrect, as it is the professional organization for Medical Record and Health Information experts. (E) is incorrect, as it is the branch of the U.S. government that oversees taxation.

176. D

Bookkeeping is the actual daily recording of the accounts or transactions of the business and is the major part of the accounting process. A day sheet (A) is used to list or post each day's charges, payments, credits, and adjustments: the daily financial transactions. Charges (B) are the fees for services rendered. Accounts receivable (C) is the amount owed to a business for services or goods supplied. A pegboard system (E) consists of day sheets, ledger cards, charge slips, and receipt forms.

177. B

Software is not one of the physical components of a computer.

178. D

Giving a superbill at the time of service is the most effective way to receive money. It is also the least expensive because a bill will not have to be generated for payment. A cycle billing system (A) is when all accounts are divided alphabetically into groups, with each group billed at a different time. A ledger card (B) is a record of charges, payments, and adjustments for an individual patient or family. Computerized mailed statements (C) can be easy to generate, but this would not be the cheapest method of billing. It may be difficult to receive payment via phone calls (E) because patients are not always available.

179. B

Experts recommend keeping the record of appointments for three years in case the information is needed in a legal case.

180. E

A superbill is the bill the patient receives from the physician at the time of service delineating the visit, tests, diagnosis, charges, and when to return. Charge slip is another name for superbill. CMS1500 (A) is the claim form accepted by most insurance carriers. This form is prepared using words and CPT codes for procedures performed and ICD-9-CM codes for diagnoses. A claim (B) is a demand for payment. Subrogation (C) is the right of an insurer to collect monies HCFA Common Procedure Coding System (HCPCS) is used by Medicare as a supplement to the CPT codes (D).

181. B

Asking the purpose of the visit is a way to control the schedule. You can accurately schedule appointments so that patients are not waiting to be seen.

182. B

The ICD-10-CM system is intended to improve the specificity and efficiency of medical coding and billing. (A) is incorrect because it is not a rationale for implementing the new system. (C) is true, but simply adding more codes was not a major intent of this transition. (D) is also technically true, but it is not a major intent of the implementation of this system. (E) is incorrect and does not apply to the use of the new coding system.

183. C

CMS1500 is the claim form accepted by most insurance carriers. This form is prepared using words and CPT codes for procedures performed and ICD-9-CM codes for diagnoses. A claim register (A) is a diary or register of claims submitted to each insurance carrier. When payment is received, the date and amount of payment is entered in the register. A superbill (B) is the bill the patient receives from the physician at the time of service delineating the visit, tests, diagnoses, charges, and when to return. A diagnosis code (D) is the numerical designation for a specific illness, injury, or disease. Modifiers (E) are two-digit numerical codes that indicate unusual procedural services.

184. E

The correct answer is (E), medical information. (A) includes facts about the patient, such as name, address, and date of birth. Health history (B) is part of the medical record in the patient's chart, as is (C), chief complaint. DRG (D) refers to the diagnostic related group assigned to the Medicare patient for an inpatient stay and is used for Medicare billing.

185. A

Codes will be expanded to seven digits. (B) is incorrect, as the codes will be indexed in alphabetical order. (C) is incorrect because the anatomic site is included in the digits of the code. (D) is incorrect because the codes will include both numbers and an alphabetical character. (E) is incorrect, as the E and V codes have been eliminated under ICD-10.

186. E

Gynecology is not a section in the *Current Procedural Terminology* book. The seven sections are: 1. Evaluation and Management, 2. Anesthesia, 3. Surgery, 4. Radiology, Nuclear Medicine, and Diagnostic Ultrasound, 5. Pathology, 6. Laboratory, and 7. Medicine.

187. B

Items that are sent via registered mail, certified mail, or overnight mail have top priority. The next level of priority includes personal or confidential mail (D), and the following level includes priority mail (A), airmail (E), and first-class mail (C).

188. E

Only authorized employees can take money from petty cash. An authorized person should be in charge of purchasing because too many different people ordering can cause confusion (A). All receipts of goods need to be recorded so a record of the goods can be kept (B). It is best to purchase goods of high quality at the lowest possible price (C). All shipments received need to be checked against the packing slip to ensure that supplies ordered were received (D).

189. D

Once the overdue account has reached 90 days, it is considered serious.

190. C

The way to properly correct any written error in the medical record is to draw a single line through the error and make the correction above the error. This method is used so the error can be seen in this legal record.

191. B

A voucher check contains a detachable voucher form. The voucher portion is used to itemize the purpose of the check, deductions, or other information. A bank draft (A) is a check written by a bank against its funds in another bank. A limited check (C) is issued on a special check form that displays a preprinted maximum dollar amount for which the check can be written. A certified check (D) is written on the payer's own check form and verified by the bank with an official stamp. A cashier's check (E) is written using the bank's own check form and signed by a bank representative.

192. B

It is very difficult to get payment from a patient who does not want to pay. Such a patient may have a reason for believing that a payment does not have to be made. A patient who has forgotten to pay (A) can be reminded by receiving a payment statement or a telephone call. A person having financial hardship (C) may not be able to pay the entire amount but is often willing to make small payments to clear the debt. A patient who has no insurance (D) can be put on a monthly payment plan. Most patients who owe money will pay their bills (E).

193. E

Monthly billing is the method that sends all bills out at the same time each month, usually around the 25th of the month. Past due is when services are rendered and a balance is owed but has not been paid past 30 days (A). Account aging is a method used to determine how long an account is overdue (B). In the cycle billing system, all accounts are divided alphabetically into groups, and each group billed at a different time (C). Wave scheduling is a method of scheduling appointments and is not related to billing (D).

194. D

Each appointment day should have times allotted for emergency appointments. Wave scheduling (A), where several patients are scheduled for the top of the hour, is based on the idea that some patients will be late and other patients require more time with the doctor. When double booking (B), more than one patient is scheduled at the same appointment time. Open-hours scheduling (C) is the system in which patients arrive at their own convenience with the understanding that they will be seen on a first-come, first-seen basis, unless it is an emergency. Physicians who see pharmaceutical representatives often block out certain times and days when they can be seen.

195. D

A medical file drawer is labeled on the outside so it is easy to locate the correct file. If the drawer is labeled inside the drawer (A), it would be difficult to locate the correct drawer. The side of the drawer (B) would be difficult to see. A tickler file (C) is a reminder file for active documents. Keeping the drawers listed in the office database would not be helpful. The drawer itself needs to be labeled so files can be located quickly (E).

196. B

The correct answer is hospitals. (A) is incorrect, as it is only a component of a hospital. (C) is incorrect, as physicians' offices will continue to use CPT and HCPC codes for their services. (D) is incorrect, as the codes will not be used in pharmacies. (E) is also incorrect, as they will apply exclusively to inpatient hospitals.

197. A

Minutes are the official record of a professional meeting. They include the date, time, location, and topic of the meeting, as well as those attending, those absent, topics discussed, and time of adjournment. The agenda (B) lists the order in which business is to be conducted during a meeting. Bylaws (C) are the rules established to provide guidance as to the structure and business practices of a company. An itinerary (D) is a list of travel information. A resolution (E) is an order of business or action taken by the governing body of an organization.

198. E

The address of the office should not be included in a job description. All other items should be part of a job description.

199. A

An inventory of equipment should be taken at least once a year.

200. A

Conditioning is the first step in the filing process. It is followed by releasing, indexing, sorting, and storing.

Part III—Clinical

201. A

Sterilization means that all organisms have been removed from an object by either gas or chemical sterilization or by autoclave. Disinfection is removal of all pathogens (B). Removal of debris with soap and water is called sanitization (C). Boiling (D) does not sterilize, and ultrasonic cleaning (E) is a method of sanitization for delicate instruments.

202. B

Disposable thermometers become inaccurate after their expiration dates. As the thermometers have not been used before, sterilization and probe covers are not required.

203. B

Personal opinion of the medical staff is not to be placed in the patient's chart. Only facts are to be documented. Direct quotations from the patient may be included and quotation marks used to specify these quotes (D). Medication history (E) would be documented to give information about past medications that have been used and the effect of those medications. This includes medication allergies. Legal history (C) and patient report of drug use (A) are included, as this information is used to assess risk of disease.

204. B

Mensuration is the process of measuring something. Auscultation (A) involves listening, as in evaluation of the bowel sounds using a stethoscope. Palpation (C) and percussion (D) both use touch; palpation would be using the hands to feel the temperature of the skin and percussion is tapping in order to hear different sounds. Observation (E) is visually evaluating the patient.

205. D

Commonly called the SST (serum separator tubes), the red/gray tubes and the gold Hemogard closure tubes contain a clot activator and separation gel. After inverting the tube five times, the clot activator shortens the time required for the formation of a clot. The separation gel in the bottom of the tube changes viscosity and will migrate up and form a barrier between the serum and blood cells. One minute (A) may seem like a familiar number during the routine phlebotomy procedure because of the typical time restraint associated with tourniquet application. Five minutes (B) is associated with an accelerated clotting time seen with the use of the yellow/gray stopper tubes or orange Hemogard closure tubes. These tubes contain thrombin, which is activated after the filled tube is inverted eight times. These tubes are used for stat serum chemistry testing. Fifteen minutes (C) is the customary time for centrifuging a serum separator tube. Sixty minutes (E) is the normal amount of time for a blood sample to clot in a tube that contains no additive. Red stopper tubes are then centrifuged to yield a separated sample of serum from blood cells.

206. C

The vastus lateralis is the preferred site for an infant who is not yet walking. The gluteus muscles are not well developed until the child is walking (A). The deltoid (B) is too small and underdeveloped in the infant. The injection is to be given in the muscle so the subcutaneous route is not acceptable (D).

207. B

Have ready a speculum for visualization and a water-soluble lubricant. You would not need to dilate the cervix in order to do the procedure (A). A suture removal tray would not be needed for a vaginal exam (C). Sterile gloves are not necessary for the routine procedure (E). The Hemoccult card (D) would only be necessary if the physician is also doing a rectal exam.

208. C

The goal of emergency treatment is to stop the burning in the skin. By cooling the area, the heat is dissipated. A cool cloth will also decrease pain. Care needs to be taken to not break the blisters (B) and to maintain the skin integrity to prevent infection (D). A bandage, if necessary, should be applied loosely (A). The physician may order silver sulfadiazine cream, which has bacteriostatic properties after the burn has been assessed (E).

209. B

Prone position, which is lying flat on the abdomen, would offer the best access to the spine. Knee-chest (A) is used for proctologic exams. Supine (C) is lying flat on the back. Lithotomy (D) is used for vaginal exams and Pap tests. Trendelenburg (E) is the shock position with the legs positioned higher than the heart. It is used in patients who have a low blood pressure or feel faint.

210. C

By providing a quiet and private area, the patient will feel comfortable sharing information with the medical assistant. Questions should be asked in person so that answers can be clarified (A). If a form is given to the patient to fill out, it should be followed up with a personal review of the information. You should not pressure the patient to answer any questions that they do not want to but can reassure them that their answers will be confidential (E). The physician may have additional questions to ask the patient but you should not leave history items for the physician to address unless the patient requests this (D).

211. C

When circulating substances such as glucose rise to an unhealthy level, the body will attempt to expel the excess via the kidneys. The renal threshold of glucose is 160–180 mg/dl. Glucose found in the urine can be associated with diabetes mellitus or pancreatic pathology. Supernatant (A) is the clear upper portion of a urine specimen that is poured off before staining the remainder for visualization under the microscope. Refractive index (B) is the method in which specific gravity is measured by the refractometer. The refractometer measures the refraction of light through sediment in the liquid. Micturition (D) is the act of voiding or emptying the bladder. After assessing the volume of a 24-hour timed urine specimen, a well-mixed portion called aliquot (E) is removed for testing. The remainder of the specimen is stored or discarded.

212. B

Coumadin is an anticoagulant and causes thinning of the blood. The blood levels must be monitored to ensure there is no abnormal bleeding due to overmedication.

213. C

A fomite is an object that can harbor pathogens such as the exam table, blood pressure cuff, or stethoscope. Disinfection is the method that is used to remove pathogens from the surface of objects (B). A vector is an animal or insect that can transmit disease (A). Ultrasonic sanitization is the method of sanitization that is used on objects that cannot be scrubbed with soap and water (E).

214. D

You should first look for the universal sign of choking: the placement of hands at the throat. You will ask the patient if he is able to speak and will not intervene if the patient is able to speak or cough. If his airway is obstructed, you should place your hands around the victim from behind and make a fist with the thumb side of the first in the space below the ribcage and above the navel. Quick, upward thrusts are made until the object is removed. The patient should not be placed on the floor while he conscious (B). There is no need to check the pulse prior to trying to remove the airway obstruction while the patient is still conscious (C). Checking for a foreign body in the patient's mouth would be inappropriate at this time (A).

215. D

The Ishihara test is used to test colorblindness. Myopia (A) is nearsightedness. Hyperopia (B) is farsightedness. Presbyopia (C) refers to changes in the vision as the eye ages and brings about the need for reading glasses (E).

216. E

You must start over again preparing the sterile field. Any instruments that are in the sterile field must be sanitized and re-sterilized before use. Once the non-sterile item is on the sterile field, the field is contaminated and should be redone.

217. C

Sanitization is the process of using soap and water scrubbing to remove blood and tissue from medical instruments. Asepsis (A) is the absence of disease. Disinfection (B) is the process of removing pathogens from objects. Sterilization (D) is the absence of all living forms from objects. Boiling (E) is a method of disinfection but cannot kill spores.

218. B

The 1-minute time limit was set forth by the Clinical and Laboratory Standards Institute (formerly NCCLS). Leaving the tourniquet on longer than 60 seconds may change the hemoconcentration of certain substances due to the passage of plasma into tissues. Thirty seconds (A) may be considered a safe amount of time but usually does not allow enough time to complete the venipuncture. The remaining choices exceed a safe and effective time limit to have a tourniquet tied in place.

219. E

The correct answer is (E), all of the above. (D) is incorrect, as (A), (B), and (C) are all important considerations if a disaster or disease outbreak occurs.

220. A

This information is found in the social history. This section may also include sexual history, drug use, recreational activities, and present family status. The chief complaint (B) is where you will find the reason for the patient coming to see the doctor this visit. The review of systems (C) is data that is collected as each of the body systems is reviewed and evaluated. Medical history (D) will include the past medical history and immunization history. Family history (E) is the medical status of the patient's family and any genetic or familial illnesses.

221. D

Hydrochlorothizide is a diuretic. Cipro (E) and amoxicillin (A) are both antibiotics. Robitussin (C) is an antitussive. Albuterol (B) is a bronchodilator.

222. A

The condenser is found within the diaphragm of the microscope and is responsible for collecting and concentrating light rays onto the object on the slide. The stage is responsible for holding and moving the slide (B). The iris is responsible for controlling the amount of light focused on the object (C). The coarse and fine adjustments will bring the object into focus (D). Water evaporation (E) is not a function of the microscope.

223. C

Disturbance in vision, headache, difficulty in speaking or understanding spoken words, and weakness on one side of the body are all signs of neurological problems. Referred pain from a heart attack can be experienced in the back, shoulder, arms, jaw, and abdomen.

224. E

The yellow-stoppered tube contains sodium polyanetholesulfonate and is used for blood cultures. When a yellow-stoppered tube is among the tubes to be used in a blood draw, it is always drawn first, so the other four choices (A, B, C, and D) are incorrect. The purpose of the order of draw is to prevent mixing and potential contamination of additives.

225. D

Waived tests have been approved by the FDA for home use or are simple lab exams and procedures that have insignificant risk of error. Pregnancy tests are low complexity tests that can be performed in a clinical laboratory or by a patient at home. Microscopic examination of urine (A) is considered a moderate-complexity test that requires laboratory equipment such as the centrifuge, microscope, specialized stain, and urine specimen slides. Gram staining (B) is a moderate-complexity test. Blood chemistry (C) is a moderate-complexity test. Pap smear (E) is considered a high-complexity test.

226. C

The normal respiratory rate for an adult is 12 to 20 breaths per minute.

227. C

The first thing that you should do is check to make sure the autoclave process was successful by checking the indicator tape or strips in bags. The packs should be marked before being put in the autoclave (D). Placing the newly sterilized packs under the older ones (A) and discarding outdated packs (B) are things to be done, but not until you are sure that the packs have been sterilized. Once a pack is sterilized, it is sterile for 28 days, as long as it remains intact.

228. E

Prozac is used to treat depression. Lanoxin (A) is a cardiotonic medication. Lasix (B) is a diuretic. Potassium chloride (C) is frequently prescribed in addition to Lasix, which can deplete the potassium in the body. Lisinopril (D) is a medication given to control blood pressure.

229. C

It is very important for the medical assistant to be prepared for an office emergency by reviewing the office policies about emergencies and making sure that she is familiar with all the available equipment that might be used in an emergency. The medical assistant must do this when she is new to an area and not rely on more experienced staff or emergency services to respond to situations (B). While it is a good idea to make a phone list and to keep policies in an area where they can be reached easily (E), this does not replace the need to be familiar with policies and emergency equipment.

230. C

Tubular gauze is a bandage that is placed over areas that are hard to bandage. Bandages hold dressings in place, maintain even pressure, support, and protect a wound from contamination or further injury. All other examples are dressings.

231. E

Sensitivity testing involves the use of the disc-diffusion method. Commercially prepared discs with known concentrations of various antibiotics are dropped on the surface of a solid culture medium in the Petri plate inoculated with the pathogen. If the pathogen is "sensitive" to an antibiotic, there is a clear or kill zone without bacterial growth around the disc. Blood agar (A) is a common additive to Petri dishes serving as a culture medium. Culturing (B) involves inoculating the specimen on a Petri dish or other growth medium and incubating at favorable temperatures that allow for optimal growth. Morphology (C) is the study of a microorganism's shape. Liquid culture medium (D) can be utilized to keep a specimen alive until it reaches the lab or can be processed.

232. D

A "blind" weight is done when you do not want the patient to know exactly what their weight is. This may be done if the patient is anorexic or overly concerned about weight gain during pregnancy so that the patient will not decrease their intake due to an increase in weight according to the scale. It is inappropriate not to record a weight in the chart (A) or to ask a patient to weigh himself at home and not weigh them at the office (B). Patients who are in danger of rapid weight gain due to fluid retention may be asked to weigh themselves at home and report weight gain of more than two pounds in one day to prevent complications of their disease.

233. B

Each practice should evaluate its unique patient population and specialty areas of practice to determine which forms of patient emergencies are most likely to occur during office hours. Directing very sick patients to the emergency room (ER) (A) is not always a proper use of ER services. A physician may not always be available in the medical office (C), so this answer is also incorrect. While having a first aid kit (D) is helpful, it may not meet the needs of more critical emergency situations—such as cardiac arrest—that can occur in a medical office. Poison control contact information (E) is also effective only in a certain type of emergency and is not the correct answer.

234. D

Choice (D), sending patients to the emergency room, would NOT be an approach used by medical practice offices during a large-scale act of bioterrorism, and the practice office should be able to make this diagnosis. (A) is incorrect, as offices would be in communication with local public health offices in this situation. (B) is incorrect, as offices should provide vaccines or immunizations, as needed. (C) is incorrect, as offices should know what signs and symptoms of diseases to look for to properly respond in a bioterrorism attack. (E) is incorrect, as offices would need to ensure patient and staff safety by proper infection control and hazardous waste disposal during a bioterrorism occurrence.

235. B

The Snellen test is used to screen for visual acuity. The eye chart is read by the patient from a distance of 20 feet and the results are compared to the normal findings of 20/20 vision. An accucheck will give blood sugar results (A). Ability to hear vibratory sound is called the Rinne test (C). Ability to distinguish color is measured by the Ishihara test (E).

236. B

The occluded airway would receive the first priority, as the body is unable to go without available oxygen for more than a few minutes before brain damage will occur. It will always be the priority situation when there is a medical problem.

237. B

The medical assistant must make sure that the patient understands the procedure that will be done and has had her questions about the procedure answered before signing the consent. The medical assistant can then have the patient sign the form and witness the signature (D). If the patient has not had the benefits and risks (A) and any alternative treatments available (E) explained or has further questions (C), the medical assistant must refer the patient back to the physician and have the patient sign the consent after this is done.

238. D

Littauer scissors are fashioned with a hook to make it easier to pick up the suture and cut it. Bandage scissors (E) are fashioned in order to cut clothing and dressings without cutting skin. Mayo scissors (B) are a type of operating scissors. A Senn retractor (C) is used to hold back tissue in an incision and a Kelly hemostat (A) is used to clamp and hold tissue.

239. D

The medical assistant would want to wear gloves when cleaning up the spill, but they would not need to be sterile gloves (E). It is appropriate to clean up the spill with a disposable paper towel and to place the paper towel in the biohazardous waste as it is unclear what the spill is. It is not appropriate to ask the patient what the spill is (A). It should be placed in the biohazard garbage, as it is unclear as to what the spill is. It should not be left for someone else to clean up (C) but would be appropriate for you to disinfect the area of the floor, or ask a housekeeper to do this if one is available after the spill is cleaned up. (B) fails to mention the use of gloves in the cleanup of an unknown liquid. It may be a bodily fluid and thus biohazardous.

240. C

Antibiotic treatment is not used for viral infections unless there is a secondary bacterial infection. The viral infection can be spread in a number of ways, including droplets (A). It may resolve quickly or can last for the lifetime of the patient (B). Tuberculosis is caused by a bacterial infection (D). While vaccinations are available for some viruses, they are not for all (E).

241. B

Generic and brand name medications must have the same active ingredients. Drug doses are calculated based on a body weight of 150 pounds (A). The effect will be increased or decreased if the weight is more or less than 150 pounds. The elderly and the young may be more sensitive to medication than adults are (D). The difference in the fat-to-muscle ratio of body composition between males and females (C) may make a difference in drug action.

242. D

Autoclaved items are considered sterile for 28 days. After that time, they must not be used and must be re-sterilized. They must be repackaged in the appropriate manner in order to make sure that the sterilization cycle has been effective.

243. E

Symptoms of insulin shock or low blood sugar is sudden and symptoms include diaphoresis, tremulousness, confusion, hunger, and tachycardia. Hyperglycemia or diabetic coma come on slowly and cause lethargy, thirst, rapid and weak pulse, and a fruity or acetone odor to the breath.

244. A

The correct answer is (A). The best way to prepare for a patient emergency is to have an emergency plan and protocol in the office. (B) is incorrect, as practices regularly treat seriously ill patients. (C) is incorrect, as many offices are not located near hospital emergency rooms. (D) is incorrect, as it is not practical to disperse patients in the office during the emergency. (E) is incorrect, because it is useful only for a narrow range of patient emergency situations, such as cardiac arrest.

245. C

The medical assistant should take a careful allergy history from the patient so that the possibility of an allergic reaction can be minimized. The medical assistant would not administer a test dose (A). While medication used in the past is useful for information, the same medication may not be appropriate for this procedure (B). The patient will not be sedated or put to sleep for a minor procedure, so a person to drive would not be necessary for that reason (D).

246. A

The knee-chest position is used for proctologic exams and sigmoidoscopy. The patient is positioned on his knees with the chest on the exam table. The patient is on the exam table on his knees, in a bowing position with the chest down, leaning on his elbows or hands. Vaginal exams are usually performed in the lithotomy position (B). Exams of the chest and the upper torso are best accomplished in the Fowler's position (C). This position is also used for patients who have difficulty breathing (D). Trendelenburg position is used for patients that have hypotension (E).

247. B

Lithotomy is the standard position for a vaginal exam. Sims position (C) is on the left side and usually used for rectal exams. Prone (A) is lying face down. Both Fowler's (D) and semi-Fowler's (E) position the patient in the sitting position with the head up and are frequently used to aid respiratory effort.

248. E

You should first reposition the airway to make sure that it is not occluded by tissue in the respiratory tract. After the airway has been opened using a jaw-thrust method, you should check again to see if there are breathing efforts (E). If not, then you would give rescue breaths and then check the circulation (A). It is inappropriate to start CPR before checking the carotid pulse (C). The pulse is not checked until you have assessed the breathing situation. Rolling the patient onto the left side into the rescue position is not appropriate if the patient is not breathing (B).

249. B

Sterile packs that have been damaged in any way must be discarded or unwrapped and re-sterilized. They can be damaged by water, dropping them onto the floor, or any break in the packaging. Sterile packs are good for 28 days. Packs that will expire the earliest should be used first. Sterile packs may be sealed in plastic to extend the time that they may be used, but this must be done at the time of sterilization and not when they are due to be re-sterilized. The sterile packs are considered sterile until they are opened for use or contaminated in some way.

250. A

Placing sutures is the one procedure listed that must be performed with sterile gloves in a normal situation. All other scenarios necessitate the use of non-sterile exam gloves and are not sterile procedures.

251. B

The normal range for specific gravity of urine is between 1.003 and 1.030. Most urine samples fall between the range of 1.010 and 1.025 making (B) the correct choice. The specific gravity of distilled water is 1.000 (A). Specific gravity measurements above 1.030 (C, D, and E) exceed the normal range and may indicate severe UTI, dehydration (associated with fever or prolonged vomiting and diarrhea), congestive heart failure, adrenal dysfunction, or hepatic disease.

252. B

Capillary or micropipettes are small glass or plastic tubes designed to hold a measured amount of blood. These tubes are used primarily for hematocrit determination. The tube is placed at the edge of the blood droplet and fills through capillary action. Microcollection (A) or microtainer tubes are small plastic tubes that have a wider opening that allows blood to flow quickly into the tube. These tubes have different-colored tops that correspond to the additives they contain. Reagent tubes (C) are a distracter. There is no such item. Serum separator tubes (D) are tubes utilized for the vacuum method of venipuncture. Evacuated glass tubes (E) are used for venipuncture if a large sample of blood is needed.

253. C

Aricept is administered for mild to moderate Alzheimer's disease, which you would not expect to be ordered for a 52-year-old patient. Premarin (A) and Provera (B) are female hormones. Calcium citrate (D) and multivitamins (E) may be ordered to prevent bone loss and vitamin deficiency.

254. B

Bleach and water mixed in a 1:10 solution makes a cheap and very effective disinfectant solution.

255. C

The tuning fork is used to screen for hearing acuity and bone conduction of sound and results and can lead to further testing for the patient. The tuning fork is struck on the palm of the hand of the practitioner, which causes it to vibrate. The tuning fork emits a low frequency sound and vibration that can be felt and heard by the patient. An otoscope (A) is used to examine the inside of the ear canal. The ophthalmoscope (B) is used to look at the structure of the eye. The Snellen test (D) measures visual acuity. The reflex hammer (E) is used for neurological testing of reflexes.

256. D

When performing the CCMS or midvoid specimen collection, females should clean the urinary meatus from *front to back* to avoid contaminating the area. The most common urinary contaminant is *E. coli* from the anal opening. Students often misread this choice. Removing the undergarments (A) allows for freedom of movement and accessibility of the area. The patient should not touch the inside of the container (B) to avoid contamination of the specimen. Female patients should continue to hold the labia apart (C) ensuring that the cleansed area does not become contaminated during urination. Touching the specimen container (E) leads to contamination and erroneous test results.

257. B

You should suspect a problem with the patient's blood glucose. By giving a form of glucose, you may fix the immediate problem. Even if the blood glucose is high, it will not do any damage and if the blood glucose is low, the patient will improve. Once glucose is given, you should immediately draw a blood sugar or do an accucheck (C). This will confirm the blood sugar. It would not be appropriate to spend time questioning the patient if he is confused and disoriented (E). The vital signs would be checked after these steps would be taken (A). If the patient is conscious, it would not be appropriate to check for respirations (D).

258. B

You would not expect to do a lung biopsy in the office as a minor procedure. Minor procedures are done for superficial lesions, cyst removal, suture of lacerations, and incision and drainage of superficial wounds. These procedures have little chance of major complications.

259. A

The sounds that are heard when the blood pressure is being auscultated using a stethoscope and a sphygmomanometer are called the Korotkoff sounds. Rinne (B) is the name of a test of hearing. The Snellen (C), Jeager (E), and Isahara (D) tests are all names of eye exams.

260. B

The popliteal pulse is located behind the knee and most easily located by bending the knee and palpating in the crease behind the knee joint. The radial pulse is located on the thumb side of the wrist (A). The dorsalis pedis is located on the dorsal surface of the foot (C). The apical pulse is located at the apex of the heart (D). The femoral pulse is located in the inner aspect of the leg at the groin (E).

261. C

While all of these things are important, hand washing is the single most effective thing that you can do to prevent the spread of infectious material. Hand washing can be accomplished with soap and water or with an alcohol-based hand sanitizer. Good hand wash practices will prevent the spread of pathogens between patients.

262. B

First-voided morning urine specimens contain the greatest concentration of certain substances. This specimen is utilized for pregnancy testing, nitrite and protein determination, bacterial culture, and microscopic examination.

Most urinalysis is performed on freshly voided random (A) urine samples collected in clean containers. A clean-catch midstream specimen (C) may be collected if a bacterial infection is suspected. An untainted specimen is needed for urine culture. The only other method of collection for a noncontaminated specimen is through catheterization. A 24-hour specimen (D) is utilized for quantitative chemical analysis such as hormone levels. Second-voided specimens (E) are usually collected to test for glucose levels.

263. **D**

The object should be assessed prior to the lift so you have a plan and can ask for help if you are unable to lift it alone. You should not try to lift an object if you have any doubts about its size or your ability. You should always bend at the knees and keep the back straight with the load close to the body. Never lift a heavy object that is located above your base of support. It is always better to ask for assistance or use assistive equipment to prevent injury to yourself.

264. **E**

The soiled paper should be gathered inward and away from clothing to prevent contamination of clothing. The exam table must be cleaned with disinfectant prior to pulling down the unused paper. Gloves should be changed between cleaning the table and pulling down the unused paper to prevent recontamination of the clean area.

265. **C**

The brachial artery is the preferred pulse site in the infant. If circulation is limited, the peripheral pulses such as the radial (B) or temporal (E) may not be palpable. The body fat composition of the infant may make it difficult to find the carotid (A) and femoral (D) pulses. The brachial artery is easily accessible as it is located in the inner aspect of the upper arm.

266. **B**

Lipitor's generic name is altorvastatin calcium. Atenolol (A) is the generic for Tenormin. Plavix is the trade name for clopidogrel bisulfate (C) and furosemide (D) is the generic for Lasix. Amlodipine (E) is the generic name for Norvasc.

267. **A**

It is normal for a person to be confused and very drowsy after a seizure. Usually there is no problem with the airway (D) after the seizure unless the patient has vomited. If this occurs, rolling the patient to the side will usually take care of this. You would expect the pulse rate and blood pressure to be elevated (C) due to the muscle activity. Immediate transfer to the hospital (E) should not be necessary unless the patient has never had a seizure, has repeated seizures, or does not regain consciousness.

268. **B**

Fowler's position is sitting upright and is the most appropriate for patients who have respiratory problems. Trendelenberg's position (A) is the head lower than the rest of the body and is used most frequently for hypotension or shock. Lithotomy position (C) is used for vaginal examination. Dorsal recumbent (D) is lying on the back with legs bent and up on the same level as the body. Prone (E) is lying flat on the abdomen.

269. **C**

The hepatic vein is a large, deep vessel responsible for draining the digestive tract and liver. The median cubital vein (A) is the most common vein utilized for venipuncture. This vessel serves as a connection between the cephalic and the basilic veins and is less likely to roll. The brachial vein (B) is located on the medial aspect of the upper arm and may be utilized for venipuncture. The cephalic vein (D) is located on the lateral aspect of the arm and is a good choice for phlebotomy. The basilic vein (E) extends from the median basilic vein up the inside of the arm. This vessel tends to roll and the medial assistant must anchor it well.

270. **C**

A nonsterile person who enters the room but does not approach the sterile field will not interfere with the sterile field in a minor procedure. Members of the sterile team should have their hair pulled back (B) and should avoid talking over the sterile field (A). Once a nonsterile item is added to the field, it is considered contaminated (D). A tear in the glove must be changed immediately in order to prevent contamination of the sterile field (E).

271. **C**

The primary function of draping is to preserve the privacy and dignity of the patient. Draping is done differently for different exams (E) but the patient should be adequately covered no matter what the position is. Draping material may be helpful in keeping the undressed patient comfortable (B) but if the patient is cold, the room temperature should be adjusted. While convenience of the medical staff is important (A and D), it is not the primary reason for draping.

272. B

The correct level for the arm to be is at or near heart level. The cuff must be the correct fit for the patient's arm. Markings are on the cuff for minimum and maximum arm size. If the fit is not correct, you will not receive an accurate reading. Normally you cannot hear any sound when the stethoscope is placed on the brachial artery. The cuff should be positioned so that the artery marking is at the brachial artery. The air should be released slowly so you do not miss the beginning sounds.

273. B

Anaphylactic shock is due to a severe allergic reaction and a massive immune response by the body. It causes difficulty breathing and swelling of the respiratory tract. There can also be cardiovascular symptoms such as hypotension and cardiovascular collapse. It can be fatal. An asthma attack (E) will cause difficulty breathing but is a chronic condition usually controlled by medication. Cardiogenic shock (D) is caused by inability of the cardiac system to pump enough blood to supply the body and does not cause swelling of the respiratory system. A myocardial infarction (A) is a heart attack. Obstructive airway disease (C) is a chronic condition of the respiratory system.

274. C

Induration is an indication of TB exposure but not necessarily disease; follow-up testing is necessary for diagnosis. The other four choices (A, B, D, and E) are all true statements regarding tuberculin testing.

275. C

The reagent strips should be held horizontally to avoid chemical reagents from each testing pad from mixing. This may cause aberrant color changes and give questionable results. Holding the testing strips vertically will also allow urine to drip onto the medical assistant's hand. Recapping the testing strip bottle quickly (A) helps preserve the integrity of the testing strips. The testing strips are sensitive to light, heat, and moisture. Touching the testing the strips with your fingers (B) may influence the effectiveness of the chemical reagents, giving false results. The testing strips need complete immersion into the urine sample (D). Discolored strips should be discarded (E). Multistix strip results are determined by assessing color changes to the reagent pads when in contact with urine.

276. C

Zoloft is from the antidepressant category, which is used to treat depression. All of the other choices are antianxiety medications, although they are used for depression in certain cases.

277. E

Ordinarily a speculum would not be needed for a simple cyst removal. The scalpel (A) would be used to cut the skin. The Senn retractor (C) would be used to pull the skin back after the incision is made. The needle holder (B) would be used to suture the incision after the surgery is done and the dressing forceps (D) would be used to apply the dressing after the procedure is done.

278. E

By asking open-ended questions, you allow the patient to answer fully and you may get more information that will in turn make the interview go more quickly. If you appear to be in a hurry (D), the patient may not offer important information. Yes and no answers (A) will not allow the patient to answer fully. Not all elderly are hard of hearing (C) nor do they need family to answer questions for them (B). This can offend the patient, which will affect the amount of information that you get from them.

279. D

Human chorionic gonadotropin hormone (hCG) is produced by the placenta and presents in the urine during pregnancy. After implantation of the fertilized egg in the uterus, the hCG levels in serum double every few days. This occurs for about 7 weeks and then begins to decline. Pregnancy tests can detect the presence of hCG as early as 1 week after implantation or 4 to 5 days before a missed menstrual period. Human growth hormone (B) is released by the anterior pituitary gland. The purpose of this hormone is to stimulate musculoskeletal growth. Antidiuretic hormone (A) is released from the posterior pituitary gland. The hormone acts to control the body's fluid balance. Heterphile antibody (C) is released into bloodstream in a patient with infectious mononucleosis and can be detected within 6 to 10 days of illness in an individual. Phenylketonuria (E) is an inherited condition in which a baby lacks phenylalanine, an essential enzyme necessary to metabolize amino acids.

280. B

Trendelenburg positioning places the patient's head lower than the body and raises the lower extremities. This helps to raise the blood pressure. Fowler's position (E) raises the head at a 90-degree angle and is used to ease respiratory problems. Lithotomy position (C) is usually used for vaginal exams. Prone (A) is lying face downward. Supine (D) is lying on the back.

281. B

The correct dosage is 250 mg. It is calculated by dividing the 75-lb. weight of the child by the 150-lb. weight of the adult (which would be 1/2), and then multiplying 1/2 by the 500-mg dosage.

282. B

While all of these factors could influence the tracing, the status of the patient is the first variable that should be checked to make sure that there is not a significant problem.

283. D

For a surgical hand wash, you would hold your fingers higher than your elbows so that water runs off the elbow area instead of the hands. This is opposite of the way that you do with a medical hand wash (B). A 60-second wash (A) would be appropriate for aseptic technique, not surgical technique. You must dry your hands with a sterile towel (C). Ideally you will have foot controls for the water but if you do not, you should turn off the water with the sterile towel after you have dried your hands and do not touch the faucet with your bare hands (E).

284. C

Lyme disease is a bacterial disease that initially causes a rash with a characteristic bull's eye and flu symptoms. If the symptoms are mild, the infection may be missed and not treated with antibiotic therapy. It then continues as a chronic infection and affects the musculoskeletal and nervous systems.

285. C

Application of ice to the area would be the first treatment, along with rest and elevation of the ankle. Exercise (B) is inappropriate as it might cause further injury at the time of the injury. Massage (D) would also be inappropriate at this time for the same reason. Ice (C) will decrease the circulation to the area, which will decrease bleeding into damaged tissues. The ice will also decrease pain. It should only be applied in 20-minute intervals to prevent cold injury to the tissues. Heat is applied only after 48 hours has passed after the injury (A). Application of an air cast (E) may be appropriate after the assessment is done but not as an initial treatment.

286. B

Nitrites occur in urine when bacteria convert or reduce nitrates to nitrites. A sufficient amount of incubation time in the bladder must pass for this conversion to take place. A positive reagent strip test may indicate the presence of a bacterial urinary tract infection. *Escherichia coli* bacterium is the most common cause of UTIs and can reduce nitrate to nitrite. Glucose (A) present in a urine sample would signify the body's inability to process carbohydrates. Ketones (C) are by-products of fat metabolism in the body and include three types: beta hydroxybutyric, acetoacetic acid, and acetone. Ketosis occurs when fat is used for energy and the muscles cannot handle the accumulation of ketones. The ketones will accrue in the body tissues and fluids. Ketonuria is observed with diabetes mellitus, low-carbohydrate diets, excessive vomiting, and starvation. Bilirubin (D) is a bile pigment not normally found in urine. Bilirubinuria is an indication of liver disease and can result from gallstones, hepatitis, and cirrhosis. Urine becomes yellow-brown or greenish and foam appears when shaken. Protein (E) should not be detected in the urine. Proteinuria is one of the first signs of renal disease. Protein excretion in high amount can be caused by unusually high stress or strenuous exercise.

287. B

Palpation is using the fingers to feel the pulse. Usually the radial artery is used in the adult patient for a routine pulse rate. A stethoscope (A) would be used in a young child or infant. The temporal pulse is located in the temporal area of the skull (C). The carotid pulse is located in the side of the neck and usually used in emergencies and to evaluate the effectiveness of CPR (D). The femoral pulse is located in the groin (E).

288. A

By placing the indicator strips in the bags and packs and using autoclave tape to secure packs, the medical assistant will be able to make sure that the instruments are sterile and ready to use in a sterile procedure. It is not necessary to open a pack and check it (C). The time needed to make sure that a pack is sterile is dependent upon the manufacturers' instructions and the material that you are sterilizing (B). It is not appropriate to leave an open area in the pack (D). You should not remove the packs from the autoclave until the drying cycle is over (E). Moisture will encourage the migration of pathogens.

289. B

Supine positioning requires the patient to lie on his back. Prone (A) requires the patient to lie face down. Oblique (C) positioning has the patient at an angle to the radiogram. Lateral (D) imaging is taking the picture from the side of the patient. Posteroanterior (E) allows the x-ray beam to penetrate the patient from back to front.

290. B

A level less than 200 mg/dl is desirable. Cholesterol is necessary in the body for several reasons. A level of 0 mg/dl (A) would be detrimental to the body. Levels 200–239 mg/dl are considered borderline high (C). Levels of 240 mg/dl and above are considered high (D and E).

291. A

Surgical asepsis is removing all organisms prior to entering the body. This is done by using sterile technique and sterile instruments in a procedure. Medical asepsis (C) is disposing of organisms after they leave the body, as in the correct disposal of biohazardous waste. Sterilization (B) is the removal of all organisms from objects, not people. Sanitization (E) is the removal of debris from objects. Personal protective equipment or PPE are items such as gloves, masks, gowns, and eye protection (D).

292. C

Equipment that serves as protection for health care workers is called personal protective equipment. This includes gowns, gloves, face masks, eye protection, shields, and hair and shoe covers.

293. A

An elastic or ACE wrap is an example of bandaging. The function of bandaging in this case would be to provide even pressure and support to the ankle by applying a bandage made of elastic cloth.

294. B

A 15-degree angle is optimal for placing the needle in the center of the selected vein. A 5-degree angle (A) is utilized when seating the needle during placement of a butterfly-winged infusion device. A 30-degree angle (C) is too much for venipuncture. This angle may cause the needle to go through the vein by puncturing the posterior wall resulting in a hematoma. A 45-degree angle (D) is utilized for subcutaneous injections. A 90-degree angle (E) is utilized during an intramuscular injection.

295. A

Staphylo- is a Greek term that denotes "bunch of grapes." *Staphylococci* are round bacteria that grow in grapelike clusters. *Neisseria meningitidis* (B) is a gram-negative bacterium. *Mycobacterium tuberculosis* (C) has a straight, curved, or branched rod shape and requires an acid-fast stain. *Escherichia coli* (D) is a gram-negative bacillus. *Streptococcus pneumoniae* (E) is a gram-positive bacterium, but this species grows in chains.

296. A

A scraping of the superficial layer of skin is called an abrasion. An avulsion (B) is a flap of skin that is forcibly torn or separated. A laceration (C) is a jagged or irregular tear of the tissues due to trauma. An incision (D) is a clean cut with a sharp object. A contusion (E) is an injury involving bleeding into the tissues without breaking the skin.

297. B

You should wash the skin with an antiseptic soap in a circular manner from the inside to the outside, not going back once you have moved further out. Up and down (A) is inappropriate direction. You would not use alcohol (C) or a disinfectant solution (E), and sterile gloves (D) are not necessary for this procedure.

KAPLAN

298. C

Venereal disease research laboratory (VDRL) and rapid plasma regain (RPR) are both serological tests that detect syphilis. Hepatitis (A) detection utilizes a serological test. Mononucleosis (B) testing detects the heterophil antibody within 6 to 10 days of the disease. Rheumatoid arthritis (D) can be detected by testing for rheumatoid factor. Systemic lupus (E) diagnosis requires antinucleotide antibody.

299. E

If a tear is noted, the assistant needs to replace the gloves. Putting tape over the tear (A) will not restore sterility. Continuing the procedure (D) is an unlikely option since most procedures require two hands. Involving a coworker (C) is unnecessary in a routine procedure. Alerting the physician (B) may not be needed if the physician is present for the procedure.

300. E

Hemoglobin is measured by weight and is expressed in grams per deciliter (g/dl). A spirometer (A) is a device used to measure lung capacity by tracking the volume and flow of exhaled air. The specific gravity of urine (B) is part of the physical examination of urine. Erythrocyte sedimentation rate, or ESR (C), measures the time it takes for red blood cells to settle in a specimen and is expressed in millimeters per hour (mm/hr); elevated times are associated with inflammatory processes. Hematocrit (D) is measured after centrifuging a specimen and is expressed as a percentage of red blood cells in a specimen; normal adult hematocrit values are 36–55 percent.

PART FIVE

Resources

Employment Resources

If you will be graduating from a Medical Assistant program soon or recently graduated, you are entering a challenging transition period as you seek a setting where you might want to work. This section discusses the job-seeking process and steps you'll need to take to present yourself well to prospective employers.

ESTABLISHING A PERMANENT CREDENTIALS FILE

Applying for positions involves not only completing application forms and sending cover letters, but also preparing and sending your professional resume to prospective employers. Other documents you'll want to keep safe and handy for the application process include:

- School transcripts
- Copies of letters of recommendation
- A list of references and their contact information
- Any other certifications related to clinical practice, such as basic or advanced life-support training, certifications of proficiency on medical apparatus, EMT certification, etc.

As time passes, you should update your resume to keep it current, rather than having to write a new one years from now when you decide to change positions. Storing it electronically will help you update it easily. Also, many employers now routinely ask candidates to email their application documents or apply on the employer website rather than using the U.S. Postal Service.

WRITING YOUR PROFESSIONAL RESUME

This is an important document in obtaining a position, so it should be carefully drafted and then shared with experienced reviewers for feedback before finalizing. There are commercial services that will help you prepare a resume, but the cost tends to be high and using this type of service is not necessary if you are willing to spend the time to develop your own.

Scrutinize a Sample Version

There are published guides to writing resumes, many containing useful examples that will show what a good resume contains and how it should be formatted. If you are still in school, you may want to ask Student Affairs staff or a faculty advisor if they have some examples you can look at.

Once you have looked at some good example resumes, note how they are organized using headings such as Educational Experience, Work Experience, Honors, Research Experience, Publications & Presentations, and Other Interests. These headings make it easier for employers to review a candidate's qualifications quickly. Another aspect to note is that within each category, entries are listed from most recent to least recent (i.e., in reverse chronology).

Piece Together Your Information

At this point, you are ready to begin jotting down information about your own educational experiences, previous job history, and other medically related activities, such as certifications, volunteer activities, etc. Once you have listed what you might want to include under the major headings, make sure you list starting and ending dates, as well as institution names and locations for each educational experience, work history, and activity you want to include. Follow the formatting and organization of a good example. Once the document has been drafted, scrutinize it very carefully to be sure that it contains no typographic or spelling errors. Then check to ensure that all time intervals are accounted for. Unaccounted-for gaps in time always raise questions in the minds of prospective employers.

RESEARCHING THE JOB MARKET

If you haven't already decided on exactly which factors you want most from a position, it's a good idea to spend some quiet time now thinking about what is most essential to you and what is optional among all the aspects that make up a particular job situation. Some factors to consider include:

- The diversity of the patient mix you want to work with
- The type of clinical setting you prefer (rural or urban, small or large)

A written "wish list" that you create now describing your ideal work situation is a valuable tool. With it, you'll have an easier time of identifying the job elements you feel are must-haves versus those you can be flexible about, helping to select positions you'd like to apply for, and, once the job offers come in, deciding which to accept.

Begin exploring job opportunities through your school's placement or alumni office, state AAMA or AMT chapters, professional organization websites and newsletters, journal classifieds, local classifieds, and any job postings available on the Internet. Medical clinics and hospitals where you did your internship are also good places to begin inquiring about job opportunities.

Do research on employment aspects that will come up repeatedly during job interviews so that you will understand what job benefits are typically offered and what's included in a standard job contract. Have relevant questions to ask potential employers.

Interview Preparation

Contact your school's alumni or placement office to ask if they have materials on interviewing skills or if they have compiled a list of the types of questions you should be prepared to answer at a job interview. Many schools also sponsor or participate in job fairs, which bring graduating students and prospective employers together. If your school doesn't offer these services, ask your student organization to organize a job fair or bring in a speaker from a local health care institution to discuss their interviewing and hiring process. At a minimum, find a good book on interviewing skills. If you want to present yourself well at a job interview, you have to prepare in advance.

Once you have been offered an interview, find out as much as you can about the hiring organization. They may have a website that will tell you a great deal about the clinical services they provide, the patient mix they serve, and any new areas of health research or community outreach in which they are involved. Knowing this kind of information about a prospective employer is extremely useful during the interview; it allows you to appear knowledgeable and also to ask questions specific to their institution's goals and mission. This wins points for any job applicant and increases the chances that you will be offered a position.

Professional Organizations

AMERICAN ASSOCIATION OF MEDICAL ASSISTANTS

Website: aama-ntl.org

This association, formed in 1955, strives to improve health care and protect the rights and improve the careers of CMAs. There are separate organizations related to the American Association of Medical Assistants—the current list of societies with contact information is accessible on the AAMA website.

AMERICAN MEDICAL TECHNOLOGISTS

Website: americanmedtech.org

RMAs also have the opportunity to become involved in state societies. As members of the AMT, RMAs can network, promote their profession, and remain current on medical assisting initiatives.

Case Studies

As a medical assistant, you will have to multitask, perform triage, educate patients, document findings, and think critically. Improving these skills takes a wealth of experience gained over multiple patient and provider encounters. Throughout your education, you likely learned about these skills individually. Putting them into practice together, in a clinical setting, is the next step.

The case studies presented in this section allow you to test your knowledge across multiple aspects of medical assisting at once. Each scenario gives you the opportunity to use critical thinking skills and to incorporate your legal, professional, medical, and administrative knowledge.

Read each case study and the questions that follow. On a separate sheet of paper, write your best answer to each question. At the end of the section, detailed answer explanations will enhance your knowledge about handling real-life situations such as these. As you review each answer explanation, take note of the medical assisting content areas in which you missed any questions. You may need additional study time in those areas to prepare for your credentialing examination.

Case Study #1: Did I Do That?

Sally Carter is a 60-year-old woman with a family history of melanoma. She takes daily doses of Synthroid and Minipress, plus a daily vitamin. Ms. Carter is scheduled to come to the office for the removal of a mole located inferior to the left mid-scapula. The day before Ms. Carter's 9:00 AM appointment, the medical assistant calls to instruct her to have nothing to eat or drink after midnight, avoid taking all medications, and wear loose clothing. The MA also reviews instructions and checks all chart documentation.

When Ms. Carter arrives at the office, the MA sets up the sterile field and then accompanies Ms. Carter from the waiting room to the treatment room, where the MA obtains her TPR, BP, and weight. The MA then provides Ms. Carter a gown, instructs her to put the opening in the back, and leaves the treatment room. Once Ms. Carter is gowned, the MA returns and assists her into a supine position. Dr. Iacono enters the room and undertakes the scheduled procedure.

Based on this scenario, answer the following questions.

1. What is melanoma?

2. Evaluate the MA's instructions when reminding Ms. Carter of the appointment. What could be improved?

3. The MA put Ms. Carter in the supine position. Why was this the incorrect position, and what position should have been used?

4. What principle of sterile procedure did the MA violate?

5. Who is responsible for obtaining informed consent from the patient?

Case Study #2: See No Evil, Hear No Evil, Speak No Evil

Gabby McGowan has been an established patient at Dr. Vladich's office for many years. Ms. McGowan knows all the medical assistants and loves to stand at the front desk and socialize when she arrives for an appointment. The office is arranged so patients sign in at the front window on a sheet listing their name and time of arrival. When a patient signs in and is checked in by the front desk MA, her name is crossed off. Also located in the office area are the telephones where two MAs manage incoming calls. Finally, there is a sliding glass window at the front office.

Ms. McGowan stands at the desk chatting with the front desk MA when she overhears a phone MA state, "Ms. Jackson, it sounds like you may have an infection, and you should see the doctor as soon as possible." Ms. McGowan asks, "Was that my neighbor Judy Jackson? I know Judy doesn't do a good job of washing her hands, and I bet she has food poisoning! Is Judy a patient at the office?" In response, the front desk MA states, "That really isn't any of your business." Ms. McGowan walks away from the window and sits next to another patient, complaining about how rude the office staff was to her.

Based on this scenario, answer the following questions.

1. What parts of this front desk setup are means of protecting patient confidentiality?

2. Evaluate the phone MA's interaction with Ms. Jackson. How might it be improved to enhance patient confidentiality?

3. Evaluate the front desk MA's response to Ms. McGowan's inquiry about Ms. Jackson. How might it be improved?

4. What is white noise? What impact might it have in the office setup described in the scenario?

5. Knowing that Ms. McGowan likes to stand at the desk and socialize, what strategies could the MAs incorporate to minimize the risk of sharing information while accommodating her desire to chat?

Case Study #3: This Won't Hurt a Bit

Suzy Stick is a medical assistant working in a medical office laboratory. She collects blood specimens that are sent to the reference lab and CLIA-waived testing. Last week, she asked her supervisor for the day off, but her request was declined due to limited staffing on the day she requested. She reports to work but is not happy. Suzy proceeds to her station to take care of the first patient, Jane. Jane is a 40-year-old woman who hates to have her blood drawn but has agreed to have all the testing done at one time as requested by her provider. She needs specimens drawn for a CBC, lipid profile, and evaluation of clotting factors.

Suzy calls Jane to the lab, prepares the equipment, and asks the patient to extend her right arm. She finds a vein and starts the procedure, following standard precautions. After running into trouble filling all the tubes, Suzy moves the needle. Jane complains of pain and reports feeling weak and sweaty. Suzy responds that it will just be another moment and continues with the process. After filling the tubes, she removes the tourniquet and needle and applies pressure to the site. She applies a bandage within 30 seconds of finishing the draw, dismisses Jane, and continues with her work. At the checkout desk, Jane asks for a release of information form. She wants to transfer to another provider.

Based on this scenario, answer the following questions.

1. Jane is having several lab tests done. What tubes should be used, and what order of draw should be used?

2. What key step did Suzy neglect to do after calling Jane to the lab?

3. What should Suzy have done when Jane reported feeling weak and sweaty?

4. What should the medical assistant at checkout do when Jane asks for a release of information form?

5. What role does a medical assistant serving as the lab supervisor or office manager have when approaching Suzy about this incident?

Case Study #4: A Slip and Fall

James has been a medical assistant in a provider's office for many years. He is considered a leader and mentor for many of the other MAs, and he prides himself on ensuring that the office runs smoothly through preparation and anticipation of provider needs.

Upon arriving at work on a snowy day, James opens the office by disarming the alarm system, turning on the lights, and heading to his workstation to prepare for patients. As patients are escorted to the exam rooms, James notes that the floor is getting wet. Because it is clear this will be an issue throughout the day due to the snow and because he doesn't want the schedule to fall behind, James decides to continue with his usual program of work. Later, James is walking ahead of an elderly patient to show her to the examination room when she slips and falls, complaining of hip pain. James tries to help her up to walk to the room but cannot get her to stand. James summons the provider, and an ambulance is called. It is later determined that the patient has suffered a hip fracture.

Based on this scenario, answer the following questions.

1. What should James have done when he noticed the floor was wet?

2. When calling the elderly patient to the examination room, what else could James have done to ensure her safety?

3. Who is held liable for injuries sustained in the office?

4. What document must James complete to address the accident?

5. James made several mistakes throughout this scenario that endangered patient safety and welfare. Which error was in violation of first aid training?

Case Study Answers and Explanations

Case Study #1: Did I Do That?

1. **What is melanoma?**

   Answer: Melanoma is an aggressive form of skin cancer that can be life-threatening if left untreated. It is mainly caused by ultraviolet radiation and is commonly associated with exposure to the sun's rays and tanning beds.

2. **Evaluate the MA's instructions when reminding Ms. Carter of the appointment. What could be improved?**

   Answer: The following aspects of the MA's instructions could be improved:

   - Instructing the patient to avoid all food is unnecessary because a mole is removed under local anesthetic. Instead, it would be advantageous to suggest a light breakfast or liquids to help the patient avoid nausea.

   - Instructing the patient to avoid taking her regular medications is incorrect. This patient's medications are necessary for thyroid function and blood pressure control and should be taken as usual.

   - Although instructing the patient to wear loose clothing does no harm, it has no benefit either. Since the patient is getting undressed, loose clothing really has no effect on the procedure or preparation.

3. **The MA put Ms. Carter in the supine position. Why was this the incorrect position, and what position should have been used?**

   Answer: In the supine position, the patient is lying on her back. Since Ms. Carter's mole is inferior to the left mid-scapula—that is, on her back—she must be placed on her abdomen in the prone position to allow easy access to the treatment site.

4. **What principle of sterile procedure did the MA violate?**

   Answer: A sterile field that is left unsupervised cannot be guaranteed as free of contamination. Do not turn your back on a sterile field. Although the assistant should gather items together in advance, setup should not occur until the field can be supervised continuously—which is usually immediately before the procedure.

5. **Who is responsible for obtaining informed consent from the patient?**

   Answer: The provider is always responsible for both informing the patient about the procedure's risks and benefits and obtaining signed consent. The MA is able to sign the form as a witness, but this only documents that the MA saw the patient sign his name. The MA is an important member of the team with regard to consent: MAs make sure the patient has had all questions answered and assist in clarifying information as needed.

Case Study #2: See No Evil, Hear No Evil, Speak No Evil

1. **What parts of this front desk setup are means of protecting patient confidentiality?**

   Answer: The privacy window is a good way to prevent unwanted information from being shared outside the administrative area. The medical assistant must ensure that it is kept closed except when a patient is checking in. The sign-in sheet is an acceptable means of checking patients in, as there is no personally identifiable information being shared on this document. Additionally, crossing the name off of the sign-in sheet with a solid marker serves as a means of avoiding sharing patient names.

2. **Evaluate the phone MA's interaction with Ms. Jackson. How might it be improved to enhance patient confidentiality?**

   Answer: It is important to avoid divulging any personally identifiable patient information when speaking on the phone around other patients. The phone MA appropriately addressed the patient and did not use her full name. But because MAs are not qualified to diagnose, telling Ms. Jackson "you may have an infection" was inappropriate. It would have been better to say, "It sounds like you need to see the doctor. I can offer you an appointment."

3. **Evaluate the front desk MA's response to Ms. McGowan's inquiry about Ms. Jackson. How might it be improved?**

   Answer: "That is none of your business" is a confrontational statement that angered Ms. McGowan, who went on to complain to another patient. It is an unprofessional response that reflects poorly on the practice and the MA. When communicating with patients, it is important to present yourself professionally at all times. A better answer to a question like Ms. McGowan's is something like, "I'm not allowed to share that information; we do our very best to protect the privacy and confidentiality of all our patients." This response is less intimidating and could even comfort the patient asking the question, because it shows that the office will protect her privacy as well.

4. **What is white noise? What impact might it have in the office setup described in the scenario?**

   Answer: White noise is background noise, such as soft music, that can be used in an office to obscure the conversations held in patient areas. Used in combination with other security measures (such as keeping the window closed when not working with patients), white noise can help minimize breaches of patient confidentiality.

5. **Knowing that Ms. McGowan likes to stand at the desk and socialize, what strategies could the MAs incorporate to minimize the risk of sharing information while accommodating her desire to chat?**

   Answer: Scheduling strategies are often beneficial. For instance, scheduling Ms. McGowan at the end of the day or at a time when her wait will likely be short may be helpful. Offering a nice greeting to Ms. McGowan, having a short conversation when she arrives, and then inviting her to have a seat while waiting presents an expectation and overall positive direction that doesn't lead to intimidation and defensiveness. It is also beneficial to acknowledge Ms. McGowan and wish her well as she leaves the office. This shows concern for her as a patient and leaves her with a good feeling about the practice.

Case Study #3: This Won't Hurt a Bit

1. **Jane is having several lab tests done. What tubes should be used, and what order of draw should be used?**

    Answer: Three tubes will be drawn. The CBC requires a lavender tube, the clotting factors require a light blue tube, and the lipid profile requires the tiger-stoppered tube (also known as serum separator tube). The order of draw should be: first, the light blue–stoppered tube; next, the tiger-stoppered tube; and finally, the lavender-stoppered tube.

2. **What key step did Suzy neglect to do after calling Jane to the lab?**

    Answer: Patient identity must always be confirmed. The MA should have asked the patient to state her name.

3. **What should Suzy have done when Jane reported feeling weak and sweaty?**

    Answer: Jane reported symptoms of syncope; she was at risk of fainting. Suzy should have made the patient's health and safety the top priority and immediately removed the tourniquet and needle to care for her. Moving the needle around in the arm is not an acceptable practice, and it is possible that the resulting pain caused the patient's reaction. Responding to patient signs and symptoms are the priority in this situation. Finally, before dismissing Jane, Suzy should have ensured that Jane was feeling better.

4. **What should the medical assistant at checkout do when Jane asks for a release of information form?**

    Answer: While it is important to comply with the patient's request, the medical assistant also needs to consider what may be the underlying cause of this request. In this situation, the MA should tell Jane she is sorry to see her leaving the practice and ask if there is a concern she can help with. If Jane is willing to share the reason for her frustration and sudden choice to transfer to another provider, the MA should refer her to the office manager for a more detailed conversation.

5. **What role does a medical assistant serving as the lab supervisor or office manager have when approaching Suzy about this incident?**

    Answer: All health care professionals must take care to prevent personal issues from interfering with their work duties. Suzy was obviously unhappy about being required to work; her attitude might have affected her customer service. It is the supervisor's responsibility to counsel Suzy on her actions and issue a verbal warning if this is Suzy's first performance incident. If a similar incident has occurred in the past, a written warning may be required—or even suspension or dismissal, depending on office policies and procedures.

Case Study #4: A Slip and Fall

1. **What should James have done when he noticed the floor was wet?**

    Answer: The medical assistant is responsible for maximizing patient safety. James should have cleaned up the wet floor, placed a "Caution: Wet Floor" marker at the site, and also placed a wet floor marker at the door to alert patients. These actions make sure safety is maximized. Clearing outside sidewalks of snow would also reduce the amount of snow tracked into the office.

2. **When calling the elderly patient to the examination room, what else could James have done to ensure her safety?**

    Answer: Again, safety is the key issue. Any patient who needs assistance should receive it. James failed to recognize that an elderly person may need an extra arm to hold on to or a device such as a cane or walker. A family member may also help if warranted. Simply asking the patient if she would like assistance or offering his arm for stability may have prevented this fall.

3. **Who is held liable for injuries sustained in the office?**

    Answer: The provider or owner of the office is held liable for negligence under the doctrine of *respondeat superior* ("let the master answer"). This incident could possibly be considered an act of nonfeasance, or failure to do something to prevent injury.

4. **What document must James complete to address the accident?**

    Answer: James will need to fill out an incident report that objectively describes the incident without adding anything personal. It should clearly state the date, time, and location of the incident and an objective account of what happened.

5. **James made several mistakes throughout this scenario that endangered patient safety and welfare. Which error was in violation of first aid training?**

    Answer: One should never move a patient who may be injured before determining the potential extent of the injury. James tried to get the patient to her feet. Instead, he should have instructed the patient not to move until help arrived or an evaluation was completed. Always stabilize the injury before trying to move the patient. The appropriate action in this scenario would be to instruct the patient not to move, then bring the provider to evaluate the patient.

KAPLAN